Pancreatic Cancer and Periampullary Neoplasms

Editor

JEFFREY M. HARDACRE

SURGICAL CLINICS
OF NORTH AMERICA

www.surgical.theclinics.com

Consulting Editor
RONALD F. MARTIN

December 2016 • Volume 96 • Number 6

ELSEVIER

1600 John F. Kennedy Boulevard • Suite 1800 • Philadelphia, Pennsylvania, 19103-2899

http://www.surgical.theclinics.com

SURGICAL CLINICS OF NORTH AMERICA Volume 96, Number 6
December 2016 ISSN 0039–6109, ISBN-13: 978-0-323-47752-9

Editor: John Vassallo, j.vassallo@elsevier.com
Developmental Editor: Colleen Viola

Surgical Clinics of North America (ISSN 0039–6109) is published bimonthly by Elsevier Inc., 360 Park Avenue South, New York, NY 10010-1710. Months of publication are February, April, June, August, October, and December. Business and Editorial Offices: 1600 John F. Kennedy Blvd., Suite 1800, Philadelphia, PA 19103-2899. Periodicals postage paid at New York, NY and additional mailing offices. Subscription prices are $375.00 per year for US individuals, $707.00 per year for US institutions, $100.00 per year for US students and residents, $455.00 per year for Canadian individuals, $895.00 per year for Canadian institutions, $510.00 for international individuals, $895.00 per year for international institutions and $250.00 per year for Canadian and foreign students/residents. To receive student/resident rate, orders must be accompanied by name of affiliated institution, date of term, and the *signature* of program/residency coordinator on institution letterhead. Orders will be billed at individual rate until proof of status is received. Foreign air speed delivery is included in all *Clinics* subscription prices. All prices are subject to change without notice. POSTMASTER: Send address changes to *Surgical Clinics*, Elsevier Health Sciences Division, Subscription Customer Service, 3251 Riverport Lane, Maryland Heights, MO 63043. **Customer Service (orders, claims, online, change of address): Telephone: 1-800-654-2452 (U.S. and Canada); 314-447-8871 (outside U.S. and Canada). Fax: 314-447-8029. E-mail: journalscustomerservice-usa@elsevier.com (for print support); journalsonline support-usa@elsevier.com (for online support).**

Reprints. For copies of 100 or more, of articles in this publication, please contact the Commercial Reprints Department, Elsevier Inc., 360 Park Avenue South, New York, New York 10010-1710. Tel. 212-633-3874, Fax: 212-633-3820, E-mail: reprints@elsevier.com.

The Surgical Clinics of North America is also published in Spanish by McGraw-Hill Interamericana Editores S.A., P.O. Box 5-237 06500 Mexico D.F. Mexico; and in Portuguese by Interlivros Edicoes Ltda., Rua Comandante Coelho 1085, CEP 21250, Rio de Janeiro, Brazil; and in Greek by Paschalidis Medical Publications, Athens Greece.

The Surgical Clinics of North America is covered in *MEDLINE/PubMed (Index Medicus), EMBASE/Excerpta Medica, Current Contents/Clinical Medicine, Current Contents/Life Sciences, Science Citation Index,* and *ISI/BIOMED.*

Contributors

CONSULTING EDITOR

RONALD F. MARTIN, MD, FACS
Lead Surgeon, York Hospital, Maine; Colonel (ret.), United States Army Reserve, York Hospital, York, Maine

EDITOR

JEFFREY M. HARDACRE, MD, FACS
Associate Professor of Surgery; Division of Surgical Oncology, University Hospitals Cleveland Medical Center, Cleveland, Ohio

AUTHORS

JOHN B. AMMORI, MD
Division of Surgical Oncology, University Hospitals Cleveland Medical Center, Cleveland, Ohio

MARSHALL S. BAKER, MD, MBA, FACS
Department of Surgery, University of Chicago Hospitals, Chicago, Illinois; Division of Surgical Oncology, Department of Surgery, NorthShore University Health System, Evanston, Illinois

JOSHUA G. BARTON, MD, FACS
Center for Pancreatic and Liver Diseases, St. Luke's Mountain States Tumor Institute, Boise, Idaho

MARCIA IRENE CANTO, MD, MHS
Division of Gastroenterology and Hepatology, Johns Hopkins Hospital, Johns Hopkins Medical Institutions, Baltimore, Maryland

AHMAD R. CHEEMA, MD
Icahn School of Medicine at Mount Sinai, Mount Sinai St. Luke's-West Hospital Center, New York, New York

KEVIN CHOONG, MD
Division of Surgical Oncology, University Hospitals Cleveland Medical Center, Cleveland, Ohio

KATHLEEN K. CHRISTIANS, MD
Division of Surgical Oncology, Department of Surgery, Medical College of Wisconsin, Milwaukee, Wisconsin

JASON W. DENBO, MD
Fellow in Complex General Surgical Oncology, Department of Surgical Oncology, MD Anderson Cancer Center, Houston, Texas

JENNIFER R. EADS, MD
Assistant Professor of Medicine, Division of Hematology and Oncology, University Hospitals Seidman Cancer Center, Case Comprehensive Cancer Center, Case Western Reserve University, Cleveland, Ohio

DOUGLAS B. EVANS, MD
Chairman, Department of Surgery, Medical College of Wisconsin, Milwaukee, Wisconsin

ASHLEY L. FAULX, MD
Division of Gastroenterology and Hepatology, Case Western Reserve University, Cleveland, Ohio

MYRA KAY FELDMAN, MD
Assistant Professor of Radiology, Cleveland Clinic Lerner College of Medicine of Case Western Reserve University; Staff Radiologist, Section of Abdominal Imaging, Imaging Institute, Cleveland Clinic, Cleveland, Ohio

CARLOS FERNÁNDEZ-DEL CASTILLO, MD
Department of Surgery, Massachusetts General Hospital, Harvard Medical School, Boston, Massachusetts

JASON B. FLEMING, MD
Professor, Department of Surgical Oncology, MD Anderson Cancer Center, Houston, Texas

ZHI VEN FONG, MD
Department of Surgery, Massachusetts General Hospital, Harvard Medical School, Boston, Massachusetts

NAMITA SHARMA GANDHI, MD
Assistant Professor of Radiology, Cleveland Clinic Lerner College of Medicine of Case Western Reserve University; Staff Radiologist, Section of Abdominal Imaging, Imaging Institute, Cleveland Clinic, Cleveland, Ohio

JEFFREY M. HARDACRE, MD, FACS
Associate Professor of Surgery; Division of Surgical Oncology, University Hospitals Cleveland Medical Center, Cleveland, Ohio

STEPHANIE M. KIM, MD
Division of Hematology and Oncology, University Hospitals Seidman Cancer Center, Case Comprehensive Cancer Center, Case Western Reserve University, Cleveland, Ohio

JASON B. LIU, MD
Department of Surgery, University of Chicago Hospitals, Chicago, Illinois

GIUSEPPE MALLEO, MD, PhD
Unit of General and Pancreatic Surgery, Department of Surgery and Oncology, The Pancreas Institute, University of Verona Hospital Trust, Verona, Italy

ROBERT C.G. MARTIN II, MD, PhD, FACS
Sam & Lolita Weakley Endowed Chair; Director, Division of Surgical Oncology; Professor of Surgery; Director, Upper GI & HPB Multi-Disciplinary Clinic; Academic Advisory Dean, University of Louisville, Louisville, Kentucky

SAOWANEE NGAMRUENGPHONG, MD
Division of Gastroenterology and Hepatology, Johns Hopkins Hospital, Johns Hopkins Medical Institutions, Baltimore, Maryland

EILEEN M. O'REILLY, MD
Associate Director, Rubenstein Center for Pancreatic Cancer Research; Attending Physician; Member, Memorial Sloan Kettering Cancer Center; Professor of Medicine, Weill Cornell Medical College, New York, New York

KELLY OLINO, MD
Assistant Professor, Department of Surgery, The University of Texas Medical Branch, Galveston, Texas

JENNIFER A. PERONE, MD
General Surgery Resident, Department of Surgery, The University of Texas Medical Branch, Galveston, Texas

TAYLOR S. RIALL, MD, PhD
Professor, Department of Surgery, Banner-University Medical Center, University of Arizona, Tucson, Arizona

AJAYPAL SINGH, MD
Division of Gastroenterology and Hepatology, Case Western Reserve University, Cleveland, Ohio

TALAR TATARIAN, MD
General Surgery Resident, Department of Surgery, The Jefferson Pancreas, Biliary and Related Cancer Center, Sidney Kimmel Medical College, Thomas Jefferson University Hospital, Philadelphia, Pennsylvania

SUSAN TSAI, MD, MHS
Division of Surgical Oncology, Department of Surgery, Medical College of Wisconsin, Milwaukee, Wisconsin

CHARLES M. VOLLMER Jr, MD
Department of Surgery, University of Pennsylvania Perelman School of Medicine, Philadelphia, Pennsylvania

JORDAN M. WINTER, MD, FACS
Associate Professor, Department of Surgery, The Jefferson Pancreas, Biliary and Related Cancer Center, Sidney Kimmel Medical College, Thomas Jefferson University, Philadelphia, Pennsylvania

GEORGE YOUNAN, MD
Division of Surgical Oncology, Department of Surgery, Medical College of Wisconsin, Milwaukee, Wisconsin

Contents

Over the past decade, emerging technologies have provided new insights into the genomic landscape of pancreatic ductal adenocarcinoma (PDA). In addition to the commonly recognized genetic drivers of pancreatic carcinogenesis (KRAS, CDKN2A, TP53, SMAD4), new genes and pathways have been implicated. However, these efforts have not identified any new high-frequency actionable mutations, limiting the success of mutation-targeted therapy in PDA. This article provides a report on the current landscape of pancreas cancer genetics and targeted therapeutics.

Pancreatic cancer (PC) is a highly fatal disease that can only be cured by complete surgical resection. However, most patients with PC have unresectable disease at the time of diagnosis, highlighting the need to detect PC and its precursor lesions earlier in asymptomatic patients. Screening is not cost-effective for population-based screening of PC. Individuals with genetic risk factors for PC based on family history or known PC-associated genetic syndromes, however, can be a potential target for PC screening programs. This article provides an overview of the epidemiology and genetic background of familial PC and discusses diagnostic and management approaches.

Imaging studies are critical for the detection, characterization, initial staging, management, and monitoring of pancreatic cancer cases. Treatment of pancreatic cancer requires a multidisciplinary approach. Ideally, assessing resectablility with imaging and subsequent treatment decisions should be made at a high-volume center of excellence with a multidisciplinary team. This article reviews the major imaging modalities used to evaluate pancreatic neoplasms, with an emphasis on pancreatic imaging protocols. The imaging appearance of solid pancreatic neoplasms and the imaging criteria used to stage and determine resectability for pancreatic ductal adenocarcinoma are described. An approach to standardized radiologic reporting is also reviewed.

Early diagnosis and accurate staging of pancreatic cancer is very important to plan optimal management strategy. Endoscopy plays an important role in the diagnosis and management of pancreatic cancer. Endoscopic ultrasound imaging (EUS) is the most sensitive modality for diagnosis, especially for small pancreatic tumors; it also allows tissue acquisition for histological diagnosis. Computed tomography scanning and EUS play complementary roles in staging and are comparable in determining resectability. Endoscopic retrograde cholangiopancreatography allows tissue sampling but is limited to palliative biliary drainage in most cases. In this article, we review the role of endoscopy in the diagnosis and management of pancreatic adenocarcinoma, with special emphasis on the use of endoscopic ultrasound and endoscopic retrograde cholangiopancreatography (ERCP).

Surgery is the key component of treatment for pancreatic and periampullary cancers. Pancreatectomy is complex, and there are numerous perioperative and intraoperative factors that are important for achieving optimal outcomes. This article focuses specifically on key aspects of the surgical management of periampullary and pancreatic cancers.

Pancreatic adenocarcinoma is a relatively uncommon malignancy associated with a high rate of cancer-related mortality despite best efforts to perform curative surgery. Adjuvant therapy in patients after surgical resection is associated with improved overall survival. Adjuvant treatment approaches may include either chemotherapy alone or a combination of chemotherapy and radiation therapy. Neoadjuvant approaches, also including either chemotherapy alone or a combination of chemotherapy and radiation therapy, are under investigation. Periampullary cancers constitute a rare and heterogeneous group of tumors that are typically treated as pancreatic cancers given their histologic similarities and tumor location.

Enhanced recovery after surgery (ERAS) protocols were first introduced to help recovery after colorectal surgery. They have now been applied to multiple surgical specialties, including pancreatic surgery. ERAS protocols in pancreatic surgery have been shown to decrease length of stay and possibly postoperative morbidity.

Although mortality rates after pancreatectomy have decreased, the incidence of postoperative morbidity remains high. The major procedure-related complications are pancreatic fistula, delayed gastric emptying, and postpancreatectomy hemorrhage. The International Study Group of Pancreatic Surgery defined leading complications in a standardized fashion, allowing unbiased comparison of operative results and management strategies. Risk factors for postoperative complications have been investigated and quantitative scoring systems established to estimate patient-specific risks. Management of postpancreatectomy complications has shifted from an operative to a conservative approach. Nevertheless, postoperative morbidities may have a profound impact on patient recovery and length of hospital stay and are associated with increased hospital costs.

Patients with localized pancreatic ductal adenocarcinoma seek potentially curative treatment, but this group represents a spectrum of disease. Patients with borderline resectable primary tumors are a unique subset whose successful therapy requires a care team with expertise in medical care, imaging, surgery, medical oncology, and radiation oncology. This team must identify patients with borderline tumors, then carefully prescribe and execute a combined treatment strategy with the highest possibility of cure. This article addresses the issues of clinical evaluation, imaging techniques, and criteria, as well as multidisciplinary treatment of patients with borderline resectable pancreatic ductal adenocarcinoma.

Multimodality therapy has become the standard approach for the treatment of pancreatic cancer. With improved response rates to newer chemotherapeutic agents, tumors that used to be considered unresectable are now being considered for operation. Neoadjuvant therapy for borderline resectable pancreatic cancer is considered standard of care and venous resection/reconstruction is no longer controversial. Arterial resection and reconstruction in select patients has also proven to be safe when done in highly specialized centers by high-volume surgeons. This article reviews indications for, and technical aspects of, vascular resection/reconstruction and shunting procedures during pancreatectomy, including critical elements of perioperative care.

> The diagnosis for locally advanced pancreatic cancer is based on high-quality cross-sectional imaging, which shows tumor invasion into the celiac/superior mesenteric arteries and/or superior mesenteric/portal venous system that is not reconstructable. The optimal management of these patients is evolving quickly with the advent of newer chemotherapeutics, radiation, and nonthermal ablation modalities. This article presents the current status of initial chemotherapy, surgical therapy, ablative therapy, and radiation therapy for patients with nonmetastatic locally advanced unresectable pancreatic cancer. Surgical resection offers the best chance of long-term disease control and the only chance for cure for patients with nonmetastatic exocrine pancreatic cancer.

> Pancreatic ductal adenocarcinoma (PDAC) is one of the most lethal and clinically challenging malignancies to treat, with an estimated 5-year survival rate of approximately 7%. At the time of initial presentation, a majority of patients have metastatic disease. The median overall survival in these patients with good performance status is 8.5 to 11.1 months and in patients with significantly impaired performance status, even less. Strategies to integrate novel agents with traditional cytotoxic therapies are under investigation and hold promise for improving outcomes in patients with metastatic PDAC. This article focuses on the current management options and novel therapeutics for metastatic PDAC.

> Most patients with pancreatic cancer will present with metastatic or locally advanced disease. Unfortunately, most patients with localized disease will experience recurrence even after multimodality therapy. As such, pancreatic cancer patients arrive at a common endpoint where decisions pertaining to palliative care come to the forefront. This article summarizes surgical, endoscopic, and other palliative techniques for relief of obstructive jaundice, relief of duodenal or gastric outlet obstruction, and relief of pain due to invasion of the celiac plexus. It also introduces the utility of the palliative care triangle in clarifying a patient's and family's goals to guide decision making.

> The incidence of intraductal papillary mucinous neoplasms (IPMNs) of the pancreas has been rising in the past two decades, driven mainly by the widespread use of cross-sectional imaging. IPMNs are intraductal mucin-producing neoplasms that involve the main pancreatic duct or its side branches and lack the ovarian stroma typically seen in mucinous cystic neoplasms. The International Association of Pancreatology released consensus guidelines in 2006 and 2012 providing clinical algorithms based

on IPMN features and risk of malignancy. In this article, we review the different classifications of IPMNs, their natural history, and clinical management and address recent controversies in the literature.

Pancreatic neuroendocrine tumors (PNETs) are a rare, heterogeneous group of neoplasms infamous for their endocrinopathies. Up to 90% of PNETs, however, are nonfunctional and are frequently detected incidentally on axial imaging during the evaluation of vague abdominal symptoms. Surgery remains the mainstay of therapy for patients diagnosed with both functional and nonfunctional PNETs. However, the multifaceted nature of PNETs challenges treatment decision making. In general, resection is recommended for patients with acceptable perioperative risk and amenable lesions.

SURGICAL CLINICS
OF NORTH AMERICA

Foreword

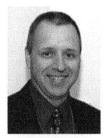

Ronald F. Martin, MD, FACS
Consulting Editor

If you are a practicing surgeon, there is a pretty good chance that you have been under pressure to increase value for some time now. It has been a clarion call for many, mainly because it is the kind of advice that is impossible to refute or dislike but equally as impossible to deliver. Please don't misinterpret that as a condemnation of improving value; rather, it is a plea for someone or some organization with authority to define exactly what that means.

The economic definition of value is fairly straightforward: quality divided by cost equals value. That is pretty hard to argue against. Where things get dicey is when we try to assign to whom the cost goes and to whom the quality goes. In a third-party payer world, the patient gets the "quality" and the payer pays the "price." In effect, that dislocates the value proposition from the onset: at least in the case of one patient whose bills are paid, or substantially paid, by a third party. As if this weren't complicated enough at the patient level, we then have to expand the notion to the collective group of insured persons. At this level, we have to factor in the collective "quality" of services delivered and the cumulative "price" paid. To even further complicate the issue, we must add the effect of this more expanded value proposition on the resultant premiums to the insured members (or their employers, states, or country) as that price point to some extent defines the sustainability of having an insured group. A fairly recent example of cumulative effects of premium shift affecting others is the recent withdrawal of large insurance products from certain state insurance exchanges created by the Patient Protection and Affordable Care Act.

When we get beyond the private insurers, and to some extent the government insurance programs, we are left with a sizable group of people with either no insurance or insurance plans with deductibles that will cause the "underinsured" person to function as if he or she has no insurance. The net result is either the failure to use needed services, whether therapeutic or preventive, or to use services that aren't paid for and subsequently yield cost shifting to those who are insured.

While not trying to state the obvious, it is a far more complex system than most are willing to admit. I would add that trying to fix the value proposition in our system's current form is either impossible or highly improbable—simply because the various

Surg Clin N Am 96 (2016) xiii–xv
http://dx.doi.org/10.1016/j.suc.2016.09.002
0039-6109/16/© 2016 Published by Elsevier Inc.

surgical.theclinics.com

stakeholders have mutually exclusive goals that are not resolvable under the current constructs.

There are clearly examples of where we could have success in improving value in any system. We could find a way to cut the cost of making a therapeutic item and deliver the same care with less cost. It sounds simple enough. However, when one starts looking at the supply chain and who keeps what part of the theoretical savings, it gets a little more complicated. Alternatively, the idea of payers simply paying less for the same (or more) services and materials philosophically borders somewhere between naive and extortionist. There is only so much downward purchase pressure we can apply before the supplier stops supplying either by choice or by necessity.

At the end of the day, or at least the end of just another day, we must accept something that is difficult: the only way to improve the global value equation for health care (and I confine my comments to health care in the United States for now) is to decide what services will and won't be available for everybody and then figure out the purchase price on those services we preserve. Of course, we could fudge it by making anything available off the "common market" and let those who can pay go there on their own nickel, though that would have significant political implications in a quasi-egalitarian society. In short, our society, through its collective decision-making bodies, needs to decide what it can pay for and what it will pay for. Then, we can work on the value side of those services.

You might ask yourself, why write about this economic material in the foreword to an issue on pancreatic surgery? I would suggest because much of pancreatic surgery is truly emblematic of the above set of dilemmas. Operations for pancreatic disorders benefit a relatively small subset of society and cost a fair amount of money. That can be said of lots of other things as well so pancreatic disorders are hardly alone in this regard. Still, pancreatic operations and their subsequent care are frequently resource and cost intensive. To the individual with the problem, say pancreatic cancer, the quality of what we can do is mostly all that matters. Without question, we have significantly improved the quality and value of what we can deliver for pancreatic problems over the last several decades. To the payers, however, the cost is still high, though not as high as it might have been, and the downstream payoff, whether measured by survival (not necessarily the best benchmark of success for a payer) or reduction in need for additional services, may not be where they would like it.

Many of us who provide these services feel the public is not receiving this care to the degree it should. In this case, we may be playing our roles as advocates or we may be self-promoting—or both. Regardless of whether we are tending toward advocacy or zealotry when we make such assertions, the claim itself that "more pancreatic services should be delivered to people" cannot stand in a vacuum. Claims like this should be compared against what other services we could provide people that may benefit them: services that would otherwise have to be curtailed as a result. This rationale, of course, applies to everything that we do, not just to pancreatic care. Unless we have an unlimited resource pool, we will have to make decisions that prioritize where we focus our limited efforts and resources.

In order that we as providers of this care may intelligently contribute to the larger conversation and understand in ourselves what we are saying that may be considered advocacy versus self-promotion, we need to understand the basis and foundations upon which we build our claims. To that end, we have Dr Hardacre and his colleagues to thank deeply for this issue of the *Surgical Clinics of North America*. Those interested in the care of patients with pancreatic disorders and pancreatology in general tend to be a driven and committed bunch. Many of them are members of the Pancreas Club. This group has been dedicated to learning about matters related to the pancreas and sharing their knowledge freely for decades. The contributors to this issue are largely derived from that pool of talented and dedicated people. I am grateful to each of them for their contributions past and present to our knowledge base.

We should all strive to give the best value we can. While the "big" value questions are political and societal, the everyday value questions are personal and professional. I believe this issue should help one give better value on both scales.

Ronald F. Martin, MD, FACS
York Hospital, Maine
Colonel (ret.), United States Army Reserve
York Hospital
16 Hospital Drive, Suite A
York, ME 03909, USA

E-mail address:
rmartin@yorkhospital.com

Preface

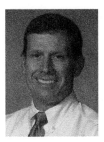

Jeffrey M. Hardacre, MD, FACS
Editor

This issue of the *Surgical Clinics of North America* provides a comprehensive review of virtually all aspects of care for the patient with pancreatic adenocarcinoma. It also provides contemporary reviews on the management of pancreatic neuroendocrine tumors as well as intraductal papillary mucinous neoplasms. The authors come from a number of specialties and from a variety of institutions across the country.

Beginning with detailed discussions of the genetics of pancreatic adenocarcinoma and inherited pancreatic cancer, the reader is walked through the imaging and endoscopic workup of pancreatic cancer. Such evaluation is critical to classifying patients as resectable, borderline resectable, locally advanced/unresectable, or metastatic so that appropriate treatment can be planned and delivered. Subsequent articles then review state-of-the-art therapy for each subset of patients. Along the way, articles are included on enhanced recovery pathways as well as the management of postpancreatectomy complications.

The care of patients with pancreatic adenocarcinoma is truly a multidisciplinary endeavor. Knowledge of not only the surgical therapy but also the nonsurgical therapy is critical for the surgeon to help guide patients on their cancer care journey. Quite often, surgeons are the gatekeepers for patients with pancreatic cancer and the ones to whom patients turn for advice on all components of their care.

I would like to thank all of the authors for their contributions to this issue. They made my work as guest editor intellectually stimulating and educational. I would also like to thank those who inspired me to become a surgeon and to pursue a career in gastrointestinal surgery: Jerry Hardacre I (my Dad), Jerry Hardacre II (my brother), along with the surgical faculty at Duke University and Johns Hopkins University Schools of Medicine. Finally, I would like to thank all the members of the Pancreas Club for sharing their knowledge and expertise through the years.

Surg Clin N Am 96 (2016) xvii–xviii
http://dx.doi.org/10.1016/j.suc.2016.09.001
0039-6109/16/© 2016 Published by Elsevier Inc.

I hope this issue serves as a useful reference for senior surgical residents and fellows as well as practicing surgeons. It has been an honor to be a part of this project.

Jeffrey M. Hardacre, MD, FACS
Associate Professor of Surgery
University Hospitals Cleveland Medical Center
11100 Euclid Avenue
Cleveland, OH 44106, USA

E-mail address:
jeffrey.hardacre@uhhospitals.org

Genetics of Pancreatic Cancer and Its Implications on Therapy

Talar Tatarian, MD[a], Jordan M. Winter, MD[b],*

KEYWORDS

- Pancreatic cancer • Genetics • Personalized medicine • Targeted therapy

KEY POINTS

- Recognized genetic drivers of pancreatic carcinogenesis include KRAS, CDKN2A, TP53, SMAD4, as well as genes involved in DNA damage repair, cell cycle regulation, chromatin modification, and axon guidance.
- Whole-exome sequencing and next-generation sequencing strategies have provided new insights into the genomic landscape of pancreas cancer, but have not identified any new high-frequency driver mutations.
- Genomic sequencing studies are affected by the low cellularity and high stromal content of pancreatic cancer, leading to variability in detected rates of driver mutations across tissue sources.
- Despite ongoing trials, there is currently a void in effective targeted therapies for pancreatic cancer.

INTRODUCTION

Pancreas cancer is a deadly disease with a 5-year survival rate of 8%.[1] It is already the third leading cause of cancer-related death in the United States, and is projected to be the second leading cause by 2020.[2] This mortality is attributable to multiple factors, including the aging demographic, ineffective treatments, and the lack of a proven method for screening or early detection. Most patients present with unresectable and incurable disease. The therapeutic mainstay of pancreatic cancer treatment remains conventional, cytotoxic therapy. Unlike other cancer types, and despite

Disclosure: The authors have nothing to disclose.
[a] Department of Surgery, The Jefferson Pancreas, Biliary and Related Cancer Center, Sidney Kimmel Medical College, Thomas Jefferson University Hospital, 1015 Walnut Street, Suite 620, Philadelphia, PA 19107, USA; [b] Department of Surgery, The Jefferson Pancreas, Biliary and Related Cancer Center, Sidney Kimmel Medical College, Thomas Jefferson University, 1025 Walnut Street, Suite 605, Philadelphia, PA 19107, USA
* Corresponding author.
E-mail address: Jordan.Winter@jefferson.edu

http://dx.doi.org/10.1016/j.suc.2016.07.014
0039-6109/16/© 2016 Elsevier Inc. All rights reserved.
surgical.theclinics.com

substantial research efforts, there are no targeted marker-based therapies that are routinely used to treat pancreatic cancer in 2016. This article reports on the current landscape of pancreas cancer genetics and targeted therapeutics.

GENETICS OF PANCREAS CANCER

Pancreatic ductal adenocarcinomas (PDAs) show numerous genetic changes that accumulate over time and drive histologic progression through pancreatic intraepithelial stages (pancreatic intraepithelial neoplasia [PanIN] 1–3) and then adenocarcinoma (**Fig. 1**).[3] These genetic changes can be classified as chromosomal alterations, microsatellite instability, epigenetic silencing, and intragenic mutations.[4,5] On a global level, large areas of chromosome loss or gain occur in virtually all PDAs, with losses occurring more frequently than gains. Chromosome instability can lead to the loss of as much as 30% of the PDA genome, with the most common regions of loss focused at the following loci: 9p, 17p, 18q, 3p, 8p, and 6q. Several of these regions correspond with areas of known PDA tumor suppressor genes.[6–8] Thus, loss of these loci (ie, loss of heterozygosity), combined with genetic mutations at the paired locus, leads to loss of function of critical proteins, including CDKN2A (9p), TP53 (17p) and SMAD4 (18q).[9] **Table 1** provides a summary of the current understanding of pancreas cancer and the most commonly altered genes.

Common Genetic Abnormalities in Pancreatic Ductal Adenocarcinoma

Historically, there have been 4 recognized genetic drivers of pancreatic carcinogenesis. *KRAS2* (12p) is an oncogene mutated in up to 95% of PDAs.[10,11] A point mutation in codon 12, 13, or 61 results in a permanently activated RAS protein, which leads to activation of downstream pathways involved in cellular proliferation and survival (ie, Raf-1, Rac, Rho, or phosphoinositide 3-kinase).[12] *KRAS* mutations are thought to occur early in PDA tumorigenesis, because they have been identified in PDA precursor lesions (PanINs).[13]

The tumor suppressor gene *CDKN2A* (p16) is also inactivated in 95% of tumors.[11] Homozygous deletions, single-allele loss combined with intragenic mutation in the second allele, or promoter hypermethylation all contribute to functional deactivation of the p16 protein. This deactivation in turn leads to increased phosphorylation

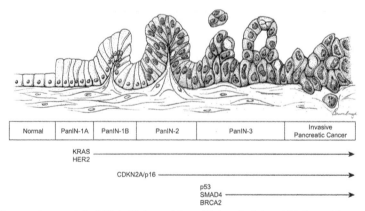

Fig. 1. Progression model of PDA. (*Adapted from* Maitra A, Adsay NV, Argani P, et al. Multicomponent analysis of the pancreatic adenocarcinoma progression model using a pancreatic intraepithelial neoplasia tissue microarray. Mod Pathol 2003;16(9):909; with permission.)

Table 1
The most common genetic abnormalities in PDA, and affected pathways

Pathway/Gene	Chromosome Location	Rate of Mutation in PDA (%)
KRAS Signaling		
KRAS2	12p	95
BRAF	7q	3
PIK3CA	3q	3
TGF-β Signaling		
SMAD4	18q	55
TGFBR2	3p	4
ACVR1B	12q	6
P53 Signaling		
TP53	17p	75
Cell Cycle Regulation		
CDKN2A	9p	95
CCND1	11q	10
CDK4	12q	10
Chromatin Modification		
KDM6A	Xp	18
ARID1A	1p	5
ARID2	12q	3
EPC1	10p	3
DNA Damage Repair		
BRCA1	17q	5
BRCA2	13q	7–10
ATM	11q	6
FANCC	9q	6
FANCG	9p	3
MLH1	3p	3
PALB2	16p	3
WNT/NOTCH Signaling		
RNF43	17q	10
MYC	8q	10
NOTCH1	9q	10
NOTCH2	1p	6
NOTCH3	19p	6
Axon Guidance		
SLIT2	4p	3
ROBO2	3p	2
Other		
PREX2	8q	10
MLL3	7q	8
ERBB	17q	4

Abbreviation: TGF-β, transforming growth factor beta.

(and deactivation) of Rb-1, progression through the G_1-S cell cycle checkpoint, and increased cell proliferation.[14,15] *TP53* is mutated in 75% of pancreas cancers.[11] Loss of heterozygosity coupled with an intragenic mutation in the remaining allele typically inactivates the tumor suppressor gene, allowing damaged cells to bypass the G_1-S checkpoint.[16] *SMAD4* encodes a transcription factor in the transforming growth factor beta (TGF-β) signaling pathway.[17,18] Homozygous deletions or loss of heterozygosity coupled with an intragenic point mutation inactivates the tumor suppressor gene and also causes failure of the G_1-S checkpoint in 55% of tumors.[11] These mutations occur late in PDA tumorigenesis and may contribute to its metastatic potential.[19] Moreover, SMAD4 loss is associated with a distant pattern of failure in advanced PDA.[20,21] Thus, oncologists have proposed that locally advanced PDA with retention of SMAD4 expression may be most suitable for chemoradiation, whereas patients harboring PDAs with expression loss are unlikely to benefit from intensified local therapy. One study of resected PDAs revealed that SMAD4 expression was uninformative with respect to pattern of failure or recurrence in patients after resection.[22]

Over the past decade, emerging technologies, such as whole-exome sequencing, and in particular next-generation sequencing strategies, have provided certain new insights into the genomic landscape of pancreas cancer. However, it should be emphasized that these high-throughput studies did not identify any new high-frequency driver mutations. Jones and colleagues[23] reported the first whole-exome genetic analysis of PDA. Samples from 24 cell lines and xenografts derived from human PDA underwent polymerase chain reaction amplification, and whole-exome Sanger sequencing of 20,661 genes. These tumors had an average of 63 genetic alterations, most of which were point mutations but that also included deletions and amplifications. These alterations naturally identified mutations in the classic oncogene, *KRAS2*, and tumor suppressor genes *CDKN2A* (p16), *TP53*, and SMAD4 (DPC4). This study also identified new genes that were mutated reproducibly, but at lower frequencies, including *ARID1A*, *MLL3*, *SF3B1*, and *TGFBR2*. The absence of apparent actionable mutations (abnormal genes that may be susceptible to pharmacologic targeting) was disappointing, and prompted investigators to group the mutated genes into 12 core-signaling pathways that were genetically altered in two-thirds of PDAs. This data clustering provides a more practical template for experimental therapeutic research, because these molecular signaling pathways are so frequently dysregulated in PDA. In fact, several pathways were genetically altered in 100% of the tumor samples (apoptosis, G_1/S regulation, hedgehog signaling, KRAS signaling, TGF-β signaling, Wnt/Notch signaling).

Biankin and colleagues[24] (of the Australian Pancreatic Cancer Genome Initiative [APCGI]) performed next-generation whole-exome sequencing and copy number analysis for a cohort of 99 patients with early-stage PDA. Unlike Jones and colleagues'[23] project, which was based on enriched tumor samples (cell lines and patient-derived xenografts), this study used primary frozen PDAs, but required tumors with greater than 20% cellularity. The technical challenge here was that frozen primary tissues contain abundant amounts of contaminating wild-type DNA from the admixed stromal component (xenografts and cell lines are almost exclusively neoplastic epithelia). The investigators identified an average of 26 mutations per patient, revealing a common but underappreciated theme: sequencing of primary PDA tissue has a lower sensitivity for mutation detection because of the low levels of neoplastic DNA. These efforts reaffirmed the importance of previously identified driver genes implicated in pancreatic carcinogenesis (KRAS, CDKN2A, TP53, SMAD4), but the effort also identified new cancer genes, including genes involved chromatin modification (*EPC1* and *ARID2*), DNA damage repair (*ATM*), as well as other diverse genes (*ZIM2*, *MAP2K4*, *NALCN*, *SLC16A4*, and *MAGEA6*). Pathway analysis identified abnormalities in axon guidance through SLIT/ROBO signaling (*SLIT2*, *ROBO1*, *ROBO2*, *ROBO3*), as a novel pathway defect implicated in pancreatic cancer.

More recently, Waddell and colleagues[25] (also part of the APCGI) performed whole-genome sequencing and copy number variation analysis of 100 PDAs. Again, frozen tissues were used for DNA extraction. These efforts led to the discovery of novel genes not previously identified in human pancreas cancer, including *KDM6A* (18%), *PREX2* (10%), *RNF43* (10%). Note that, RNF43 had been identified previously as an E3 ubiquitin ligase that was frequently mutated in mucinous pancreatic cystic tumors (eg, intraductal papillary mucinous neoplasms and mucinous cystic neoplasms).[26] Additional oncogenes with genetic mutations at a lower rate included *ERBB2*, *MET*, *CDK6*, *PIK3CA*, and *PIK3R3*.[25]

Fig. 2 provides a review of the genes and functional pathways implicated in pancreas cancer.

Validity of Current Mutation Studies

Genomic sequencing studies that are used by some clinicians as part of clinical care (eg, Caris Life Sciences, Foundation Medicine) are performed principally on formalin-fixed paraffin-embedded (FFPE) primary tumors. From a technical standpoint, these genetic analyses are flawed, compared with frozen tumors, which form the basis of

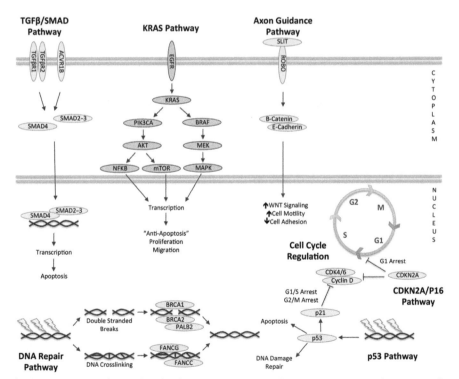

Fig. 2. Common pathways involved in pancreatic tumorigenesis. Represented are normally functioning pathways. Mutations in any number of genes can contribute to deregulation of the pathway and subsequent tumorigenesis. mTOR, mammalian target of rapamycin; NFKB, nuclear factor kappa B.

the abovementioned studies, and certainly compared with more enriched samples like cell lines and xenografts. Mutation artifacts (false-positive) are commonly seen in molecular profiling studies of FFPE tissues because of DNA damage from tissue processing.[27] In addition, the exceedingly low levels of tumor DNA from these samples and low neoplastic cellularity compromise detection capabilities.[28,29] Molecular analyses beyond genetics, including gene expression and protein expression studies, are also subject to RNA or protein degradation, as well as changes in expression levels with warm ischemia.[30–32]

Next-generation sequencing is able to overcome some of the detection limits that are caused by the low neoplastic cellularity of FFPE PDA tissues, but significant limitations for mutation detection remain. Variability in detected rates of driver mutations across tissue sources is readily apparent when studies are compared (**Table 2**). For example, the observed rates of driver mutations in primary frozen tumors or fine-needle aspiration samples were much lower than expected compared with xenografts and cell line models.[23,24,33] As a point of emphasis, the mutation rates observed in the tissue source with the enriched neoplastic component (cell lines and xenograft) were measured using older direct Sanger sequencing technology. The latter studies were performed using next-generation sequencing, revealing that the tissue source is the most critical factor for mutation detection. This factor is an under-recognized technological barrier to effective mutation-targeted therapy to treat pancreatic cancer: high stromal content in PDAs interferes with technical aspects of mutation detection. Therefore, routine clinical testing of PDA for mutations would be challenged, even if actionable abnormalities existed (eg, genetic defects that can be targeted with effective drugs).

PANCREAS CANCER AND THERAPEUTIC TARGETS

Although technical challenges to mutation detection for routine clinical use remain, the most daunting barrier to mutation-targeted therapy for PDA is a void in effective targeted therapies. Significant discoveries have been made with this approach for non-pancreatic cancers, such as trastuzumab for HER2+ (human epidermal growth factor receptor-2–positive) breast cancer and imatinib for KIT+ gastrointestinal stromal tumors (GISTs) or Ph+ chronic myeloid leukemia (CML). In order to understand the potential (or lack thereof) for a mutation-targeted approach to treat PDA, it is useful to briefly survey the precision medicine landscape in clinical oncology to provide context and a practical benchmark.

Precision Medicine in Clinical Oncology

The best, and one of the earliest examples of, successful targeted therapy in clinical oncology is imatinib and Philadelphia chromosome-positive CML. Compared with

Table 2			
Comparison of detected driver mutation rates (%) in different PDA models			
Gene	Cell Line/Xenograft[23]	Primary Frozen Tumor[24]	Endoscopic FNA[33]
KRAS	100	95	82
TP53	88	33	53
SMAD4	26	16	35
CDKN2A	30	2	7

Abbreviation: FNA, fine-needle aspiration.
  Data from Refs.[23,24,33]

conventional chemotherapy, imatinib improved survival by almost 2 years (median overall survival [OS], 72 vs 52 months; 6-year survival, 50% vs 29%; P = .002).[34] Imatinib had a similar impact on c-kit mutation–positive GIST, and was later approved for the neoadjuvant and adjuvant settings. Precision medicine has also been highly successful in breast cancer and melanoma. HER2 overexpression is seen in up to 30% of breast cancers.[35] Patients with HER2+ breast cancers have shown a significant survival benefit when treated with first-line trastuzumab and docetaxel versus docetaxel alone (progression-free survival [PFS], 11.7 vs 6.1 months; P = .0001. OS, 31.2 vs 22.7 months; P = .0325).[36] Even better results are seen when pertuzumab is added to trastuzumab and docetaxel (PFS, 18.7 vs 12.4 months with placebo; P<.001. OS, 56.5 vs 40.8 months; P<.001).[37] Therefore, combination HER2 inhibition likely adds 2 years of life to women with advanced HER2+ breast cancer. In melanoma, combination therapies targeting BRAF mutations have been nearly as promising. In patients with metastatic or unresectable BRAF mutant melanoma, combination dabrafenib and trametinib has shown superior results to vemurafenib monotherapy (PFS, 12.6 vs 7.3 months; P<.001. OS, 25.6 vs 18 months; P<.001).[38] Before BRAF targeting, these patients were surviving less than 9 months.[39]

Activating mutations in the EGFR gene are seen in approximately 23% of lung cancers, with higher rates in nonsmokers and Asian populations.[40,41] These mutations are best targeted by the small-molecule tyrosine kinase inhibitors, like erlotinib. A randomized, multicenter, phase III trial in patients with non–small cell lung cancer (NSCLC) showed a significant difference in median PFS (13.1 vs 4.6 months; P<.0001) compared with standard chemotherapy, although there was no benefit in OS.[42]

Although specific examples of successful mutation-targeted therapies are apparent in certain other cancer types, successful examples are surprisingly few. **Table 3** lists all US Food and Drug Administration (FDA)–approved drugs for mutation-targeted therapy. Importantly, hopes of repurposing these drugs for the management of PDA are low, because the target mutations are generally rare events in PDA. Thus, the magnitude of the benefit of mutation-targeted therapy is often overstated, and there is almost no relevance for patients with pancreatic cancer.

Target Genes in Pancreatic Ductal Adenocarcinoma

Despite advances in the understanding of the pathogenesis and genetics of pancreas cancer, efforts to exploit discovered targets have provided minimal return in clinical

Table 3
US Food and Drug Administration–approved drugs for mutation-targeted therapies, and the indicated tumor type

Mutated Gene Target	Drug	Principal Tumor Type	% Mutated in PDA
BRCA2	Olaparib	Ovarian	5
KRAS WT	Cetuximab	Colon	5
HER2	Trastuzumab, pertuzumab, lapatinib	Breast	3
BRAF	Trametinib, dabrafenib, vemurafenib	Melanoma	1
KIT	Imatinib	GIST	0
ABL	Imatinib, bosutinib, dasatinib, nilotinib	CML	0
EGFR	Gefitinib, erlotinib, afatinib	Lung	0
ALK	Crizotinib, ceritinib	Lung	0

Abbreviation: WT, wild type.

outcomes of patients with PDA to date. As stated, the library of mutated genes in PDA are generally not actionable. First, most of the mutated genes in PDA are tumor suppressor genes. Mutation-targeted therapy generally requires a gain-of-function mutation that is susceptible to pharmacologic inhibition. In contrast, inactivated tumor suppressor genes cannot be targeted by inhibitory compounds; their function needs to be restored. Second, there are no high-frequency mutations in tyrosine kinases (eg, KIT, EGFR), which historically are the easiest protein class to target pharmacologically. Third, the high number of genetically altered genes in each PDA poses the question of whether or not a clinical benefit is consistently achievable through targeting just 1 of these abnormally altered genes. Even if an oncogene can be inhibited, the average PDA has greater than 40 other mutated genes that likely contribute to the pathobiology of the tumor.

Attempts have been made to target a few genetically abnormal genes and pathways in PDA, with minimal success. These examples are discussed here.

HER2/ERBB2

HER2 (or ERBB2) is amplified in only 4% of pancreas cancers.[43] The FDA-approved drug trastuzumab is a monoclonal antibody that inhibits HER2-mediated signaling,[44] and is effective in the treatment of invasive breast and gastric/gastroesophageal cancers, in which HER2 overexpression is seen in up to 30% of patients in these tumor types.[35,45] Clinical trials in patients with pancreas cancer have been far less promising. A multicenter phase II trial of trastuzumab in patients with pancreatic cancer with HER2 amplification found no improvement in survival compared with standard chemotherapy.[46]

EGFR

Unlike lung cancer, trials targeting EGFR mutations have been unsuccessful for pancreas cancer. The National Cancer Institute of Canada Clinical Trials Group performed a phase III trial randomizing patients with locally advanced or metastatic pancreas cancer to gemcitabine therapy with or without erlotinib. Erlotinib provided a statistical, but marginal, clinical benefit for medial OS (6.24 vs 5.91 months or just 10 days; $P = .038$) and PFS (3.75 vs 3.55 months; $P = .004$).[47] This study did not stratify by genotype, largely because EGFR mutations are so rare in PDA (see **Table 3**). More recently, a group in Taiwan performed a similar randomization and specifically evaluated the role of EGFR mutations. The study reaffirmed the marginal benefit of combined erlotinib/gemcitabine and showed prolonged survival in those with EGFR mutations (PFS, 5.9 vs 2.4 months; $P = .0004$. OS, 8.7 vs 6 months; $P = .044$).[48] However, EGFR mutations are present in 55% of Chinese patients (but in 0% of white people, in whom EGFR amplifications, and not mutations, are more prevalent).

KRAS

EGFR has also been targeted using a monoclonal antibody, cetuximab, with efficacy against metastatic colorectal cancer with wild-type KRAS. The CRYSTAL trial showed a small benefit in median PFS when cetuximab was used with FOLFIRI (folinic acid, fluorouracil, irinotecan), compared with FOLFIRI alone, as first-line treatment in KRAS wild-type metastatic colorectal cancer (9.9 vs 8.7 months; $P = .02$).[49] Historically, up to 95% of pancreas tumors have mutations in KRAS, suggesting that targeting EGFR in KRAS wild-type PDA is likely to have a marginal benefit at best.[10] Phase II trials evaluating combination cetuximab and gemcitabine adjuvant therapy in pancreas cancer found no benefit in disease-free survival or OS compared with gemcitabine alone, even when adjusted for KRAS wild-type status.[50]

KRAS has been proposed by some clinicians as a "holy grail" of mutant targeted therapy for PDA because of the high prevalence of these mutations. The National Cancer Institute has developed a RAS initiative with earmarked funds based on a widespread belief in the importance of this gene as a therapeutic target. However, efforts to inhibit this protein have failed to have a clinical impact, particularly in pancreatic cancer. Tipifarnib is a farnesyltransferase inhibitor with a downstream effect of inhibiting KRAS activity. A phase III clinical trial of gemcitabine with and without tipifarnib found no improvement in median PFS (112 vs 109 days; $P = .72$) or median OS (193 vs 182 days; $P = .75$).[51] Conceptually, it is unclear whether effective KRAS inhibition will be an important clinical achievement. KRAS mutations are an early genetic event, suggesting that the gain-of-function mutation is important in the progression of pancreatic cancer precursor lesions. This suggestion is evident in studies of patient tissues[52,53] as well as in transgenic mouse models.[54] However, the importance of the mutation has not been shown in invasive human PDAs, which contain an abundance of other molecular abnormalities, as previously described. Multiple preclinical studies have raised questions about the magnitude of the impact that would be achieved through KRAS inhibition.[55–58]

BRAF
BRAF targeted therapy has been successful in melanoma and limited nonmelanoma cancers. A recent basket trial evaluated vemurafenib monotherapy in 122 patients with BRAF V600 mutation–positive nonmelanoma tumors (colorectal, NSCLC, Langerhans cell histiocytosis, primary brain tumors, cholangiocarcinoma, anaplastic thyroid cancer, and multiple myeloma). An objective response was seen in 42% of those with NSCLC, with a median PFS of 7.3 months. No response was seen in patients with colorectal cancer.[59] This study did not include patients with BRAF mutant PDA and there have been no randomized trials to date. A small percentage of PDAs are thought to harbor BRAF mutations (<3%; see **Table 3**). These variants are of the medullary adenocarcinoma subtype.[60]

IDH1
There are several clinical trials (NCT02074839, NCT02492737, NCT02481154, NCT02073994, NCT02632708) currently underway to evaluate the role of IDH1 inhibitors (AG-120, AG-221, AG-881) in both solid tumors (gliomas) and hematologic malignancies (acute myeloid leukemia). IDH1 mutations have never been reported in pancreatic cancer; however the authors recently discovered a patient at our institution that harbored such a mutation (manuscript in preparation).

BRCA
Germline mutations in the BRCA1 and BRCA2 genes have been shown to increase the lifetime risk of developing pancreas cancer by 3.5-fold to 10-fold.[61] Mutations are typically inherited in an autosomal dominant pattern and, although rare in the general population, are seen in 11% to 17% of patients with familiar pancreatic cancer (hereditary breast and ovarian cancer syndrome). These genes encode for proteins responsible for DNA repair through homologous recombination.[62] BRCA-deficient breast and ovarian tumors have shown sensitivity to certain classes of drugs that target DNA repair or DNA integrity; namely platinum agents and poly(adenosine diphosphate ribose) polymerase (PARP) inhibitors.[63,64] For instance, there was a near doubling of PFS (4.8–8.4 months; $P<.001$) in platinum-sensitive ovarian cancer with olaparib monotherapy, and the benefit was greatest in BRCA-mutant carriers.[65] More recently, the response rate to olaparib in castration-resistant prostate cancer was 88% in

16 cancers with defects in the Fanconi anemia DNA repair pathway, as opposed to no responses in the remaining patients.[66]

Platinum therapy (ie, cisplatin) causes cross-linking of DNA, which sensitizes BRCA-deficient cells to this class of drugs.[67] Most studies of cisplatin therapy in BRCA-deficient patients with pancreas cancer have been retrospective and include small numbers of patients. Lowery and colleagues[68] retrospectively studied 15 patients with BRCA mutations who were treated for pancreas cancer. Six patients with metastatic disease received a platinum agent as first-line therapy, and 5 had a partial response based on response evaluation criteria in solid tumors (RECIST) criteria. Albeit a small sample size, this is a promising finding, because the most aggressive chemotherapy regimens reportedly achieve response rates between 20% and 30%.[69,70] A more recent study retrospectively evaluated 71 patients with BRCA1-associated or BRCA2-associated pancreas cancer. In comparing patients with stage 3 and 4 disease (n = 43), the median OS in patients receiving platinum-based therapy (n = 22) was improved compared with those receiving nonplatinum therapy (n = 21, 22 vs 9 months, $P<.039$).[71] A recent case report identified a BRCA2-deficient patient with metastatic pancreas cancer who had a complete response with combination cisplatin and gemcitabine therapy. The patient remained in remission 10 months after his last treatment.[72]

PARP inhibitors are a newer class of drugs that cause the accumulation of single-strand breaks in DNA, which BRCA-deficient cells are unable to repair; this leads to chromosome instability and cell death.[63,73] Small case series and reports have reported promising results in some patients with PDA.[68,74,75] Phase I trials have established the safety of olaparib in combination with gemcitabine for locally advanced or metastatic pancreas cancer (NCT00515866).[76] A phase II basket trial of BRCA1/2 deficient solid tumors and recurrent cancer evaluated olaparib monotherapy. In 23 patients with pancreas cancer, 5 (21.7%) showed a tumor response according to RECIST criteria, for a median duration of 4 months.[77] A phase III trial is currently evaluating the use of olaparib as maintenance therapy in BRCA-deficient patients with pancreas cancer initially treated with platinum-based drugs (NCT02184195). In addition, multiple prospective randomized phase II trials are underway to evaluate the addition of veliparib to combination cisplatin/gemcitabine as first-line therapy for locally advanced or metastatic pancreas cancer with BRCA mutations (NCT01585805).

FUTURE DIRECTIONS

Despite the advances that have been made in the past 2 decades, pancreas cancer continues to be a deadly disease, with only modest advances in the clinical arena. As the understanding of the genomics of pancreas cancer has increased, the translation to improved outcomes has been minimal. The genetic landscape has been thoroughly mapped, so it seems that precision medicine focused on mutation-targeted therapy holds little promise for PDA. The verdict is almost complete on this subject, because the likelihood that a novel actionable and high-frequency mutation in PDA will be discovered in the future remains exceedingly small. The most significant opportunity in this space clearly relates to the effect of PARP inhibition for BRCA2-deficient PDAs (~5%–10% of all PDAs), and the results of ongoing phase II and III trials are eagerly awaited. Although platinum-based drugs may be particularly effective against these tumors, the relevance of these drugs as personalized therapies may be overstated, because most patients with PDA receive a platinum agent at some point in their disease course (eg, oxaliplatin). The addition of PARP inhibitors to the treatment of BRCA-deficient PDA may improve outcomes in affected patients, with implications for 5% to 10% of all PDAs. KRAS remains the only high-frequency mutated oncogene in PDA with a potential for pharmacologic inhibition, but the clinical benefit of this strategy is uncertain for invasive PDA.

Clinical, academic, and commercial services offer genetic sequencing for PDA, but there is little evidence to support such tests at present, other than investigations to identify genetic deficiencies in DNA repair pathways (eg, BRCA1, BRCA2, PALB2). Anecdotal discoveries of actionable mutations exist, but high-level evidence is lacking.

Attempts to personalize therapy for patients with PDA will likely move beyond genetics in the near future. For instance, the authors are currently conducting a multi-institution randomized phase II clinical trial investigating molecular targeted therapy, which principally examines gene expression profiles and other molecular changes in PDA (eg, phosphoproteomics). In this study, the expression profile of putative predictive markers, such as TS (5-flurouracil), ERCC1 (oxaliplatin), and RRM1 (gemcitabine), along with other molecular analytes, will be used to guide therapy. In addition, patient-derived tumors, such as xenografts and organoids, may provide ex-vivo cancer models to empirically test drugs and combinations that can then be used to guide personal therapies in patients. There are substantial efforts designed to harness the immune system against PDA.[78–80] Combining the understanding of genetic pathways, the tumor microenvironment, and the behavior of each individual tumor will give clinicians the best chance at success.

REFERENCES

1. Siegel RL, Miller KD, Jemal A. Cancer statistics, 2016. CA Cancer J Clin 2016; 66(1):7–30.
2. Rahib L, Smith BD, Aizenberg R, et al. Projecting cancer incidence and deaths to 2030: the unexpected burden of thyroid, liver, and pancreas cancers in the United States. Cancer Res 2014;74(11):2913–21.
3. Maitra A, Adsay NV, Argani P, et al. Multicomponent analysis of the pancreatic adenocarcinoma progression model using a pancreatic intraepithelial neoplasia tissue microarray. Mod Pathol 2003;16(9):902–12.
4. Winter JM, Maitra A, Yeo CJ. Genetics and pathology of pancreatic cancer. HPB (Oxford) 2006;8(5):324–36.
5. Hansel DE, Kern SE, Hruban RH. Molecular pathogenesis of pancreatic cancer. Annu Rev Genomics Hum Genet 2003;4:237–56.
6. Iacobuzio-Donahue CA, van der Heijden MS, Baumgartner MR, et al. Large-scale allelotype of pancreaticobiliary carcinoma provides quantitative estimates of genome-wide allelic loss. Cancer Res 2004;64(3):871–5.
7. Mahlamaki EH, Hoglund M, Gorunova L, et al. Comparative genomic hybridization reveals frequent gains of 20q, 8q, 11q, 12p, and 17q, and losses of 18q, 9p, and 15q in pancreatic cancer. Genes Chromosomes Cancer 1997;20(4): 383–91.
8. Curtis LJ, Li Y, Gerbault-Seureau M, et al. Amplification of DNA sequences from chromosome 19q13.1 in human pancreatic cell lines. Genomics 1998;53(1): 42–55.
9. Hidalgo M, Von Hoff DD. Translational therapeutic opportunities in ductal adenocarcinoma of the pancreas. Clin Cancer Res 2012;18(16):4249–56.
10. Smit VT, Boot AJ, Smits AM, et al. KRAS codon 12 mutations occur very frequently in pancreatic adenocarcinomas. Nucleic Acids Res 1988;16(16): 7773–82.

11. Hruban RH, Iacobuzio-Donahue C, Wilentz RE, et al. Molecular pathology of pancreatic cancer. Cancer J 2001;7(4):251–8.

12. Kranenburg O. The KRAS oncogene: past, present, and future. Biochim Biophys Acta 2005;1756(2):81–2.

13. Collins MA, Pasca di Magliano M. Kras as a key oncogene and therapeutic target in pancreatic cancer. Front Physiol 2013;4:407.

14. Caldas C, Hahn SA, da Costa LT, et al. Frequent somatic mutations and homozygous deletions of the p16 (MTS1) gene in pancreatic adenocarcinoma. Nat Genet 1994;8(1):27–32.

15. Schutte M, Hruban RH, Geradts J, et al. Abrogation of the Rb/p16 tumor-suppressive pathway in virtually all pancreatic carcinomas. Cancer Res 1997; 57(15):3126–30.

16. Taylor WR, Stark GR. Regulation of the G2/M transition by p53. Oncogene 2001; 20(15):1803–15.

17. Hahn SA, Schutte M, Hoque AT, et al. DPC4, a candidate tumor suppressor gene at human chromosome 18q21.1. Science 1996;271(5247):350–3.

18. Yoo J, Ghiassi M, Jirmanova L, et al. Transforming growth factor-beta-induced apoptosis is mediated by Smad-dependent expression of GADD45b through p38 activation. J Biol Chem 2003;278(44):43001–7.

19. Embuscado EE, Laheru D, Ricci F, et al. Immortalizing the complexity of cancer metastasis: genetic features of lethal metastatic pancreatic cancer obtained from rapid autopsy. Cancer Biol Ther 2005;4(5):548–54.

20. Crane CH, Varadhachary GR, Yordy JS, et al. Phase II trial of cetuximab, gemcitabine, and oxaliplatin followed by chemoradiation with cetuximab for locally advanced (T4) pancreatic adenocarcinoma: correlation of Smad4(Dpc4) immunostaining with pattern of disease progression. J Clin Oncol 2011;29(22): 3037–43.

21. Iacobuzio-Donahue CA, Fu B, Yachida S, et al. DPC4 gene status of the primary carcinoma correlates with patterns of failure in patients with pancreatic cancer. J Clin Oncol 2009;27(11):1806–13.

22. Winter JM, Tang LH, Klimstra DS, et al. Failure patterns in resected pancreas adenocarcinoma: lack of predicted benefit to SMAD4 expression. Ann Surg 2013;258(2):331–5.

23. Jones S, Zhang X, Parsons DW, et al. Core signaling pathways in human pancreatic cancers revealed by global genomic analyses. Science 2008;321(5897): 1801–6.

24. Biankin AV, Waddell N, Kassahn KS, et al. Pancreatic cancer genomes reveal aberrations in axon guidance pathway genes. Nature 2012;491(7424):399–405.

25. Waddell N, Pajic M, Patch AM, et al. Whole genomes redefine the mutational landscape of pancreatic cancer. Nature 2015;518(7540):495–501.

26. Wu J, Jiao Y, Dal Molin M, et al. Whole-exome sequencing of neoplastic cysts of the pancreas reveals recurrent mutations in components of ubiquitin-dependent pathways. Proc Natl Acad Sci U S A 2011;108(52):21188–93.

27. Wong SQ, Li J, Tan AY, et al. Sequence artefacts in a prospective series of formalin-fixed tumours tested for mutations in hotspot regions by massively parallel sequencing. BMC Med Genomics 2014;7:23.

28. Kern SE, Winter JM. Elegance, silence and nonsense in the mutations literature for solid tumors. Cancer Biol Ther 2006;5(4):349–59.

29. Winter JM, Brody JR, Kern SE. Multiple-criterion evaluation of reported mutations: a proposed scoring system for the intragenic somatic mutation literature. Cancer Biol Ther 2006;5(4):360–70.

30. Ma Y, Dai H, Kong X. Impact of warm ischemia on gene expression analysis in surgically removed biosamples. Anal Biochem 2012;423(2):229–35.

31. Fleige S, Pfaffl MW. RNA integrity and the effect on the real-time qRT-PCR performance. Mol Aspects Med 2006;27(2–3):126–39.

32. Spruessel A, Steimann G, Jung M, et al. Tissue ischemia time affects gene and protein expression patterns within minutes following surgical tumor excision. Biotechniques 2004;36(6):1030–7.

33. Valero V 3rd, Saunders TJ, He J, et al. Reliable detection of somatic mutations in fine needle aspirates of pancreatic cancer with next-generation sequencing: implications for surgical management. Ann Surg 2016;263(1):153–61.

34. Interferon alfa-2a as compared with conventional chemotherapy for the treatment of chronic myeloid leukemia. The Italian Cooperative Study Group on Chronic Myeloid Leukemia. N Engl J Med 1994;330(12):820–5.

35. Iqbal N, Iqbal N. Human epidermal growth factor receptor 2 (HER2) in cancers: overexpression and therapeutic implications. Mol Biol Int 2014;2014:852748.

36. Marty M, Cognetti F, Maraninchi D, et al. Randomized phase II trial of the efficacy and safety of trastuzumab combined with docetaxel in patients with human epidermal growth factor receptor 2-positive metastatic breast cancer administered as first-line treatment: the M77001 study group. J Clin Oncol 2005;23(19):4265–74.

37. Swain SM, Baselga J, Kim SB, et al. Pertuzumab, trastuzumab, and docetaxel in HER2-positive metastatic breast cancer. N Engl J Med 2015;372(8):724–34.

38. Robert C, Karaszewska B, Schachter J, et al. Two year estimate of overall survival in COMBI-v, a randomized, open-label, phase III study comparing the combination of dabrafenib and trametinib with vemurafenib as first-line therapy in patients with unresectable or metastatic BRAF V600E/K mutation-positive cutaneous melanoma. The European Cancer Congress 2015. 2015. Available at: https://www.europeancancercongress.org/Vienna2015/Scientific-Programme/Searchable-Programme?trackid=00181-anchorScpr. Accessed February 26, 2016.

39. Chapman PB, Hauschild A, Robert C, et al. Improved survival with vemurafenib in melanoma with BRAF V600E mutation. N Engl J Med 2011;364(26):2507–16.

40. Shigematsu H, Lin L, Takahashi T, et al. Clinical and biological features associated with epidermal growth factor receptor gene mutations in lung cancers. J Natl Cancer Inst 2005;97(5):339–46.

41. Prabhakar CN. Epidermal growth factor receptor in non-small cell lung cancer. Transl Lung Cancer Res 2015;4(2):110–8.

42. Zhou C, Wu YL, Chen G, et al. Erlotinib versus chemotherapy as first-line treatment for patients with advanced EGFR mutation-positive non-small-cell lung cancer (OPTIMAL, CTONG-0802): a multicentre, open-label, randomised, phase 3 study. Lancet Oncol 2011;12(8):735–42.

43. Menard S, Casalini P, Campiglio M, et al. HER2 overexpression in various tumor types, focussing on its relationship to the development of invasive breast cancer. Ann Oncol 2001;12(Suppl 1):S15–9.

44. Hudis CA. Trastuzumab–mechanism of action and use in clinical practice. N Engl J Med 2007;357(1):39–51.

45. Bang YJ, Van Cutsem E, Feyereislova A, et al. Trastuzumab in combination with chemotherapy versus chemotherapy alone for treatment of HER2-positive advanced gastric or gastro-oesophageal junction cancer (ToGA): a phase 3, open-label, randomised controlled trial. Lancet 2010;376(9742):687–97.

46. Harder J, Ihorst G, Heinemann V, et al. Multicentre phase II trial of trastuzumab and capecitabine in patients with HER2 overexpressing metastatic pancreatic cancer. Br J Cancer 2012;106(6):1033–8.
47. Moore MJ, Goldstein D, Hamm J, et al. Erlotinib plus gemcitabine compared with gemcitabine alone in patients with advanced pancreatic cancer: a phase III trial of the National Cancer Institute of Canada Clinical Trials Group. J Clin Oncol 2007;25(15):1960–6.
48. Wang JP, Wu CY, Yeh YC, et al. Erlotinib is effective in pancreatic cancer with epidermal growth factor receptor mutations: a randomized, open-label, prospective trial. Oncotarget 2015;6(20):18162–73.
49. Van Cutsem E, Kohne CH, Hitre E, et al. Cetuximab and chemotherapy as initial treatment for metastatic colorectal cancer. N Engl J Med 2009;360(14):1408–17.
50. Fensterer H, Schade-Brittinger C, Muller HH, et al. Multicenter phase II trial to investigate safety and efficacy of gemcitabine combined with cetuximab as adjuvant therapy in pancreatic cancer (ATIP). Ann Oncol 2013;24(10):2576–81.
51. Van Cutsem E, van de Velde H, Karasek P, et al. Phase III trial of gemcitabine plus tipifarnib compared with gemcitabine plus placebo in advanced pancreatic cancer. J Clin Oncol 2004;22(8):1430–8.
52. Moskaluk CA, Hruban RH, Kern SE. p16 and K-ras gene mutations in the intraductal precursors of human pancreatic adenocarcinoma. Cancer Res 1997; 57(11):2140–3.
53. Hruban RH, Wilentz RE, Kern SE. Genetic progression in the pancreatic ducts. Am J Pathol 2000;156(6):1821–5.
54. Hingorani SR, Wang L, Multani AS, et al. Trp53R172H and KrasG12D cooperate to promote chromosomal instability and widely metastatic pancreatic ductal adenocarcinoma in mice. Cancer Cell 2005;7(5):469–83.
55. Mologni L, Dekhil H, Ceccon M, et al. Colorectal tumors are effectively eradicated by combined inhibition of {beta}-catenin, KRAS, and the oncogenic transcription factor ITF2. Cancer Res 2010;70(18):7253–63.
56. Pecot CV, Wu SY, Bellister S, et al. Therapeutic silencing of KRAS using systemically delivered siRNAs. Mol Cancer Ther 2014;13(12):2876–85.
57. Zorde Khvalevsky E, Gabai R, Rachmut IH, et al. Mutant KRAS is a druggable target for pancreatic cancer. Proc Natl Acad Sci U S A 2013;110(51):20723–8.
58. Shi XH, Liang ZY, Ren XY, et al. Combined silencing of K-ras and Akt2 oncogenes achieves synergistic effects in inhibiting pancreatic cancer cell growth in vitro and in vivo. Cancer Gene Ther 2009;16(3):227–36.
59. Hyman DM, Puzanov I, Subbiah V, et al. Vemurafenib in multiple nonmelanoma cancers with BRAF V600 mutations. N Engl J Med 2015;373(8):726–36.
60. Calhoun ES, Jones JB, Ashfaq R, et al. BRAF and FBXW7 (CDC4, FBW7, AGO, SEL10) mutations in distinct subsets of pancreatic cancer: potential therapeutic targets. Am J Pathol 2003;163(4):1255–60.
61. Hahn SA, Greenhalf B, Ellis I, et al. BRCA2 germline mutations in familial pancreatic carcinoma. J Natl Cancer Inst 2003;95(3):214–21.
62. Farmer H, McCabe N, Lord CJ, et al. Targeting the DNA repair defect in BRCA mutant cells as a therapeutic strategy. Nature 2005;434(7035):917–21.
63. Ashworth A. A synthetic lethal therapeutic approach: poly(ADP) ribose polymerase inhibitors for the treatment of cancers deficient in DNA double-strand break repair. J Clin Oncol 2008;26(22):3785–90.
64. Hucl T, Rago C, Gallmeier E, et al. A syngeneic variance library for functional annotation of human variation: application to BRCA2. Cancer Res 2008;68(13): 5023–30.

65. Ledermann J, Harter P, Gourley C, et al. Olaparib maintenance therapy in platinum-sensitive relapsed ovarian cancer. N Engl J Med 2012;366(15):1382–92.

66. Mateo J, Carreira S, Sandhu S, et al. DNA-repair defects and olaparib in metastatic prostate cancer. N Engl J Med 2015;373(18):1697–708.

67. van der Heijden MS, Brody JR, Dezentje DA, et al. In vivo therapeutic responses contingent on Fanconi anemia/BRCA2 status of the tumor. Clin Cancer Res 2005; 11(20):7508–15.

68. Lowery MA, Kelsen DP, Stadler ZK, et al. An emerging entity: pancreatic adenocarcinoma associated with a known BRCA mutation: clinical descriptors, treatment implications, and future directions. Oncologist 2011;16(10):1397–402.

69. Conroy T, Desseigne F, Ychou M, et al. FOLFIRINOX versus gemcitabine for metastatic pancreatic cancer. N Engl J Med 2011;364(19):1817–25.

70. Von Hoff DD, Ervin T, Arena FP, et al. Increased survival in pancreatic cancer with nab-paclitaxel plus gemcitabine. N Engl J Med 2013;369(18):1691–703.

71. Golan T, Kanji ZS, Epelbaum R, et al. Overall survival and clinical characteristics of pancreatic cancer in BRCA mutation carriers. Br J Cancer 2014;111(6): 1132–8.

72. Sonnenblick A, Kadouri L, Appelbaum L, et al. Complete remission, in BRCA2 mutation carrier with metastatic pancreatic adenocarcinoma, treated with cisplatin based therapy. Cancer Biol Ther 2011;12(3):165–8.

73. Benafif S, Hall M. An update on PARP inhibitors for the treatment of cancer. Onco Targets Ther 2015;8:519–28.

74. Lowery M, Shah MA, Smyth E, et al. A 67-year-old woman with BRCA 1 mutation associated with pancreatic adenocarcinoma. J Gastrointest Cancer 2011;42(3): 160–4.

75. Vyas O, Leung K, Ledbetter L, et al. Clinical outcomes in pancreatic adenocarcinoma associated with BRCA-2 mutation. Anticancer Drugs 2015;26(2):224–6.

76. Bendell J, O'Reilly EM, Middleton MR, et al. Phase I study of olaparib plus gemcitabine in patients with advanced solid tumours and comparison with gemcitabine alone in patients with locally advanced/metastatic pancreatic cancer. Ann Oncol 2015;26(4):804–11.

77. Kaufman B, Shapira-Frommer R, Schmutzler RK, et al. Olaparib monotherapy in patients with advanced cancer and a germline BRCA1/2 mutation. J Clin Oncol 2015;33(3):244–50.

78. Nomi T, Sho M, Akahori T, et al. Clinical significant and therapeutic potential of the programmed death-1 ligand/programmed death-1 pathway in human pancreatic cancer. Clin Cancer Res 2007;13(7):2151–7.

79. Beatty GL, Chiorean EG, Fishman MP, et al. CD40 agonists alter tumor stroma and show efficacy against pancreatic carcinoma in mice and humans. Science 2011;331(6024):1612–6.

80. Stromnes IM, Schmitt TM, Hulbert A, et al. T cells engineered against a native antigen can surmount immunologic and physical barriers to treat pancreatic ductal adenocarcinoma. Cancer Cell 2015;28(5):638–52.

Screening for Pancreatic Cancer

Saowanee Ngamruengphong, MD, Marcia Irene Canto, MD, MHS*

KEYWORDS

- Familial pancreatic cancer • Pancreatic cancer • Pancreatic cyst
- Pancreatic intraepithelial neoplasia • Intraductal papillary mucinous neoplasm
- Screening

KEY POINTS

- Individuals with an inherited predisposition for pancreatic cancer (high-risk individuals) based on their family history or known pancreatic cancer-associated genetic mutation are at higher risk to develop pancreatic cancer.
- Noninvasive precursor lesions for pancreatic cancer are more common and of a higher grade in familial pancreatic cancer patients than in patients with sporadic disease. High-grade precursor duct lesions and small early stage pancreatic cancer are the targets for screening.
- Screening should include endoscopic ultrasonography and/or MRI/magnetic resonance cholangiopancreatography, ideally in a multidisciplinary setting. Computed tomography scan can be used to further characterize a solid lesion if it is found on the screening imaging.
- Surgery should be performed at centers with expertise in pancreatic surgery when there is a concerning solid lesion, cysts that are 2 cm or larger, mural nodule or solid component, or a dilated main pancreatic duct.

INTRODUCTION

Pancreatic cancer (PC) is a highly fatal disease. In the United States, approximately 53,070 new cases of PC were projected to occur in 2016, accompanied by an estimated 41,780 cancer deaths.[1] PC can only be cured by complete surgical resection. However, most patients with PC have unresectable disease at the time of diagnosis. Therefore, there is a need to detect PC and its precursor lesions earlier in asymptomatic patients before disease progression so that a cure can more likely be achieved.

Because of the low incidence of PC, screening is not cost-effective for population-based screening. Individuals with genetic risk factors for PC based on their family

Disclosures: No relevant financial disclosures.
Division of Gastroenterology and Hepatology, Johns Hopkins Hospital, Johns Hopkins Medical Institutions, Blalock 407, Baltimore, MD 21287, USA
* Corresponding author.
E-mail address: mcanto1@jhmi.edu

Surg Clin N Am 96 (2016) 1223–1233
http://dx.doi.org/10.1016/j.suc.2016.07.016
0039-6109/16/© 2016 Elsevier Inc. All rights reserved.

history or known PC-associated genetic syndromes are at high risk to develop PC. Thus, these high-risk individuals (HRIs) can be a potential target for PC screening programs. This article provides an overview of the epidemiology and genetic background of familial PC and discusses the diagnostic and management approaches for these patients.

EPIDEMIOLOGY AND RISK FACTORS FOR FAMILIAL PANCREATIC CANCER

About 5% to 10% of individuals with PC have a family history of the disease.[2,3] Hereditary risk for PC can be categorized into 2 groups: (1) hereditary cancer syndromes and (2) familial pancreatic cancer. The former refers to patients with defined inherited cancer syndromes in which patients are at increased risk for a number of malignancies, including pancreatic cancer. On the other hand, familial PC is defined as those having at least a pair of affected first-degree relatives (FDRs) with PC (**Box 1**).

Nongenetic factors also contribute to the increased risk associated with a family history of PC. Smoking is an independent risk factor for familial PC (odds ratio [OR], 3.7; 95% confidence interval [CI], 1.8–7.6). The age of onset of familial PC is similar to that of sporadic PC (>60 years).[4] Smoking lowers the age of onset by approximately 20 years in hereditary pancreatitis and decreases age of onset of PC in familial kindreds.[5,6] Members of familial PC kindreds should be counseled not to smoke.[7]

GENETIC PREDISPOSITION FOR PANCREATIC CANCER

Several genetic predispositions have been described to be associated with PC. Although most genetic defects causing hereditary PC remain to be discovered, several genetic cancer syndromes associated with PC have been described.

Patients with inherited cancer syndromes such as hereditary pancreatitis, Peutz-Jeghers syndrome (PJS), familial atypical multiple mole melanoma, Lynch syndrome (hereditary nonpolyposis colorectal cancer), ataxia telangiectasia, and Li-Fraumeni syndrome have an increased risk of developing PC (**Table 1**). It should be noted

---

Box 1
High-risk individuals for pancreatic cancer screening

- Individuals with 3 or more affected blood relatives with PC, including at least 2 related by first degree (familial PC), with at least one of the affected related to the at-risk relative by first degree (parent, sibling, child)
- Individuals with at least 2 affected FDRs with PC
- All patients with Peutz–Jeghers syndrome should be screened, regardless of family history of PC
- p16 (CDKN2A) gene mutation carriers with 1 affected FDR
- BRCA2 gene mutation carriers with 1 affected FDR
- BRCA2 gene mutation carriers with 2 affected family members (no FDR) with PC
- PALB2 gene mutation carriers with 1 affected FDR
- ATM gene mutation carriers
- Mismatch repair gene mutation carriers (Lynch syndrome) with 1 affected FDR

Data from Canto MI, Harinck F, Hruban RH, et al. International Cancer of the Pancreas Screening (CAPS) Consortium summit on the management of patients with increased risk for familial pancreatic cancer. Gut 2013;62(3):339–47.

Table 1
Inherited cancer syndromes associated with increased risk of pancreatic cancer

Syndrome	Gene(s)	Locus	Lifetime Risk of PC, Percent
Hereditary breast/ovarian cancer	BRCA2, BRCA1	13q	3–5
	PALB2	16p	Unknown
Familial atypical multiple mole melanoma syndrome	CDKN2A	9p	10–19
Peutz-Jeghers syndrome	STK 11	19p	11–36
Familial adenomatous polyposis	APC	5q	Unknown
Hereditary nonpolyposis colon cancer (Lynch II)	DNA mismatch repair genes	2p, 3p, 7p	4
Hereditary pancreatitis	PRSS1, SPINK1	7q, 5q	25–40
Ataxia telangiectasia	ATM	11q	Unknown
Li-Fraumeni syndrome	P53	17p	Unknown

Adapted from Brentnall TA. Management strategies for patients with hereditary pancreatic cancer. Curr Treat Options Oncol 2005;6:437; with permission.

that individuals with PC gene mutations susceptible to PC may not have a family history of PC.[8] Germline mutations in the BRCA2, PALB2, p16, STK11, ATM, PRSS1, PALB2 genes, and the hereditary colon cancer genes, are associated with significantly increased risk of PC. Among these, BRCA1 and BRCA2 mutations are the most common known mutations in familial PC (12%–19%).[9,10]

Hereditary Pancreatitis

Hereditary pancreatitis is an autosomal-dominant disorder with incomplete penetrance. It is commonly associated with mutations in serine protease 1 gene (PRSS1) on chromosome 7q35, which encodes cationic trypsinogen. The International Hereditary Pancreatitis Study Group reported that the risk of PC is approximately 50 to 60 times greater than expected compared with the background population.[5] In a French case series, the standardized incidence ratio (SIR) of PC was 87 (95% CI 42–113). The cumulative risk of PC at age 50 and 75 years was 11% and 49% for men and 8% and 55% for women, respectively. Smoking and diabetes mellitus were the main associated risk factors.[11] Despite the high risk of PC, patients with hereditary pancreatitis have similar mortality risk compared with the general population.[12] The diagnostic yield and outcomes of screening for PC in this subgroup of HRIs have not been well studied.

Hereditary Breast Cancer

BRCA2 mutations are frequently found (5%–17%) in patients with familial PC.[10,13,14] The risk of PC in those with BRCA2 gene mutation is increased 3.5-fold (range 1.87–6.58).[15,16] Approximately 1% of all Ashkenazi Jews carry BRCA2 genes. Therefore, individuals with Jewish ancestry and a diagnosis of PC should be referred for BRCA gene mutation screening (6174delT), which is present in 1% of Ashkenazi Jewish individuals[17] and 4% of patients with PC.[18]

About 1% of BRCA1/BRCA2-negative breast cancer cases with PC are caused by germline defects in the PALB2 (partner and localizer of BRCA2) gene.[19,20] PALB2 mutations have been identified in 2.1% to 4.9% of familial PC kindreds.[3,21,22] PALB2 gene mutations confer an increased risk of both breast and pancreatic cancer. The lifetime risk of PC in affected individuals remains unknown. It is assumed that the risk in PALB2 mutation carriers may be comparable to that in BRCA1/BRCA2 carriers.

Peutz-Jeghers Syndrome

Peutz-Jeghers syndrome is an autosomal-dominant syndrome associated with mutations of STK11 gene. This condition is at high risk of cancers of the gastrointestinal tract, lung, breast.[23] The risk of developing PC is very high, with lifetime risk of 11% to 36% by the age of 70.[24,25]

Familial Atypical Multiple-Mole Melanoma Syndrome

Familial atypical multiple-mole melanoma (FAMMM) syndrome is caused by mutation of CDKN2A (so-called p16 or multiple tumor suppressor-1 gene). The syndrome is characterized by multiple nevi, cutaneous and ocular malignant melanomas, and PCs. A variant syndrome, so called "the FAMMM-pancreatic carcinoma syndrome," carries a cumulative risk of PC up to 17% by age 75.[26–31]

Lynch Syndrome

Individuals with the DNA mismatch repair gene mutations (MLH1, MSH2, MSH6, PMS2) have a cumulative risk of 3.7% to develop PC by the age 70 and 8.6-fold increased risk compared with the general population.[32–34] Medullary histology is a characteristic feature of a mismatch repair-deficient cancer, and individuals with PC who have this history should have further testing for Lynch syndrome.[35]

Familial Pancreatic Cancer

Familial PC (FPC) is defined as a genetic predisposition in individuals with at least a pair of FDRs with pancreatic ductal adenocarcinoma, in the absence of a known genetic susceptibility syndrome. The literature has suggested that the risk of developing PC among an individual with family history of pancreatic cancer ranges from 1.5- to 30-fold.[10–12,20,36–40] Data from a prospective registry-based study revealed that the overall risk of PC in member of FPC kindreds was a ninefold increase (95% CI: 4.5–16.1). This risk increases with the number of affected relatives: 4.6-fold increased risk (95% CI, 0.5–16.4) for 1 FDR with PC; 6.4-fold increased risk (95% CI: 1.8–16.4) for 2 FDRs with PC, and 32.0-fold increased risk (95% CI: 10.2–74.7) for 3 or more FDRs with PC.[2]

A statistical risk assessment model "PancPRO" has been developed to estimate the risk of a future PC for asymptomatic individuals based on the individual's family history.[41] In an Italian prospective study, the lifetime risk of PC was calculated by PancPro. The pedigrees of 570 families of patients presenting with pancreatic ductal adenocarcinoma were collected. Considering a tenfold risk over the general population as a threshold for including a subject in a surveillance program, 19 families (3.3%) involving 92 FDRs with age greater than 40 years would be selected in a surveillance program.[42]

SCREENING AND SURVEILLANCE OF PANCREATIC CANCER

Most PC is believed to arise from pancreatic intraepithelial neoplasia (PanIN) and intraductal papillary mucinous neoplasms (IPMNs). A pathologic study has suggested that PC developing in familial cancer kindreds arises from PanIN.[43] Patients who have curative surgery for noninvasive and small, margin-negative PC have a significantly improved long-term survival.[44]

The goal of screening and surveillance of PC is to detect and curatively resect preinvasive lesions with high-grade dysplasia (HGD). These lesions mainly are PanIN3 and IPMN with HGD, which are at high risk of malignant transformation into PC. Noninvasive precursor lesions are more common and of a higher grade (PanIN 3 and IPMN with HGD) in familial PC patients than in patients with sporadic disease.[45–47] Rate of progression of these preinvasive lesions to invasive cancer in HRIs remains to be determined. However, data from nonfamilial PC patients suggest that sporadic noninvasive IPMN takes 3 to 5 years to become an invasive PC.[48] About 2% to 7% of small branch duct IPMNs progress to invasive PC over 5 year follow-up.[49,50]

Several cohort studies have reported a diagnostic yield of screening programs for PC in HRIs ranging from 3.9% to 50%, varying depending on study populations and study endpoints.[51–60] Small pancreatic cysts, likely representing branch duct IPMNs, are the most common abnormal finding and are found in 34% to 53% of HRIs within the screening program.[60] Solid lesions are less common.

Age Initiate to Screening

The age to initiate screening and age to end screening of pancreatic lesions in HRIs remain unclear. For patients with hereditary pancreatitis, a consensus conference recommended that screening should be offered to patients who are at least 40 years of age due to young age onset of PC in affected individuals.[61] Similarly, patients with Peutz-Jeghers syndrome should begin screening earlier, at about 30 years of age or older because of younger age of onset of PCs (about 45 years). For HRIs with familial PC, a multidisciplinary international consortium recommended starting screening at age 50.[62] Some centers start screening at age 55, because the median age of onset of familial PC is 65 years, similar to that in sporadic PC. Most familial PCs are diagnosed in patients 60 years or older.

Imaging Modalities

Imaging modalities such as computed tomography (CT), endoscopic ultrasonography (EUS), and MRI with cholangiopancreatography (MRCP) have been studied for screening and surveillance of PC in HRIs.

The initial screening should include EUS and/or MRI/MRCP but not CT.[62] Pancreas protocol-enhanced CT provides high-resolution imaging of the pancreas; however, it has a lower detection rate of small pancreatic lesions in the high-risk population compared with EUS or MRI.[51,54,60,63] CT scan can be used to further characterize the solid lesion if it is found on the screening imaging.[62] MRI and CT scan also allow examination of other abdominal organs, which is important for certain genetic syndromes with elevated risk of multiple organ malignancy.

In a multicenter study involving 225 asymptomatic HRIs who underwent screening for PC, CT, MRI, and EUS detected a pancreatic lesion in 11%, 33%, and 42% of patients, respectively. The detected pancreatic lesions included 82 IPMNs and 3 pancreatic endocrine tumors.[60] In the study of patients with sporadic IPMNs, EUS was superior to transabdominal ultrasound, CT scan, and MRI in detection of IPMN-derived and -concomitant PC at diagnosis and during follow-up.[64]

Cost-Effectiveness of Screening

A few studies on cost-effectiveness of screening for PC in HRIs have been reported. In patients with Peutz-Jeghers syndrome who are at increased risk of PC, screening would cost more than $35,000 per life saved.[65] In a decision analysis comparing 1-time screening for pancreatic dysplasia with EUS versus no screening, endoscopic screening was cost-effective, with an incremental cost-effectiveness ratio of $16,885/life–year saved.[66]

Serologic Testing

It is known that serum CA 19-9 is neither sensitive nor specific for PC, and it is not appropriate for mass screening. Data on blood tests for biomarkers of PC such as serum CA19-9 in HRIs are limited. In a prospective cohort study using serum CA 19-9 in 546 individuals who had at least 1 FDR with PC, CA 19-9 was elevated in 4.9% of cases. Neoplastic or malignant findings were detected in 5 patients (0.9%), and pancreatic adenocarcinoma was detected in 1 patient (0.2%).[67]

Pancreatic Juice and Pancreatic Cyst Fluid Biomarkers

Prevalence of genetic alterations that contribute to familial PC such as mutant KRAS2 and inactivation of TP53 or SMAD4 is similar to that of sporadic PC.[68] Thus, genetic markers of sporadic pancreatic adenocarcinomas can be used to detect familial PC. Genetic markers for PC in pancreatic juice and/or pancreatic cyst fluid may improve early diagnosis of and screening for high-risk lesions that are not detectable by imaging, thus improving identification of lesions that require surgery.[69]

EUS-guided fine needle aspiration (EUS-FNA) allows sampling of the pancreatic cyst fluid and cyst wall, which can be sent for a range of tests including molecular testing. In a multicenter, retrospective study of 130 patients with resected pancreatic cystic neoplasms, cyst fluid was analyzed in order to

Identify gene mutations in pancreatic cysts (BRAF, CDKN2A, CTNNB1, GNAS, KRAS, NRAS, PIK3CA, RNF43, SMAD4, TP53, and VHL)
Identify loss of heterozygosity at CDKN2A, RNF43, SMAD4, TP53, and VHL tumor suppressor loci
Identify aneuploidy

A panel of molecular markers and clinical features can classify cyst type with 90% to100% sensitivity and 92% to 98% specificity.[69] The clinical benefit of these molecular markers in pancreatic cyst fluid in HRIs has not been well studied.

EUS-FNA is generally safe procedure; however, it can rarely cause bleeding, pancreatitis, and infection. In addition, in patients with multiple pancreatic lesions, sampling of all lesions may not be feasible. Furthermore, cytologic analyses of the FNA specimens may lead to false-positive diagnoses of pancreatic neoplasia. Routine EUS-FNA is not performed unless there is a solid lesion of any size or a mural nodule in a cyst of any size. To avoid potential adverse events and limitation related to EUS-FNA, there have been increasing interests in analysis of molecular markers in pancreatic juice collected from duodenum.

In a study of secretin-stimulated pancreatic juice collected from the duodenum during upper endoscopy by Kanda and colleagues,[70] GNAS mutations were found in 66% of IPMNs, a rate similar to that observed in cyst fluid aspirated during EUS. The same group further examined TP53 mutations, a known tumor suppressor gene that has been implicated in progression of IPMNs, in duodenal samples of pancreatic juice.[71] They identified TP53 mutations in pancreatic juice in 67% of patients with pancreatic ductal adenocarcinoma and PanIN-3 or IPMN with HGD, but not in individuals without advanced lesions. These studies suggested that pancreatic juice collected from the duodenum can potentially be used as a screening modality for PC.

MANAGEMENT OF DETECTED PANCREATIC LESIONS IN ASYMPTOMATIC HIGH-RISK INDIVIDUALS

Most pancreatic lesions in asymptomatic HRIs undergoing screening can be observed and do not require surgery.[60] Prophylactic pancreatectomy is not recommended for asymptomatic HRIs without pancreatic lesions because of morbidity and mortality related to surgery.[62] Discussions regarding the need for surgery in asymptomatic high-risk individuals with screening-detected pancreatic lesions should ideally occur in a multidisciplinary setting, similar to tumor board. Surgery should be performed in a high-volume center with expertise in pancreatic surgery.

Solid pancreatic lesions are found in 1.4% of asymptomatic HRIs.[60] According to consensus guidelines, solid lesions, particularly those seen by multiple imaging modalities, are ominous, and the threshold for surgical resection is much lower. There was no consensus on management of indeterminate smaller solid lesions (<1 cm diameter). EUS-FNA of these lesions can be considered, although the diagnostic yield is usually low.[62]

Cystic pancreatic lesions were found in 39% of HRIs within a screening program.[60] Most of these lesions appear to be low-risk branch-duct IPMNs.[62] International consensus guidelines for the management of IPMNs can be applied to HRIs with IPMNs to assess risk of HGD or malignancy.[72] In asymptomatic HRIs, surgery for suspected branch duct IPMNs can be considered for lesions 2 cm or larger or the presence of mural nodules or solid component.[62] The patient with a cyst without worrisome features of HGD or malignancy should be monitored with imaging after 6 to 12 months.[23,62] Shorter follow-up (≤3 months) should be considered for indeterminate lesions.

If main pancreatic duct strictures/dilations are detected without associated lesions in the imaging study, repeat imaging within 3 months is recommended.[62] When main pancreatic duct dilation is associated with any cystic lesion, a concern for main duct involvement should be raised, even with duct size less than 5 mm.

SUMMARY

Screening and surveillance of HRIs for early pancreatic neoplasia, including high-grade, preinvasive precursor lesions and early PC, is currently recommended. The outcomes of surveillance and treatment of screening-detected lesions remain under evaluation. Optimization of surgical criteria for resection and development and validation of biomarkers in pancreatic juice, cyst fluid, and blood are needed.

REFERENCES

1. Siegel RL, Miller KD, Jemal A. Cancer statistics, 2016. CA Cancer J Clin 2016; 66(1):7–30.
2. Klein AP, Brune KA, Petersen GM, et al. Prospective risk of pancreatic cancer in familial pancreatic cancer kindreds. Cancer Res 2004;64(7):2634–8.
3. Schneider R, Slater EP, Sina M, et al. German national case collection for familial pancreatic cancer (FaPaCa): ten years experience. Fam Cancer 2011;10(2): 323–30.
4. Tersmette AC, Petersen GM, Offerhaus GJ, et al. Increased risk of incident pancreatic cancer among first-degree relatives of patients with familial pancreatic cancer. Clin Cancer Res 2001;7(3):738–44.
5. Lowenfels AB, Maisonneuve P, Whitcomb DC. Risk factors for cancer in hereditary pancreatitis. International Hereditary Pancreatitis Study Group. Med Clin North Am 2000;84(3):565–73.
6. Yeo TP, Hruban RH, Brody J, et al. Assessment of "gene-environment" interaction in cases of familial and sporadic pancreatic cancer. J Gastrointest Surg 2009; 13(8):1487–94.

7. Rulyak SJ, Lowenfels AB, Maisonneuve P, et al. Risk factors for the development of pancreatic cancer in familial pancreatic cancer kindreds. Gastroenterology 2003;124(5):1292–9.

8. Goggins M, Schutte M, Lu J, et al. Germline BRCA2 gene mutations in patients with apparently sporadic pancreatic carcinomas. Cancer Res 1996;56(23):5360–4.

9. Lal G, Liu G, Schmocker B, et al. Inherited predisposition to pancreatic adenocarcinoma: role of family history and germ-line p16, BRCA1, and BRCA2 mutations. Cancer Res 2000;60(2):409–16.

10. Hahn SA, Greenhalf B, Ellis I, et al. BRCA2 germline mutations in familial pancreatic carcinoma. J Natl Cancer Inst 2003;95(3):214–21.

11. Rebours V, Boutron-Ruault MC, Schnee M, et al. Risk of pancreatic adenocarcinoma in patients with hereditary pancreatitis: a national exhaustive series. Am J Gastroenterol 2008;103(1):111–9.

12. Rebours V, Boutron-Ruault MC, Jooste V, et al. Mortality rate and risk factors in patients with hereditary pancreatitis: uni- and multidimensional analyses. Am J Gastroenterol 2009;104(9):2312–7.

13. Couch FJ, Johnson MR, Rabe KG, et al. The prevalence of BRCA2 mutations in familial pancreatic cancer. Cancer Epidemiol Biomarkers Prev 2007;16(2):342–6.

14. Murphy KM, Brune KA, Griffin C, et al. Evaluation of candidate genes MAP2K4, MADH4, ACVR1B, and BRCA2 in familial pancreatic cancer: deleterious BRCA2 mutations in 17%. Cancer Res 2002;62(13):3789–93.

15. Breast Cancer Linkage Consortium. Cancer risks in BRCA2 mutation carriers. J Natl Cancer Inst 1999;91(15):1310–6.

16. van Asperen CJ, Brohet RM, Meijers-Heijboer EJ, et al. Cancer risks in BRCA2 families: estimates for sites other than breast and ovary. J Med Genet 2005; 42(9):711–9.

17. Struewing JP, Abeliovich D, Peretz T, et al. The carrier frequency of the BRCA1 185delAG mutation is approximately 1 percent in Ashkenazi Jewish individuals. Nat Genet 1995;11(2):198–200.

18. Ferrone CR, Levine DA, Tang LH, et al. BRCA germline mutations in Jewish patients with pancreatic adenocarcinoma. J Clin Oncol 2009;27(3):433–8.

19. Blanco A, de la Hoya M, Osorio A, et al. Analysis of PALB2 gene in BRCA1/BRCA2 negative Spanish hereditary breast/ovarian cancer families with pancreatic cancer cases. PLoS One 2013;8(7):e67538.

20. Jones S, Hruban RH, Kamiyama M, et al. Exomic sequencing identifies PALB2 as a pancreatic cancer susceptibility gene. Science 2009;324(5924):217.

21. Slater EP, Langer P, Niemczyk E, et al. PALB2 mutations in European familial pancreatic cancer families. Clin Genet 2010;78(5):490–4.

22. Hofstatter EW, Domchek SM, Miron A, et al. PALB2 mutations in familial breast and pancreatic cancer. Fam Cancer 2011;10(2):225–31.

23. Giardiello FM, Welsh SB, Hamilton SR, et al. Increased risk of cancer in the Peutz-Jeghers syndrome. N Engl J Med 1987;316(24):1511–4.

24. Giardiello FM, Brensinger JD, Tersmette AC, et al. Very high risk of cancer in familial Peutz-Jeghers syndrome. Gastroenterology 2000;119(6):1447–53.

25. van Lier MG, Wagner A, Mathus-Vliegen EM, et al. High cancer risk in Peutz-Jeghers syndrome: a systematic review and surveillance recommendations. Am J Gastroenterol 2010;105(6):1258–64 [author reply: 1265].

26. Lynch HT, Brand RE, Hogg D, et al. Phenotypic variation in eight extended CDKN2A germline mutation familial atypical multiple mole melanoma-pancreatic carcinoma-prone families: the familial atypical mole melanoma-pancreatic carcinoma syndrome. Cancer 2002;94(1):84–96.

27. Lynch HT, Fusaro RM. Pancreatic cancer and the familial atypical multiple mole melanoma (FAMMM) syndrome. Pancreas 1991;6(2):127–31.

28. Vasen HF, Gruis NA, Frants RR, et al. Risk of developing pancreatic cancer in families with familial atypical multiple mole melanoma associated with a specific 19 deletion of p16 (p16-Leiden). Int J Cancer 2000;87(6):809–11.

29. Kluijt I, Cats A, Fockens P, et al. Atypical familial presentation of FAMMM syndrome with a high incidence of pancreatic cancer: case finding of asymptomatic individuals by EUS surveillance. J Clin Gastroenterol 2009;43(9):853–7.

30. Maker AV, Warth JA, Zinner MJ. Novel presentation of a familial pancreatic cancer syndrome. J Gastrointest Surg 2009;13(6):1151–4.

31. Goldstein AM, Fraser MC, Struewing JP, et al. Increased risk of pancreatic cancer in melanoma-prone kindreds with p16INK4 mutations. N Engl J Med 1995; 333(15):970–4.

32. Park JG, Park YJ, Wijnen JT, et al. Gene–environment interaction in hereditary nonpolyposis colorectal cancer with implications for diagnosis and genetic testing. Int J Cancer 1999;82(4):516–9.

33. Win AK, Young JP, Lindor NM, et al. Colorectal and other cancer risks for carriers and noncarriers from families with a DNA mismatch repair gene mutation: a prospective cohort study. J Clin Oncol 2012;30(9):958–64.

34. Kastrinos F, Mukherjee B, Tayob N, et al. Risk of pancreatic cancer in families with Lynch syndrome. JAMA 2009;302(16):1790–5.

35. Goggins M, Offerhaus GJ, Hilgers W, et al. Pancreatic adenocarcinomas with DNA replication errors (RER+) are associated with wild-type K-ras and characteristic histopathology. Poor differentiation, a syncytial growth pattern, and pushing borders suggest RER+. Am J Pathol 1998;152(6):1501–7.

36. Roberts NJ, Jiao Y, Yu J, et al. ATM mutations in patients with hereditary pancreatic cancer. Cancer Discov 2012;2(1):41–6.

37. Lowenfels AB, Maisonneuve P, DiMagno EP, et al. Hereditary pancreatitis and the risk of pancreatic cancer. International Hereditary Pancreatitis Study Group. J Natl Cancer Inst 1997;89(6):442–6.

38. Howes N, Lerch MM, Greenhalf W, et al. Clinical and genetic characteristics of hereditary pancreatitis in Europe. Clin Gastroenterol Hepatol 2004;2(3):252–61.

39. Whitcomb DC. Inflammation and cancer v. chronic pancreatitis and pancreatic cancer. Am J Physiol Gastrointest Liver Physiol 2004;287(2):G315–9.

40. Thompson D, Easton DF. Cancer incidence in BRCA1 mutation carriers. J Natl Cancer Inst 2002;94(18):1358–65.

41. Wang W, Chen S, Brune KA, et al. PancPRO: risk assessment for individuals with a family history of pancreatic cancer. J Clin Oncol 2007;25(11):1417–22.

42. Leonardi G, Marchi S, Falconi M, et al. "PancPro" as a tool for selecting families eligible for pancreatic cancer screening: an Italian study of incident cases. Dig Liver Dis 2012;44(7):585–8.

43. Meckler KA, Brentnall TA, Haggitt RC, et al. Familial fibrocystic pancreatic atrophy with endocrine cell hyperplasia and pancreatic carcinoma. Am J Surg Pathol 2001;25(8):1047–53.

44. Winter JM, Cameron JL, Campbell KA, et al. 1423 pancreaticoduodenectomies for pancreatic cancer: a single-institution experience. J Gastrointest Surg 2006; 10(9):1199–210 [discussion: 1210–1].

45. Wu J, Matthaei H, Maitra A, et al. Recurrent GNAS mutations define an unexpected pathway for pancreatic cyst development. Sci Transl Med 2011;3(92): 92ra66.

46. Matthaei H, Schulick RD, Hruban RH, et al. Cystic precursors to invasive pancreatic cancer. Nat Rev Gastroenterol Hepatol 2011;8(3):141–50.

47. Shi C, Klein AP, Goggins M, et al. Increased prevalence of precursor lesions in familial pancreatic cancer patients. Clin Cancer Res 2009;15(24):7737–43.

48. Sohn TA, Yeo CJ, Cameron JL, et al. Intraductal papillary mucinous neoplasms of the pancreas: an updated experience. Ann Surg 2004;239(6):788–97 [discussion: 797–9].

49. Sawai Y, Yamao K, Bhatia V, et al. Development of pancreatic cancers during long-term follow-up of side-branch intraductal papillary mucinous neoplasms. Endoscopy 2010;42(12):1077–84.

50. Uehara H, Nakaizumi A, Ishikawa O, et al. Development of ductal carcinoma of the pancreas during follow-up of branch duct intraductal papillary mucinous neoplasm of the pancreas. Gut 2008;57(11):1561–5.

51. Al-Sukhni W, Borgida A, Rothenmund H, et al. Screening for pancreatic cancer in a high-risk cohort: an eight-year experience. J Gastrointest Surg 2012;16(4):771–83.

52. Brentnall TA. Pancreatic cancer surveillance: learning as we go. Am J Gastroenterol 2011;106(5):955–6.

53. Canto MI, Goggins M, Hruban RH, et al. Screening for early pancreatic neoplasia in high-risk individuals: a prospective controlled study. Clin Gastroenterol Hepatol 2006;4(6):766–81 [quiz: 665].

54. Canto M, Goggins M, Yeo CJ, et al. Screening for pancreatic neoplasia in high-risk individuals: an EUS-based approach. Clin Gastroenterol Hepatol 2004;2(7):606–21.

55. Langer P, Kann PH, Fendrich V, et al. Five years of prospective screening of high-risk individuals from families with familial pancreatic cancer. Gut 2009;58(10):1410–8.

56. Ludwig E, Olson SH, Bayuga S, et al. Feasibility and yield of screening in relatives from familial pancreatic cancer families. Am J Gastroenterol 2011;106(5):946–54.

57. Poley JW, Kluijt I, Gouma DJ, et al. The yield of first-time endoscopic ultrasonography in screening individuals at a high risk of developing pancreatic cancer. Am J Gastroenterol 2009;104(9):2175–81.

58. Vasen HF, Wasser M, van Mil A, et al. Magnetic resonance imaging surveillance detects early-stage pancreatic cancer in carriers of a p16-Leiden mutation. Gastroenterology 2011;140(3):850–6.

59. Verna EC, Hwang C, Stevens PD, et al. Pancreatic cancer screening in a prospective cohort of high-risk patients: a comprehensive strategy of imaging and genetics. Clin Cancer Res 2010;16(20):5028–37.

60. Canto MI, Hruban RH, Fishman EK, et al. Frequent detection of pancreatic lesions in asymptomatic high-risk individuals. Gastroenterology 2012;142(4):796–804 [quiz: e14–5].

61. Ulrich CD, Consensus Committees of the European Registry of Hereditary Pancreatic Diseases, Midwest Multi-Center Pancreatic Study Group, International Association of Pancreatology. Pancreatic cancer in hereditary pancreatitis: consensus guidelines for prevention, screening and treatment. Pancreatology 2001;1(5):416–22.

62. Canto MI, Harinck F, Hruban RH, et al. International Cancer of the Pancreas Screening (CAPS) Consortium summit on the management of patients with increased risk for familial pancreatic cancer. Gut 2013;62(3):339–47.

63. Brentnall TA, Bronner MP, Byrd DR, et al. Early diagnosis and treatment of pancreatic dysplasia in patients with a family history of pancreatic cancer. Ann Intern Med 1999;131(4):247–55.

64. Kamata K, Kitano M, Kudo M, et al. Value of EUS in early detection of pancreatic ductal adenocarcinomas in patients with intraductal papillary mucinous neoplasms. Endoscopy 2014;46(1):22–9.
65. Latchford A, Greenhalf W, Vitone LJ, et al. Peutz-Jeghers syndrome and screening for pancreatic cancer. Br J Surg 2006;93(12):1446–55.
66. Rulyak SJ, Kimmey MB, Veenstra DL, et al. Cost-effectiveness of pancreatic cancer screening in familial pancreatic cancer kindreds. Gastrointest Endosc 2003; 57(1):23–9.
67. Zubarik R, Gordon SR, Lidofsky SD, et al. Screening for pancreatic cancer in a high-risk population with serum CA 19-9 and targeted EUS: a feasibility study. Gastrointest Endosc 2011;74(1):87–95.
68. Brune K, Hong SM, Li A, et al. Genetic and epigenetic alterations of familial pancreatic cancers. Cancer Epidemiol Biomarkers Prev 2008;17(12):3536–42.
69. Springer S, Wang Y, Dal Molin M, et al. A combination of molecular markers and clinical features improve the classification of pancreatic cysts. Gastroenterology 2015;149(6):1501–10.
70. Kanda M, Knight S, Topazian M, et al. Mutant GNAS detected in duodenal collections of secretin-stimulated pancreatic juice indicates the presence or emergence of pancreatic cysts. Gut 2013;62(7):1024–33.
71. Kanda M, Sadakari Y, Borges M, et al. Mutant TP53 in duodenal samples of pancreatic juice from patients with pancreatic cancer or high-grade dysplasia. Clin Gastroenterol Hepatol 2013;11(6):719–30.e5.
72. Tanaka M, Fernández-del Castillo C, Adsay V, et al. International consensus guidelines 2012 for the management of IPMN and MCN of the pancreas. Pancreatology 2012;12(3):183–97.

Imaging Evaluation of Pancreatic Cancer

Myra Kay Feldman, MD*, Namita Sharma Gandhi, MD

KEYWORDS

- Pancreatic cancer • Pancreatic imaging • Computed tomography • MRI
- Resectability • Structured radiologic reports

KEY POINTS

- Imaging techniques available for the diagnosis, staging, and management of pancreatic neoplasms include computed tomography (CT), PET-CT, MRI, and endoscopic ultrasound (EUS).
- Specialized imaging protocols tailored for evaluation of the pancreas are essential for optimal lesion detection and accurate staging and management of pancreatic neoplasms.
- Biphasic (or dual-phase) multidetector CT is the preferred imaging modality for staging and assessing the resectability of pancreatic adenocarcinoma.
- MRI is nonionizing, has a higher contrast resolution, and is used to evaluate pancreatic neoplasms if the primary tumor is not visible with CT or if patients have a contraindication to contrast-enhanced CT.
- Structured radiologic reporting with standardized terminology and format is critical to ensure that all information needed to stage and plan treatment of pancreatic adenocarcinoma is communicated to the multidisciplinary team.

INTRODUCTION

Pancreatic cancer is the tenth most common cancer in the United States, with an estimated 48,960 new cases reported in 2015. It is currently the fourth leading cause of cancer-related deaths in the United States.[1] The best hope for cure of pancreatic ductal adenocarcinoma (PDA), the most common form of pancreatic cancer, includes complete surgical resection as part of a multimodality treatment plan. However, it has been estimated that only 15% to 20% of patients present with resectable disease.[2] Patients with complete, incomplete, or margin-positive resection (R0, no residual disease; R1, residual microscopic disease; or R2, residual macroscopic disease, respectively) have progressively decreasing survival rates.[3]

Imaging studies are critical for the detection, characterization, initial staging, management, and monitoring of pancreatic cancer cases. Diagnostic imaging of the

Section of Abdominal Imaging, Imaging Institute, Cleveland Clinic, 9500 Euclid Avenue A21, Cleveland, OH 44195, USA
* Corresponding author.
E-mail address: feldmam2@ccf.org

Surg Clin N Am 96 (2016) 1235–1256
http://dx.doi.org/10.1016/j.suc.2016.07.007
0039-6109/16/© 2016 Elsevier Inc. All rights reserved.

pancreas has traditionally posed a challenge to the radiologist because of the subtle imaging appearance of some tumors, especially those that are smaller than 2 cm and those that do not cause a border deformity of the pancreas. Dedicated pancreatic imaging protocols tailored to optimize pancreatic lesion conspicuity and highlight the ductal and peripancreatic anatomy are crucial for accurate determination of resectability. As such, the National Comprehensive Cancer Network (NCCN) has established guidelines for the imaging modalities and imaging protocols used to evaluate PDA.[4]

Treatment of pancreatic cancer requires a multidisciplinary approach. Ideally, assessing resectablility with imaging and subsequent treatment decisions should be made at a high-volume center of excellence with a multidisciplinary team. Recently, a structured radiologic report using standardized nomenclature and formatting has been endorsed by radiologic and clinical specialties to appropriately communicate essential information required to accurately stage and manage pancreatic cancer. Although the use of this form of reporting is not yet universal, it has been shown to add significant value to the care of patients with PDA.[5]

This article reviews the major imaging modalities used to evaluate pancreatic neoplasms, with an emphasis on pancreatic imaging protocols. We describe the imaging appearance of solid pancreatic neoplasms, and the imaging criteria used to stage and determine resectability for PDA. An approach to standardized radiologic reporting is also reviewed.

IMAGING TECHNIQUES AND PROTOCOLS

Computed tomography (CT) and MRI are the first-line imaging modalities used to evaluate pancreatic neoplasms. The role of PET remains unclear, but this modality is most commonly used to assess for the presence of extrapancreatic metastatic disease. Endoscopic ultrasound (EUS) plays an important role in guiding fine-needle aspiration (FNA) or biopsy. Endoscopy in the evaluation of pancreatic cancer is covered in detail elsewhere in this issue. A summary of the indications, advantages, and disadvantages of each imaging modality is provided in **Table 1**.

Computed Tomography

Pancreatic protocol dual-phase CT is recommended by the NCCN guidelines as the preferred imaging study for the initial evaluation of PDA (**Table 2**).[4] CT is more widely available than MRI and is less costly. Furthermore, the spatial resolution of CT is much better than MRI allowing for more accurate assessment of subtle perivascular disease. A dual-phase study should be performed even if a single-phase standard CT scan is available, unless there is evidence of metastatic, nonresectable disease on the standard CT scan.[5] Dual-phase imaging is performed in the pancreatic (late arterial) and portal venous phases of contrast enhancement. Conspicuity of PDA is greatest in the pancreatic phase (**Fig. 1**); therefore, this phase is used to delineate the primary tumor and to evaluate arterial involvement by the tumor. The portal venous phase images are used to evaluate venous involvement by the tumor and to identify distant spread of disease.[6] Unenhanced imaging is not helpful in the initial staging of pancreatic cancer. Intravenous contrast should be injected via a power injector at a rate of at least 3.5 to 5 mL/s. The timing of imaging after contrast injection varies among scanners and is typically determined in one of two ways. Scans can be performed at a fixed time delay after contrast administration (typically 35–80 seconds for late arterial phase depending on scanner speed and 65–80 seconds for portal venous phase).[7] This method is plagued by suboptimal enhancement in some patients because of variations in circulation. Alternatively, automated bolus tracking software can trigger scans

Table 1
Imaging modalities for pancreatic cancer

Modality	Indications	Advantages	Disadvantages	Contraindications
CT	Preferred modality to stage PDA	High spatial resolution Widely available Lower cost than MRI	Tumors may not be visible because of poor contrast resolution	Intravenous contrast contraindicated in patients with severe allergy or poor renal function
MRI	Cases with high suspicion for pancreatic neoplasm and negative CT Preferred modality to evaluate pancreatic cystic lesions Alternative for those with CT contrast allergy or compromised renal function	Excellent contrast resolution Provides characterization of liver lesions (potential metastasis)	High cost Limited availability Image artifacts	Noncompatible implanted medical devices GFR <30 mL/min/1.73 m² (relative contraindication because of nephrogenic systemic fibrosis risk) Not suitable for patients who cannot lie still/hold breath or have claustrophobia
PET-CT	Role in pancreatic cancer evaluation is unclear; may be used for metastatic evaluation	Provides functional metabolic information	Poor spatial and contrast resolution High cost	Elevated glucose levels
EUS	Guide FNA for tissue sampling Cases with strong suspicion for pancreatic lesion and negative CT and MRI	Useful for cytohistopathologic sampling	Invasive Small field of view	Patient must be able to undergo conscious sedation

Abbreviations: CT, computed tomography; EUS, endoscopic ultrasound; FNA, fine-needle aspiration; GFR, glomerular filtration rate; PDA, pancreatic ductal adenocarcinoma.

Table 2
CT protocol for pancreatic imaging

Parameter	Value
CT scanner specifications	Multidetector
Oral contrast	250 mL water (or neutral contrast) while waiting for scan and 250 mL water just before scan No iodinated or high-attenuation contrast
Intravenous contrast	150 mL Omnipaque 300 (or other high-concentration contrast) 60 mL saline flush 4-mL/s injection rate
Scan acquisition timing	Pancreatic (late arterial) phase: trigger with bolus tracking Portal venous phase: trigger with bolus tracking or 70–80 s (depending on speed of scanner)
Image acquisition and reconstruction	0.6-mm collimation (thinnest) 3-mm slice thickness 1 mm × 0.8 mm for reconstruction (smallest slice with overlap)
Reconstruction	3 mm × 3 mm coronal multiplanar reformat for both phases 3D, MIP, multiplanar reformat software available to radiologists during review

Abbreviations: 3D, three-dimensional, MIP, maximum intensity projection.

to be performed once a certain threshold of contrast attenuation is reached at a set location (typically the descending or upper abdominal aorta). This corrects for variance in circulation among patients and improves the conspicuity of PDA during the pancreatic phase.[8] At our institution, automatic bolus tracking is used to time the pancreatic phase, and venous-phase imaging is then performed at a fixed time (70–80 seconds).

High-attenuation oral contrast should not be administered when evaluating the pancreas because this type of contrast in the gastric body could cause beam attenuation artifact, compromising the evaluation of the adjacent pancreas and possibly obscuring ampullary pathology. Neutral oral contrast agents, such as those used in CT enterography (Breeza, Beekley Medical, Bristol, CT), water, or milk are usually administered to the patient before imaging to distend the duodenum, thereby improving conspicuity of lesions in this location (see **Fig. 1**C). At our institution, patients drink 250 mL of water 15 minutes before the study and again just before getting on the table. Some authors advocate using larger doses of neutral contrast agents to better distend the region when ampullary pathology is suspected. Some institutions also administer glucagon or effervescent crystals to reduce peristalsis and improve distention of the duodenum.[9]

Multidetector technology allows for rapid acquisition of high-resolution isotropic images that are reviewed in multiple planes via multiplanar reformat imaging. Studies have shown that reviewing multiplanar reformat CT data in the coronal and sagittal planes allows for improved detection and staging of tumors.[6,10] Curved planar reformatted images are used to view a specific structure of interest, such as a vessel, which may lie or course in a nonstandard plane (see **Fig. 1**D, E). At our institution, the pancreatic and portal venous image sets are reviewed in axial and coronal planes. Three-dimensional (3D) software is immediately available to the interpreting physician and is used to create additional sagittal or curved planar reformatted images for further evaluation.

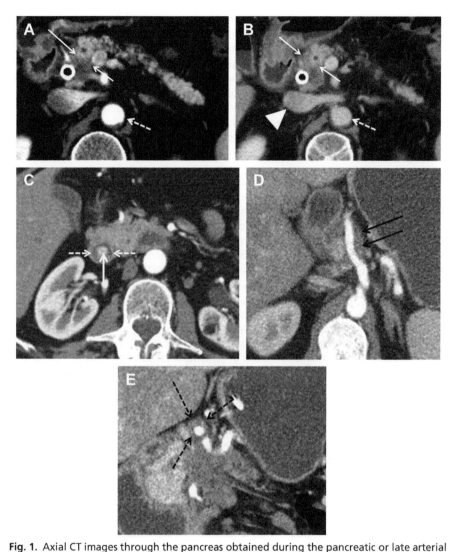

Fig. 1. Axial CT images through the pancreas obtained during the pancreatic or late arterial phase of contrast enhancement (*A*). This phase is recognized by the bright enhancement of the aorta (*dashed arrow*). The borders of the low-attenuation PDA (*solid arrows*) are well delineated in this phase compared with the background pancreatic parenchyma. A metal biliary stent is seen. Axial CT at the same level but obtained during the venous phase of contrast enhancement (*B*). The venous phase is identified by less dense enhancement of the aorta (*dashed arrow*) with similar attenuation to the inferior vena cava (*triangle*). The borders of the low-attenuation PDA (*solid arrows*) are less distinct on this phase. An axial CT image in a different patient obtained during the pancreatic phase of contrast enhancement shows a hypervascular duodenal carcinoid (*solid arrow*) (*C*). The lesion stands out against the surrounding lower-attenuation fluid (*dashed arrows*) within the duodenal lumen. An axial CT scan performed during the pancreatic phase shows soft tissue along 50% of the superior mesenteric artery (*arrows*) (*D*). The borders above and below the superior mesenteric artery are not visible in the axial plane. A coronal reformatted image obtained from the same arterial phase acquisition shows that the superior mesenteric artery is completely (100%) encased by soft tissue attenuation tumor (*dashed arrows*) (*E*).

Emerging CT technologies are also being explored for use in pancreatic imaging. Dual-energy CT scanners simultaneously image at two distinct energy levels. Dual-energy CT data can be processed to optimize images and to identify or quantify a certain material, such as iodine from contrast material. Although a thorough discussion of dual-energy CT imaging capabilities is beyond the scope of this article, studies have shown improved lesion detection, border definition, and lesion characterization, and improved evaluation of structures relevant to treatment planning with these techniques.[11] Additionally, the routine use of lower tube potential (kilovoltage) allows for better differentiation between enhancing normal parenchyma and the generally hypo-enhancing pancreatic carcinoma.

MRI

Although CT is considered the first-line imaging modality for the evaluation of PDA, MRI can offer advantages over CT in specific clinical situations. MRI has superior contrast resolution compared with CT and is thus more sensitive for the detection of non-contour-deforming pancreatic tumors. However, because the spatial resolution of MRI is less than CT, subtle perivascular and peripancreatic changes are not as readily or accurately identified. MRI is used to characterize hepatic lesions as metastatic disease.[12] MRI combined with MR cholangiopancreatography (MRCP) offers better evaluation of the pancreatic duct and can better detect and classify pancreatic cystic lesions. MRI can also be used in patients with contraindications to CT, such as intravenous contrast allergy or renal insufficiency.

Most pancreatic MRI protocols use a combination of imaging sequences obtained in different planes; these sequences are designed to highlight pancreatic parenchymal and ductal anatomy. These protocols should include a T2-weighted single-shot fast-spin-echo sequence, T1-weighted in-phase and opposed-phase gradient echo sequences, a T2-weighted fat-suppressed sequence, heavily T2-weighted 3D MRCP sequences, and 3D gradient echo T1-weighted sequences with fat suppression obtained before contrast and with dynamic postcontrast imaging to include the pancreatic (arterial) and portal venous phases of contrast enhancement. Diffusion-weighed imaging (DWI) with apparent diffusion coefficient (ADC) mapping should also be included (**Table 3**).[5,12] A noncontrast MRCP scan is not sufficient to diagnose and stage PDA.[5]

T1-weighted in-phase and opposed-phase sequences are used to assess for intracellular fat. On these sequences, fat loses signal or appears darker on the opposed-phase set of images as compared with the in-phase set of images (**Fig. 2A, B**). The precontrast T1-weighted gradient echo sequence with fat suppression is used to assess for the presence of extracellular or macroscopic fat (**Fig. 2C**). Fat-suppression imaging is important in pancreatic imaging, because prominent or asymmetric areas of pancreatic fat can be mistaken for a mass. Images from this sequence are also compared against postcontrast images. T1-weighted images are used to assess for the presence of hemorrhage, which appears as T1 hyperintense (white).[13]

All MRI protocols to evaluate pancreatic cancers should include 3D gradient echo T1-weighted dynamic postcontrast imaging through the pancreas, peripancreatic tissues, and liver. MRI contrast agents taken up by biologic tissues appear as T1 hyperintense (white). This series of postcontrast scans is crucial for detecting lesions, evaluating the vascular anatomy, and assessing metastatic disease (**Fig. 2D**).

T2-weighted sequences, sometimes referred to as "fluid-sensitive" sequences, are used to assess for the presence of fluid. Simple fluid is T2 hyperintense (white) on these sequences (**Fig. 2E**). Many tumors, including hepatic metastases, demonstrate T2 intermediate signal, making this sequence helpful for lesion detection.

Table 3
MRI protocol for pancreatic imaging

Sequence	Plane	Slice Thickness	Purpose
T2-weighted single-shot FSE or HASTE	Axial, coronal, sagittal (optional)	4 mm	Evaluate overall anatomy
T1-weighted in-phase and opposed-phase gradient echo	Axial	4 mm	Evaluate intracellular fat
T2-weighted with fat suppression	Axial	7–9 mm	Lesion detection Evaluate for fluid signal
Heavily T2-weighted 3D MRCP	Coronal, MIP reconstruction (optional)	1.1 mm 3D	Evaluate duct and cystic structures
T1-weighted 3D gradient echo with fat saturation before and after contrast to include arterial, portal venous, delayed venous, and 4-min delayed phases	Axial, coronal (optional)	2.3 mm 3D	Detect and characterize lesions, evaluate vascular involvement
DWI with ADC mapping	Axial	6 mm	Detect lesions
Offline 3D reconstructions	—	—	Characterize duct anatomy and relationship of cysts to ducts

Abbreviations: FSE, fast spin echo; HASTE, half-Fourier acquisition single-shot turbo spin echo; MIP, maximum intensity projection.

MRCP is a special type of sequence that is heavily T2 weighted so that only fluid signal is imaged. MRCP images are obtained using two-dimensional or 3D techniques. The 3D technique produces thin-slice images, which can more effectively evaluate small side branches and filling defects. These sequences are used to evaluate the pancreatic and biliary duct anatomy. MRCP imaging is also helpful for evaluating pancreatic cystic lesions (**Fig. 2F**).[13]

DWI is a functional MRI technique that assesses water motion in biologic tissues (called Brownian motion). Brownian motion is affected by tissue cellularity, viscosity of fluids, and the presence of intact cell membranes. Increased cellular density with many intact cellular membranes, a finding in many neoplastic tissues, is associated with restricted water motion. On DWI, tissues with restricted diffusion appear bright (white). The generation of ADC maps allows for quantitative assessment of this diffusion.[14] In the setting of pancreatic cancer, DWI is used to detect primary tumor and metastatic disease. Both PDA and pancreatic neuroendocrine tumors (PNET) typically demonstrate higher signal intensity than the background pancreas on DWI, along with lower ADC values (**Fig. 2G, H**). Studies have shown that adding DWI to MRI protocols increases the sensitivity for lesion detection, particularly for lesions smaller than 2 cm.[15,16] However, DWI cannot be used alone to characterize lesions, because more necrotic or less fibrous tumors may not show restricted diffusion. Additionally, benign processes, such as infection and pancreatitis, can demonstrate restricted diffusion. Current research is evaluating the use of DWI and ADC values as predictors of tumor aggressiveness and response to therapy.[17]

Newer techniques, such as MRI perfusion imaging, are also being evaluated for use in pancreatic tumor characterization and therapy monitoring.[14,18]

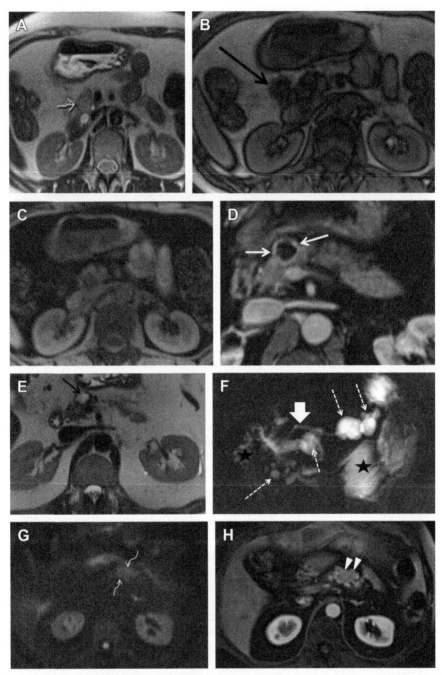

Fig. 2. Axial T2-weighted image without fat suppression shows focal T2 hyperintense lesion (*arrow*) in the pancreatic head (*A*). Subcutaneous and mesenteric fat is also hyperintense on this image. On the axial T1-weighted opposed-phase image, the pancreatic head lesion shows blooming T2 hypointense signal (*arrow*) (*B*). Axial T1 gradient echo precontrast image with fat suppression shows that the pancreatic head lesion is hypointense compared with the background pancreas (*C*). Fat in the mesentery is also hypointense.

Not every patient can undergo MRI. These studies take much longer to perform than CT examinations and thus require greater patient cooperation, with patients being required to lie still and maintain longer breath holds. Some patients cannot tolerate the examinations because of claustrophobia. Others may not be suited for MRI because of the presence of incompatible implanted devices. Finally, patients may not be eligible for the use of intravenous gadolinium-based contrast because of allergy or poor renal function (glomerular filtration rate <30 mL/min/1.73 m^2), which could lead to nephrogenic systemic fibrosis in the presence of gadolinium-based contrast.

PET

In PET, the radiotracer 18 F-fluorodeoxyglucose (FDG) is injected intravenously. In general, neoplastic cells take up proportionally more glucose than nonneoplastic tissue. FDG is trapped in the cells, because it cannot be metabolized by the usual glycolytic pathways. The radiolabeled FDG thus accumulates in neoplastic tissues and emits positrons, which are detected by the PET scanner. Radiologists use qualitative and semiquantitative data when interpreting PET studies. The quantitative standard uptake value represents the metabolic activity of an area of interest corrected for the dose of radiotracer administered and the weight of the patient.[19]

Hybrid PET-CT scanners combine low-dose CT imaging with standard PET imaging. In these studies, data from the CT scan are used for attenuation correction and radiotracer localization. The CT data are typically acquired during free respiration without oral or intravenous contrast. This results in CT images with decreased spatial resolution because of respiration motion artifact and suboptimal tissue contrast because of the lack of intravenous contrast. However, modern PET-CT scanners are now able to combine PET imaging with full-dose CT imaging and more sophisticated CT protocols, such as the dual-phase contrast-enhanced pancreas protocol described previously. This results in CT images with resolution and anatomic detail similar to those of standard CT scans with the added metabolic information provided by the PET data.

Interpreting studies on the use of PET and PET-CT in pancreatic tumors is confounded by discrepancies among protocols used in the past and those available on modern equipment. The NCCN guidelines state that the role of PET-CT in the management of PDA remains unclear but that it can be used particularly in high-risk patients, such as those with borderline resectable disease, markedly elevated tumor markers, and large tumors or lymph nodes.[5] This modality is currently most widely used for initial staging and treatment planning (**Fig. 3**). Research has demonstrated

◄───

Axial T1-weighted postcontrast image shows a cystic pancreatic neuroendocrine tumors (PNET) (*D*). The peripheral rim of solid tissue enhances more than the background pancreas (*arrows*), an imaging feature characteristic of neuroendocrine tumors. Axial T2-weighted image from the same location shows that the cystic component of the tumor is T2 hyperintense (*arrow*) (*E*). Maximum intensity projection image acquired from 3D heavily T2-weighted MRCP sequence shows multiple pancreatic cystic lesions (*dashed arrows*) that communicate with the main pancreatic duct (*thick arrow*), compatible with intraductal papillary mucinous neoplasms (*F*). Fluid signal is also present within the duodenal and gastric lumen (*asterisks*). Axial DWI in patient with increasing CA19-9 and negative CT 3 years after distal pancreatectomy for PDA (*G*). The recurrent hyperintense mass in the pancreatic body along the resection margin (*arrows*) is obvious on the DWI series (*G*) and subtle on the axial T1 gradient echo contrast-enhanced pancreatic phase images (*arrowheads*) (*H*).

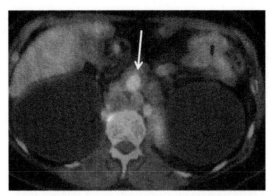

Fig. 3. Axial fused PET-CT image in a patient with newly diagnosed PDA shows FDG-avid uncinate process mass (*arrow*). PET-CT was ordered in this case because the patient had a history of lymphoma, breast cancer, and primary lung cancer.

that PET-CT also shows promise for predicting prognosis, planning radiotherapy, monitoring treatment response, and evaluating recurrent disease.[20,21]

PET-CT is generally not performed in patients with hyperglycemia (glucose levels >200 mg/100 mL) because this could cause decreased FDG uptake and thus lead to false-negative results. Contraindications for contrast agents with PET-CT are the same as those for standard CT.

PET-MRI is an emerging technology that uses MRI data for attenuation correction and spatial localization. The potential use of this modality in pancreatic cancer is yet to be determined.[22]

Endoscopic Ultrasound

EUS has become more widely available and accepted in the management of pancreatic cancer over the past decade. This modality uses a high-resolution EUS probe that is advanced to the stomach and duodenum in close proximity to the pancreas. As with all forms of ultrasound, image quality is user dependent. When performed by an expert practitioner, EUS is the most sensitive test available to evaluate for a pancreatic mass. This modality is particularly useful for lesion detection when the primary lesion is not seen by CT or MRI and when the lesion measures less than 2 cm.[23]

The main value of EUS imaging is that it is possible to introduce an FNA or core biopsy device under EUS guidance. This allows for preoperative tissue sampling, which in some cases is valuable for establishing a definitive diagnosis. EUS with FNA is an invasive procedure with inherent risks of bleeding and pancreatitis. The risk of these EUS-associated adverse effects has been estimated at 0.5% to 2%. Although very uncommon, tumor seeding has also been reported after EUS FNA.[23,24]

The American Society for Gastrointestinal Endoscopy advises the use of EUS with FNA in all cases of suspected resectable PDA.[23] The NCCN guidelines state that although EUS is not recommended as a routine staging tool, in patients with resectable disease, EUS with FNA is preferred over CT-guided biopsy because of a lower risk of tumor seeding.[5]

EUS can also be used to guide fiducial placement for use in radiation therapy, and EUS-guided fine-needle tattooing may be useful in patients with lesions that are not well visualized by other forms of abdominal imaging.[23]

IMAGING FEATURES OF SOLID PANCREATIC NEOPLASMS

PDA and PNET are the most common solid pancreatic neoplasms and are the focus of this discussion. Other solid pancreatic neoplasms include lymphoma, metastatic disease, and solid pseudopapillary tumor. Imaging features of solid pancreatic neoplasms are summarized in **Table 4**. Pancreatic cystic neoplasms are not discussed in this article because their evaluation generally follows a separate diagnostic algorithm.

Pancreatic Ductal Adenocarcinoma

Most PDA tumors are located in the pancreatic head, followed by the body and tail. On MRI, PDA tumors are hypointense to the background pancreas on T1- and T2-weighted images. PDA tumors typically restrict diffusion and appear hyperintense on DWI and hypointense on ADC maps.

On contrast-enhanced CT and contrast-enhanced MRI, PDA lesions typically enhance less than the background pancreas (**Fig. 4A**). This hypoenhancement is most evident on pancreatic phase images. Up to 10% of lesions may be isoattenuating to the background pancreas on CT, making these lesions difficult to detect.[25] However, when the primary mass cannot be identified, its presence may be inferred by the identification of ancillary imaging features including pancreatic or common bile duct obstruction, convex border deformity, or peripancreatic soft tissue infiltration. Obstruction and dilation of the pancreatic duct with abrupt duct cutoff at the level of the tumor is a commonly seen ancillary imaging feature. The "double duct sign" occurs when both the pancreatic and common bile ducts are obstructed by a pancreatic head mass. Atrophy of the pancreas proximal to the lesion may also be seen

Table 4		
Imaging features of solid pancreatic neoplasms		
Lesion	**Imaging Modality**	**Imaging Findings**
PDA	Pancreatic CT preferred for staging; pancreatic MRI if CT is contraindicated	Mass hypovascular compared with pancreas on pancreatic phase, heterogeneous enhancement on venous phase Pancreatic atrophy beyond mass Pancreatic duct dilated with cutoff at mass Common bile duct and hepatic ducts dilated if mass is in periampullary location Convex border deformity
PNET	Pancreatic CT; pancreatic MRI; octreotide scan for detection	Hypervascular T1 hypointense and T2 hyperintense Cystic change or calcifications may be present
Pancreatic lymphoma	Standard CT	Solid discrete mass or infiltrative Variable enhancement Tumor may not respect anatomic boundaries
Pancreatic parenchymal metastasis	CT or MRI	Hypervascular (renal cell carcinoma) or hypovascular Single, multifocal, or diffuse

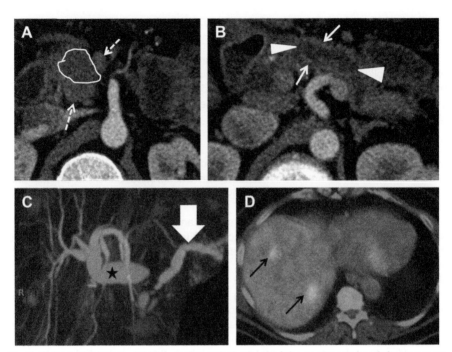

Fig. 4. Pancreatic phase axial CT scan through the level of the pancreatic head shows a mass that is hypodense (*outline*) compared with the background pancreas (*dashed arrows*) (*A*). Axial image from the same patient at a different level shows markedly dilated pancreatic duct (*arrowheads*) and atrophic pancreatic parenchyma in the body and tail (*arrows*) (*B*). Maximum intensity projection image from MRCP shows the "double duct sign," with markedly dilated common bile duct (*asterisk*), intrahepatic ducts, and pancreatic duct (*arrow*) (*C*). Axial PET-CT image from a different patient with pancreatic cancer shows FDG-avid liver metastasis (*arrows*) (*D*).

(**Fig. 4**B, C).[26,27] Vascular invasion is identified when soft tissue surrounds vessels with loss of the expected perivascular fat plane. Vessels, especially venous structures, may be effaced or displaced by surrounding soft tissue tumor. Filling defects or thrombus within vessels can also be seen. Distant metastatic disease is most commonly identified in the liver and peritoneum.

On EUS, PDA lesions are hypoechoic compared with the normal pancreas and tend to be ill defined. The field of view with EUS is narrow, limiting the evaluation of metastatic spread to locoregional lymph nodes and adjacent vessels.

PDA lesions and metastatic disease are hypermetabolic on PET (**Fig. 4**D). However, small lesions and lesions with necrosis may not be detected on this imaging modality.

Pancreatic Neuroendocrine Tumors

PNET account for 1% to 2% of all pancreatic neoplasms. They may occur at any age but are most common in the fourth to sixth decades of life. There is no sex predilection with these tumors. Although there is increased risk for PNET with some genetic syndromes, most cases of PNET occur sporadically. PNET is either benign or malignant and functioning or nonfunctioning.[28]

PNET have a varied imaging appearance. Functioning tumors that secrete peptides that cause symptoms typically present earlier than nonfunctioning tumors and are thus often smaller at presentation. On CT and MRI, functioning tumors demonstrate uniform precontrast attenuation or signal and homogeneous postcontrast enhancement (**Fig. 5**A). Nonfunctioning tumors may not be clinically diagnosed until they cause symptoms from mass effect or metastatic disease; therefore, these lesions are often larger at presentation. Nonfunctioning tumors may have areas of cystic degeneration or internal calcifications resulting in mixed attenuation or signal on precontrast images. These lesions demonstrate heterogeneous enhancement (**Fig. 5**B). Unlike PDA, PNET are typically hypervascular compared with the background pancreas.[26,28]

On MRI, PNET tend to be T1 hypointense. T2 signal is variable, with most tumors showing T2 hyperintense signal compared with the background pancreas and others showing intermediate T2 signal. As on CT, PNET typically enhance more than the background pancreas.

IN-111 octreotide scans can be used to detect suspected PNET. In these studies, radiolabeled octreotide is picked up by PNET with somatostatin receptors (**Fig. 5**C, D). This modality is not sensitive for insulinomas.[28] In PNET, PET-CT is mainly used to evaluate metastatic lesions, which appear as FDG avid.

Pancreatic Lymphoma

Pancreatic lymphoma is typically a B-cell, non-Hodgkin type of disease. Primary pancreatic lymphoma is rare, comprising less than 2% of all extranodal lymphomas.

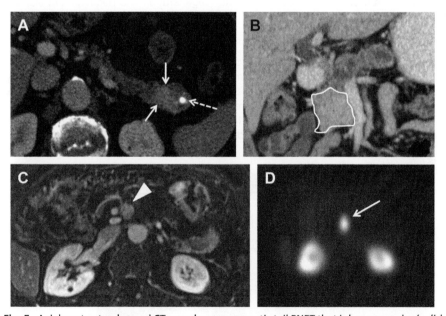

Fig. 5. Axial contrast-enhanced CT scan shows pancreatic tail PNET that is hypervascular (*solid arrows*) compared with the background pancreas (*A*). The mass contains a calcification (*dashed arrow*). Axial contrast-enhanced CT scan in another patient with pancreatic head PNET enhancing more than the background pancreas (*outline*) (*B*). Axial T1 contrast-enhanced MRI in a patient who had undergone pancreaticoduodenectomy for pancreatic head PNET with new enhancing soft tissue nodule adjacent to the superior mesenteric artery (*arrowhead*) (*C*). Axial image from IN-111 octreotide study in the same patient at the same level shows that the nodule takes up octreotide (*arrow*), compatible with recurrent/metastatic disease (*D*).

Secondary lymphoma with spread from adjacent lymph nodes is the most common form to involve the pancreas. Pancreatic lymphoma can appear as a well-circumscribed discrete mass or as infiltrative disease with enlargement of the gland. Lymphomatous masses generally enhance to the same degree of the pancreas although the enhancement pattern is variable. Untreated lymphoma does not contain calcifications. Pancreatic lymphoma does not respect anatomic boundaries, and disease may be seen in the intraperitoneal abdomen with nodal disease below the level of the renal arteries. Lymphoma can surround vasculature, as in PDA; however, the vasculature is typically not occluded by lymphoma.[29] One important feature of lymphoma is that when the pancreatic head is involved the degree of biliary and pancreatic ductal dilation is much less than one would expect for the size of the mass (**Fig. 6**).

Pancreatic Parenchymal Metastases

Metastatic disease to the pancreas is rare. Renal cell carcinoma and lung cancer are the most common neoplasms associated with pancreatic metastasis; metastatic disease from breast cancer, gastrointestinal tract malignancies, melanoma, osteosarcoma, and thyroid cancer have also been described. Metastatic disease to the pancreas can be solitary, multifocal, or diffuse. Enhancement patterns with metastases are variable. Although most metastatic lesions show peripheral or homogeneous contrast enhancement greater than the background pancreas, metastatic lesions from colon, lung, or breast cancers can be hypovascular. Renal cell carcinoma metastases are often hypervascular. Cystic degeneration and necrosis can also be seen (**Fig. 7**).[26,30]

Miscellaneous Solid Pancreatic Neoplasms

Solid pseudopapillary tumor accounts for 1% to 2% of all pancreatic tumors. This tumor exhibits a strong female predilection (9:1) and occurs in younger patients, typically occurring in the second decade of life. These lesions are well encapsulated and slow growing and thus tend to be large at presentation. The capsule is low attenuation on CT and shows hypointense signal on T1- and T2-weighted images. The center of the tumor is characterized by cystic degeneration and hemorrhage, causing a

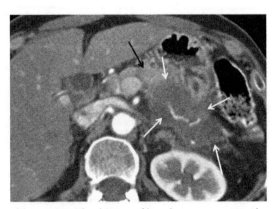

Fig. 6. In a 72-year-old woman with a history of lymphoma, contrast-enhanced CT scan shows an infiltrative pancreatic body/tail hypodense mass (*white arrows*) enhancing less than the pancreas (*black arrow*) that encases but does not occlude the splenic artery. A biopsy demonstrated B-cell lymphoma.

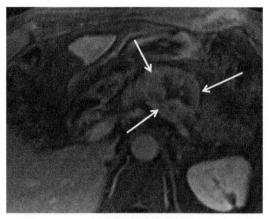

Fig. 7. In a 62-year-old man with a history of renal cell carcinoma who had undergone a right nephrectomy, MRI shows a heterogeneously enhancing pancreatic body/tail (*arrows*), indicating renal cell carcinoma metastasis.

heterogeneous appearance on MRI and CT. Postcontrast imaging shows early enhancement of the capsule with heterogeneous progressive enhancement of the center of the lesion.[31]

Other rare tumors, including pancreatoblastoma, epithelial tumors, mesenchymal tumors, and mixed tumors, can occur in the pancreas but are rare and beyond the scope of this article.

CLASSIFICATION OF RESECTABLE, BORDERLINE RESECTABLE, AND LOCALLY ADVANCED/NONRESECTABLE PANCREATIC DUCTAL ADENOCARCINOMA

PDA treatment guidelines published by the NCCN classify PDA as resectable, borderline resectable, or locally advanced/nonresectable.[5,32,33] Assessment of tumor resectability is based on tumor location, vascular involvement, and metastasis as determined by imaging **(Table 5)**. For nonmetastatic PDA, decisions regarding resectability should be made by a multidisciplinary team after acquisition of dedicated pancreatic protocol imaging and staging studies.[5]

PDA is considered resectable when there is no distant metastatic disease or lymphadenopathy. In addition, there must be a clear fat plane with no tumor contact with the surrounding arteries and either no tumor contact or less than 180° tumor contact with the superior mesenteric vein (SMV) and portal vein with no contour deformity **(Figs. 8 and 9)**. A staging laparoscopy should be selectively considered based on clinical predictors that optimize yield. These predictors include pancreatic head tumors larger than 3 cm, tumors of the pancreas body and tail, equivocal findings on CT scan, and high CA 19-9 levels (>100 U/mL).[33]

Borderline resectable pancreatic cancer represents a tumor that is confined locoregionally with no imaging or laparoscopic evidence of metastatic disease; additionally, the tumor is deemed not imminently resectable to a negative margin but potentially resectable to a negative margin by surgical criteria after trial of neoadjuvant therapy. **Table 6** summarizes the current various definitions of borderline resectable tumors used by different groups based on vascular involvement.[5,33–35] A multidisciplinary approach that can arrive at a consensus recommendation is highly recommended in the treatment of borderline resectable pancreatic cancer **(Fig. 10)**.

Table 5
PDA resectability based on NCCN 2015 guidelines

Resectability Status	Arterial Involvement	Venous Involvement
Resectable	No contact with CA, SMA, or CHA	No or <180° tumor contact with SMV/PV with no contour deformity
Borderline resectable	Pancreatic head/uncinate • Solid tumor contact with CHA, which does not extend to hepatic bifurcation or celiac axis • Solid tumor contact <180° • Solid tumor contact with variant arterial anatomy (eg, replaced SMA) Pancreatic body/tail • Solid tumor contact with CA <180° • Solid tumor contact with CA >180° with no involvement of aorta and intact GDA	• Solid tumor contact with SMV >180° but reconstructable • Solid tumor contact with IVC
Unresectable	Pancreatic head/uncinate • Solid tumor contact with SMA or CA >180° • Solid tumor contact with first jejunal branch of SMA Pancreatic body/tail • Solid tumor contact with SMA or CA >180° • Aortic involvement	• Unreconstructable venous involvement of SMV or PV • Contact with most proximal jejunal draining vein of SMV

Abbreviations: CA, celiac artery; CHA, common hepatic artery; GDA, gastroduodenal artery; IVC, inferior vena cava; PV, portal vein; SMA, superior mesenteric artery; SMV, superior mesenteric artery.

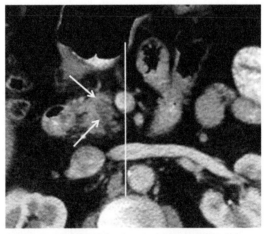

Fig. 8. In a 59-year-old man with abdominal pain, CT scan in the late arterial phase shows a hypodense pancreatic head/uncinate mass (*arrows*) to the right of the superior mesenteric vein (SMV) (*vertical line*) with no involvement of the SMV or superior mesenteric artery. This case was resectable.

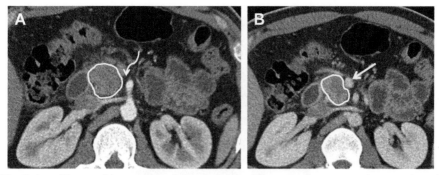

Fig. 9. In a 35-year-old man with abdominal pain, CT scan in the pancreatic parenchymal phase (*A*) and portal venous phase (*B*) shows a 3-cm pancreatic head/uncinate mass (*outlined*) abutting (<180°) the SMV (*straight arrow*) with no involvement of the superior mesenteric artery, as shown by the preserved fat plane (*curved arrow*). There were no metastasis, and this case was resectable.

PDA is considered nonresectable when metastatic disease is present, including distant metastases and nonregional nodal metastases. Common sites of distant metastatic disease from PDA are the liver and peritoneum (**Fig. 11**). PDA is also considered nonresectable when there is more than 180° solid tumor contact with the superior mesenteric artery or celiac axis or solid tumor contact with the first jejunal branch of the superior mesenteric artery. For body/tail PDA, cases of solid tumor contact greater than 180° with the celiac artery and contact with the aorta are considered nonresectable. Cases involving unreconstructable SMV/portal vein involvement and contact with the most proximal draining jejunal branch of the SMV are also nonresectable.

Table 6
Various definitions of borderline resectable PDA

VESSEL	NCCN 2015[5]	MD Anderson[35]	AHPBA/SSAT/SSO[33]	Intergroup Trial[34]
SMV-PV	Abutment[a]	Occlusion	Abutment, encasement[b]	Tumor-vessel interface >180° and/or reconstructable[c] occlusion
SMA	Abutment	Abutment	Abutment	Tumor-vessel interface <180°
CHA	Abutment or short-segment encasement	Abutment or short-segment encasement	Abutment or short-segment encasement	Reconstructable short-segment interface tumor-vessel interface
Celiac trunk	No abutment or encasement	Abutment	No abutment or encasement	Tumor-vessel interface <180°

Abbreviations: AHPBA, american hepato-pancreato-biliary association; SSAT, society for surgery of the alimentary tract; SSO, society of surgical oncology.
  [a] Abutment: tumor-vessel interface less than 180° circumference.
  [b] Encasement: tumor-vessel interface greater than 180° circumference.
  [c] Normal vein or artery proximal and distal to the site of tumor vessel involvement suitable for vascular reconstruction.
  Data from Refs.[5,33–35]

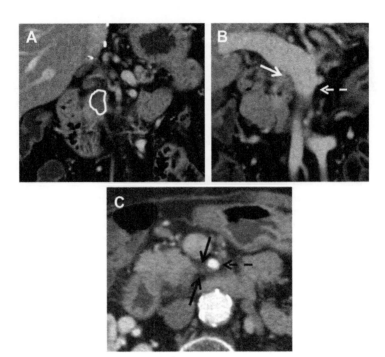

Fig. 10. In a 69-year-old woman with abdominal pain, contrast-enhanced CT scan in coronal reformats (*A, B*) and axial (*C*) shows a hypodense pancreatic head/uncinate mass (*outlined*) with less than 180° abutment (*white straight arrow*) of the SMV (*white dashed arrow*) and less than 180° abutment (*black straight arrows*) of the superior mesenteric artery (*black dashed arrow*). This case was considered borderline resectable by the multidisciplinary tumor board.

STANDARDIZATION OF RADIOLOGIC REPORTING FOR PANCREATIC DUCTAL ADENOCARCINOMA

Because imaging plays an essential role in the staging and assessment of resectability for PDA, it is imperative that radiologic reports include all information necessary to determine resectability and that this information is communicated in a clear and consistent format. Structured radiologic reports include a checklist of findings to be reported and use a standardized lexicon. This form of reporting facilitates management of PDA and allows for assessment of eligibility for clinical trials and decreases the need for repeat imaging studies. Various societies and institutions have proposed unique standardized templates and lexicons for reporting imaging findings for PDA.[36,37] The Society of Abdominal Radiology has collaborated with the American Pancreatic Association and developed a standardized structured reporting template for PDA[36]; this template has been adopted by our institution and is described next (**Tables 7–9**).

The term "head/uncinate" is defined by its location with respect to the SMV. Tumors to the right of the SMV are in the head/uncinate and if resectable, are amenable to pancreatoduodenectomy. Tumors to the left of the SMV are in the body/tail and are potentially amenable to distal pancreatectomy.

In descriptions of vascular involvement, the term "abutment" is used when there is less than 180° of contact between the solid tumor and a vessel, whereas the term

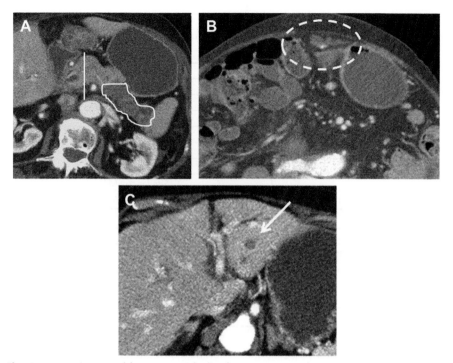

Fig. 11. In an 80-year-old woman with diarrhea, contrast-enhanced CT scan (*A*) shows a pancreatic body/tail hypoenhancing mass (left of SMV, *vertical line; outline*) (*B*). There is peritoneal carcinomatosis (*dashed circle*) and (*C*) liver metastasis (*arrow*). This case was nonresectable. With such a presentation, dual-phase CT is not needed.

"encasement" is used when there is more than 180° of contact between the solid tumor and a vessel. The presence of hazy stranding in the perivascular fat should be mentioned, because this could indicate tumor infiltration, posttreatment change (after chemoradiotherapy), or pancreatitis, especially in cases of recent FNA or biopsy.

The celiac axis, common hepatic artery and its variants, and superior mesenteric artery should be specifically evaluated and reported in all cases. Any change in contour deformity or thrombosis should also be recorded. If pertinent, the length of the vascular segment involved, the proximity of involved vascular segments to

Table 7	
Structured reporting template for PDA: morphology	
Characteristic	**Description**
Morphology (pancreatic parenchymal phase)	Hypodense/isodense
Size	Measurable disease >1 cm (give dimensions)
Location	Head/uncinate: right of SMV Body/tail: left of SMV
Pancreatic duct narrowing/cutoff	Present or absent
Biliary duct narrowing/cutoff	Present or absent

Table 8
Structured reporting template for PDA: vascular evaluation

Artery Characteristic	Description
SMA	
Degrees of solid soft tissue contact	Present or absent; <180° or >180°
Degrees of hazy attenuation/stranding	Present or absent; <180° or >180°
Focal vessel narrowing or contour deformity	Present or absent
Involvement of first jejunal branch	Present or absent
CHA	Similar to SMA
Celiac	Similar to SMA
Splenic	Similar to SMA
Variant anatomy (if present)	Similar to SMA
Veins Characteristic	**Description**
SMV	
Degrees of solid soft tissue contact	Present or absent; <180° or >180°
Degrees of hazy attenuation/stranding	Present or absent; <180° or >180°
Focal vessel narrowing or contour deformity	Present or absent
Involvement of most proximal jejunal draining vein	Present or absent
Main PV	Similar to SMV

other landmarks (branch vessels), and the presence of arterial variants involved by the tumor should be noted. The presence of celiac and superior mesenteric artery stenosis should also be recorded, because this might affect surgical management.

SMV and portal vein involvement is the most important determinant of resectability. The extent of circumferential involvement, thrombosis, and contour deformity should be described. As with arterial assessment, the extent of segmental involvement and its proximity to the nearest venous branch should also be described.

Information about invasion of adjacent structures, such as the stomach or duodenum, should also be included in the radiology report, because this may alter the surgical approach.

SUMMARY

Imaging plays an important role in the diagnosis and management of solid pancreatic neoplasms. Standardization of imaging algorithms, imaging protocols, and

Table 9
Structured reporting template for PDA: extrapancreatic evaluation

Extrapancreatic Characteristic	Description
Liver lesions	Present or absent; suspicious, indeterminate, or benign
Peritoneal/omental nodules	Present or absent
Ascites	Present or absent
Suspicious lymph nodes[a]	Present or absent; location
Invasion of adjacent structures	Present or absent

[a] Greater than 1 cm, round, heterogeneous.

radiologic reporting is important to ensure optimal patient care and disease management.

REFERENCES

1. American Cancer Society website. Cancer facts and figures 2015. Available at: www.cancer.org/research/cancerfactsstatistics/cancerfactsfigures2015/. Accessed March 9, 2016.
2. Li D, Xie K, Wolff R, et al. Pancreatic cancer. Lancet 2004;363(9414):1049–57.
3. Hernandez J, Mullinax J, Clark W, et al. Survival after pancreaticoduodenectomy is not improved by extending resections to achieve negative margins. Ann Surg 2009;250(1):76–80.
4. National Comprehensive Cancer Network website. NCCN Clinical Practice Guidelines in Oncology. Pancreatic adenocarcinoma, version 2.2015. Available at: http://www.nccn.org/professionals/physician_gls/f_guidelines.asp. Accessed March 9, 2016.
5. Brook OR, Brook A, Vollmer CM, et al. Structured reporting of multiphasic CT for pancreatic cancer: potential effect on staging and surgical planning. Radiology 2015;274(2):464–72.
6. Ichikawa T, Erturk SM, Sou H, et al. MDCT of pancreatic adenocarcinoma: optimal imaging phases and multiplanar reformatted imaging. AJR Am J Roentgenol 2006;187(6):1513–20.
7. Lall CG, Howard TJ, Skandarajah A, et al. New concepts in staging and treatment of locally advanced pancreatic head cancer. AJR Am J Roentgenol 2007;189(5): 1044–50.
8. Fukukura Y, Takumi K, Kamiyama T, et al. Pancreatic adenocarcinoma: a comparison of automatic bolus tracking and empirical scan delay. Abdom Imaging 2010; 35(5):548–55.
9. Alessandrino F, Souza D, Ivanovic AM, et al. MDCT and MRI of the ampulla of Vater. Part II: non-epithelial neoplasms, benign ampullary disorders, and pitfalls. Abdom Imaging 2015;40(8):292–312.
10. Brugel M, Link TM, Rummeny EJ, et al. Assessment of vascular invasion in pancreatic head cancer with multislice spiral CT: value of multiplanar reconstructions. Eur Radiol 2004;14(7):1188–95.
11. Agrawal MD, Pinho DF, Kulkarni NM, et al. Oncologic applications of dual-energy CT in the abdomen. Radiographics 2014;34(3):589–612.
12. Miller FH, Rini NJ, Keppke AL. MRI of adenocarcinoma of the pancreas. AJR Am J Roentgenol 2006;187(4):W365–74.
13. Sandrasegaran K, Lin C, Akisik FM, et al. State-of-the-art pancreatic MRI. AJR Am J Roentgenol 2010;195(1):42–53.
14. Luna A, Pahwa S, Bonini C, et al. Multiparametric MR imaging in abdominal malignancies. Magn Reson Imaging Clin N Am 2016;24(1):157–86.
15. Park MJ, Kim YK, Choi SY, et al. Preoperative detection of small pancreatic adenocarcinoma: value of adding diffusion-weighted imaging to conventional MR imaging for improving confidence level. Radiology 2014;273(2):433–43.
16. Matsuki M, Inada Y, Nakai G, et al. Diffusion-weighed MR imaging of pancreatic carcinoma. Abdom Imaging 2007;32(4):481–3.
17. Barral M, Taouli B, Guiu B, et al. Diffusion-weighted MR imaging of the pancreas: current status and recommendations. Radiology 2015;274(1):45–63.
18. Liu K, Xie P, Peng W, et al. Assessment of dynamic contrast-enhanced magnetic resonance imaging in the differentiation of pancreatic ductal

adenocarcinoma from other pancreatic solid lesions. J Comput Assist Tomogr 2014;38(5):681–6.

19. Kalra MK, Maher MM, Boland GW, et al. Correlation of positron emission tomography and CT in evaluating pancreatic tumors: technical and clinical implications. AJR Am J Roentgenol 2003;181(2):387–93.

20. Dibble EH, Karantanis D, Mercier G, et al. PET/CT of cancer patients: part 1, pancreatic neoplasms. AJR Am J Roentgenol 2012;199(5):952–67.

21. Chirindel A, Alluri KC, Chaudhry MA, et al. Prognostic value of FDG PET/CT-derived parameters in pancreatic adenocarcinoma at initial PET/CT staging. AJR Am J Roentgenol 2015;204(5):1093–9.

22. Huellner MW, Appenzeller P, Kuhn FP, et al. Whole-body nonenhanced PET/MR versus PET/CT in the staging and restaging of cancers: preliminary observations. Radiology 2014;273(3):859–69.

23. ASGE Standards of Practice Committee, Elobeidi MA, Decker GA, et al. The role of endoscopy in the evaluation and management of patients with solid pancreatic neoplasia. Gastrointest Endosc 2016;83(1):17–28.

24. Mizuno N, Hara K, Hijioka S, et al. Current concept of endoscopic ultrasound-guided fine needle aspiration for pancreatic cancer. Pancreatology 2011; 11(Suppl 2):40–6.

25. Prokesch RW, Chow LC, Beaulieu CF, et al. Isoattenuating pancreatic adenocarcinoma at multi-detector row CT: secondary signs. Radiology 2002;224(3):764–8.

26. Low G, Panu A, Millo N, et al. Multimodality imaging of neoplastic and nonneoplastic solid lesions of the pancreas. Radiographics 2011;31(4):993–1015.

27. Schima W, Ba-Ssalamah A, Kolblinger C, et al. Pancreatic adenocarcinoma. Eur Radiol 2007;17(3):638–49.

28. Lewis RB, Lattin GE Jr, Paal E. Pancreatic endocrine tumors: radiologic-clinicopathologic correlation. Radiographics 2010;30(6):1445–64.

29. Merkle EM, Bender GN, Brambs HJ. Imaging findings in pancreatic lymphoma: differential aspects. AJR Am J Roentgenol 2000;174(3):671–5.

30. Scatarige JC, Horton KM, Sheth S, et al. Pancreatic parenchymal metastases: observations on helical CT. AJR Am J Roentgenol 2001;176(3):695–9.

31. Cantisani V, Mortele KJ, Levy A, et al. MR imaging features of solid pseudopapillary tumor of the pancreas in adult and pediatric patients. AJR Am J Roentgenol 2003;181(2):395–401.

32. Tempero MA, Arnoletti JP, Behrman SW, et al. National Comprehensive Cancer Networks. Pancreatic adenocarcinoma, version 2.2012: featured updates to the NCCN guidelines. J Natl Compr Canc Netw 2012;10(6):703–13.

33. Callery MP, Chang KJ, Fishman EK, et al. Pretreatment assessment of resectable and borderline resectable pancreatic cancer: expert consensus statement. Ann Surg Oncol 2009;16(7):1727–33.

34. Katz MH, Marsh R, Herman JM, et al. Borderline resectable pancreatic cancer: need for standardization and methods for optimal clinical trial design. Ann Surg Oncol 2013;20(8):2787–95.

35. Varadcharary GR, Tamm EP, Abbruzzese JL, et al. Borderline resectable pancreatic cancer: definitions, management, and role of preoperative therapy. Ann Surg Oncol 2006;13(8):1035–46.

36. Al-Hawary MM, Francis IR, Chari ST, et al. Pancreatic ductal adenocarcinoma radiology reporting template: consensus statement of the Society of Abdominal Radiology and the American Pancreatic Association. Radiology 2014;270(1):248–60.

37. CT pancreatic mass staging. radreport.org. Radiological Society of North America. 2015. Available at: www.radreport.org/template/0000135. Accessed March 9, 2016.

Endoscopic Evaluation in the Workup of Pancreatic Cancer

Ajaypal Singh, MD*, Ashley L. Faulx, MD

KEYWORDS

- Pancreatic ductal adenocarcinoma (PDAC) • Endoscopic ultrasound (EUS)
- Fine-needle aspiration (FNA)
- Endoscopic retrograde cholangiopancreatography (ERCP)

KEY POINTS

- Endoscopic ultrasound (EUS) imaging is the most sensitive diagnostic modality for pancreatic cancer, especially for tumors smaller than 2 cm in size.
- EUS also allows simultaneous fine-needle aspiration for cytologic diagnosis of the malignant process.
- Endoscopic retrograde cholangiopancreatography (ERCP) brushings and biopsies have low sensitivity (but high specificity) for pancreatic cancers and should not be used primarily for diagnosis owing to high risk of complications.
- Endoscopic biliary drainage via ERCP is the first-line palliative modality for malignant biliary obstruction.
- Both computed tomography and EUS play a complementary role in staging and preoperative planning; data to indicate superiority of one over the other is lacking.

INTRODUCTION

Pancreatic cancer is a relatively rare disease and ranks 12th in terms of prevalence among cancers in the United States, but it is the fourth leading cause of cancer related deaths.[1] It is projected to become the second leading cause of cancer related mortality by 2020.[2] The overall 5-year survival for pancreatic cancer is very low at 7.2%. It is around 27% for localized disease, but 2.4% for metastatic disease. Despite multiple advances in imaging technologies, less than 10% of the cancers are diagnosed at a localized stage.[1] Much emphasis is being placed on early diagnosis of this deadly disease at a stage when curative surgical resection is possible. Owing to the low sensitivity of cross-sectional imaging to detect small tumors in the pancreas, endoscopic

Division of Gastroenterology and Hepatology, Case Western Reserve University, Wearn 247, 11100 Euclid Avenue, Cleveland, OH 44106, USA
* Corresponding author.
E-mail address: ajay749@gmail.com

Surg Clin N Am 96 (2016) 1257–1270
http://dx.doi.org/10.1016/j.suc.2016.07.006
0039-6109/16/© 2016 Elsevier Inc. All rights reserved.

surgical.theclinics.com

diagnosis by using endoscopic ultrasound (EUS) has become a mainstay for diagnosis of pancreatic cancer. EUS also provides additional benefit of tissue sampling for histologic diagnosis. In this article, we review the clinical presentation of pancreatic cancer and the modalities available for diagnosis with special emphasis on the use of EUS and endoscopic retrograde cholangiopancreatography (ERCP).

CLINICAL PRESENTATION

Clinical presentation in patients with pancreatic adenocarcinoma is variable and depends on the location and stage of the disease. Owing to improving resolution and more frequent use of imaging, more patients are being diagnosed with smaller tumors that are discovered incidentally on scans done for unrelated reasons. Patients with symptomatic cancer can present with obstructive jaundice, abdominal pain, weight loss, acute pancreatitis, new-onset diabetes, worsening of long-standing diabetes, or paraneoplastic symptoms usually related to coagulopathy. Pancreatic head tumors usually present early with obstructive jaundice, but the diagnosis of pancreatic body and tail cancers is often delayed because these do not produce early symptoms and are commonly recognized when symptoms are produced by a nonlocalized disease process. Physical examination findings may include muscle wasting, jaundice, lymphadenopathy, and hepatomegaly. Many patients with pancreatic cancer have a normal physical examination on initial presentation. The laboratory characteristics include elevated bilirubin and alkaline phosphatase in patients with biliary obstruction. CA 19-9 is the only available serum biomarker for pancreatic cancer, but is limited by its low sensitivity and specificity.[3] It is often used to monitor the progression or recurrence of disease after surgery and/or neoadjuvant therapy.[4] The use of CA 19-9 for diagnostic purposes is not recommended.

DIAGNOSTIC MODALITIES

The diagnosis of pancreatic cancer usually involves cross-sectional imaging and endoscopy in the appropriate clinical setting. Surgical exploration for diagnosis is rarely needed with modern imaging and endoscopy. We briefly review imaging modalities for the diagnosis of pancreatic cancer (reviewed in detail elsewhere in this issue) and then focus on the role of endoscopy for diagnosis, with particular focus on EUS.

TRANSABDOMINAL ULTRASOUND IMAGING

Transabdominal ultrasound imaging is the most commonly used study in patients with jaundice and right upper quadrant pain owing to its low cost, easy availability, and lack of any radiation exposure. It has very high sensitivity in detecting biliary dilatation and also the level of obstruction, but in addition to being user dependent it has a very low sensitivity for actual detection of pancreatic masses.[5,6] In patients with suspected pancreatic malignancy, computed tomography (CT) scanning is the most commonly used initial study and the usefulness of abdominal ultrasound imaging in these patients is very limited.

CROSS-SECTIONAL IMAGING: COMPUTED TOMOGRAPHY AND MRI

CT is the most commonly used initial imaging modality in patients with suspected pancreatic malignancy. With the advent of multidetector CT (MDCT) imaging, the sensitivity of CT for diagnosing pancreatic cancer is reported to be greater than 80%.[7] However, the sensitivity of MDCT for diagnosing small pancreatic tumors (<20 mm in size) is still relatively low (around 50%).[8,9] With availability of EUS-guided fine-needle aspiration (FNA), CT-guided percutaneous needle biopsy is currently not used as the first line method for tissue acquisition owing to the risk of needle tract seeding (discussed in detail in EUS section).[10,11] One major advantage of CT imaging is that it provides information about localized as well as distant staging of pancreatic cancer. Data have shown that CT imaging is the best available imaging modality to assess local vascular involvement and hence resectability.[12] Pancreas protocol CT scans, which include an arterial phase (scanning at 35–50 seconds after contrast injection) to allow detection of pancreatic masses and a portal phase (60–90 seconds after contrast injection) to allow for evaluation of vasculature and surrounding structures, are very important in surgical planning.

Contrast-enhanced MRI has sensitivity and accuracy approaching that of MDCT for diagnosis and staging of pancreatic cancer, but it is more costly and less readily available than MDCT. The image quality may be affected by respiratory artifact. There are some emerging data to suggest that MRI might be able to diagnose small pancreatic cancers before CT imaging owing to detection of subtle changes in pancreatic parenchyma.[13–15]

ROLE OF ENDOSCOPY IN DIAGNOSIS OF PANCREATIC CANCER
Endoscopic Ultrasound Imaging

EUS involves passage of an endoscope with an ultrasound transducer at its tip into the gastrointestinal tract. EUS provides detailed sonographic images of the gastrointestinal tract lining and the surrounding structures. The common types of echoendoscopes available are radial (sector array) and linear (convex array), although forward viewing echoendoscopes have been developed recently. The radial array echoendoscopes provide circumferential (360°) views in a plane perpendicular to the shaft of the endoscope; hence, ultrasound images are similar in orientation to those of CT scans. The linear echoendoscopes provide images in the same plane as the long axis of the endoscope, more similar to those obtained on transabdominal ultrasound imaging. Pancreatic adenocarcinoma typically appears as an irregular, hypoechoic mass in the pancreatic parenchyma with poorly defined margins on EUS. Upstream pancreatic duct dilatation and parenchymal atrophy, if present, are also more indicative of a malignant process. Malignant lymph nodes usually are round and hypoechoic with well-defined margins, and more than 1 cm in size, where as benign lymph nodes usually are triangular or oval, hypoechoic, and have poorly defined margins (**Fig. 1**). The linear array echoendoscopes provide the additional ability to perform needle sampling of the desired lesions through the working channel (**Fig. 2**). Because of this advantage,

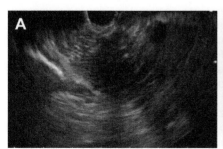 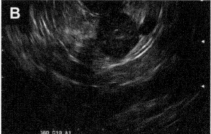

Fig. 1. Endosonographic appearance of an adenocarcinoma (*A*) and a neuroendocrine tumor (*B*) in the tail of pancreas. The adenocarcinoma has poorly defined irregular margins compared with the well-defined round contour of the neuroendocrine tumor.

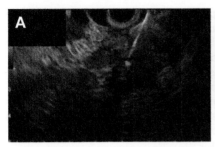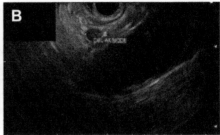

Fig. 2. Patient with newly diagnosed pancreatic head mass. (*A*) Endoscopic ultrasound imaging–guided fine-needle aspiration of the irregular, hypoechoic mass was done, cytology confirmed the diagnosis of adenocarcinoma. (*B*) A malignant appearing hypoechoic, round celiac axis lymph node with well-defined margins was also noted.

linear scopes are more commonly used for the workup of suspected pancreatic masses.

Accuracy

EUS is the most sensitive imaging modality for diagnosis of pancreatic cancer with reported sensitivity ranging from 87% to 100%.[7,16–18] Published studies have shown superiority of EUS over transabdominal ultrasound imaging, CT scanning, and MRI for diagnosis of pancreatic cancer. Although most of the data regarding superiority of EUS for pancreatic cancer diagnosis compare it with conventional CT scans, some of the published studies have shown that EUS is more sensitive than the MDCT imaging as well. Agarwal and colleagues[18] retrospectively compared EUS and pancreas protocol MDCT in 81 consecutive patients with suspected pancreatic cancer and showed that the accuracy of EUS for diagnosing pancreatic cancer was significantly higher compared with MDCT (94% vs 74%). These findings were confirmed by a prospective, observational cohort study by DeWitt and colleagues.[7] They compared EUS with MDCT in 120 patients with suspected pancreatic cancer and showed that EUS was superior to MDCT for diagnosing pancreatic masses (sensitivity 98% vs 86%; $P = .012$). In a systematic review, Dewitt and colleagues[8] reviewed 9 studies comparing CT and EUS imaging for pancreatic tumor detection and concluded that EUS was more sensitive than CT and the specificity of EUS was either superior or equivalent to that of CT imaging for diagnosis of pancreatic malignancy.

The most important predictor for survival in patients with pancreatic cancer is the stage at diagnosis and fewer than 10% of the pancreatic cancers are diagnosed at a localized stage.[1] Studies have shown that surgical resection rates and overall survival are better for smaller tumors. However, cross-sectional imaging is not very sensitive at diagnosing smaller tumors, especially those less than 2 cm in size. Published data have shown that more than 80% of pancreatic cancers were not identified on CT scan at a mean interval of 13.2 months before final diagnosis.[19] The improved sensitivity of EUS for detecting pancreatic masses is of particular significance for tumors less than 3 cm in size. One of the earlier studies comparing EUS imaging, CT scanning, and MRI for diagnosis of pancreatic cancer, showed that EUS had a sensitivity of 93% for diagnosing cancers less than 3 cm in size compared with 53% for CT and 67% for MRI.[20] More recent data are limited but also support the superiority of EUS over MDCT for detection of small pancreatic masses. In a retrospective review of 116 patients with clinical suspicion for pancreatic cancer but absence of a definite mass seen on MDCT, EUS was shown to have a sensitivity of 87% and more than 90% accuracy in diagnosing pancreatic tumors.[21]

Many patients undergo EUS to evaluate for pancreatic cancer when there is high clinical suspicion, but a definite pancreatic mass is not seen on cross-sectional imaging. It is very important in these situations for EUS to have a high negative predictive value (NPV). Studies have shown that in the setting of a normal EUS examination in patients with clinical suspicion of pancreatic malignancy, the NPV is 100% after a follow-up period of 2 years.[22,23] It should, however, be noted that this high NPV is applicable when the pancreatic parenchyma is normal, because the usefulness of EUS in the setting of parenchymal and ductal changes as seen in chronic pancreatitis is limited. The sensitivity of EUS in diagnosing pancreatic cancer in chronic pancreatitis is around 60% to 70%, but it remains superior to cross-sectional imaging.[24,25] Emerging technologies that can further improve the diagnostic capability of EUS include contrast-enhanced EUS and elastography.[26–28] Contrast-enhanced EUS is currently available in Europe but not yet in the United States.

In addition to its high sensitivity, another major advantage of EUS is the ability to perform needle sampling of the target tissue for histologic diagnosis. EUS-guided FNA of pancreatic masses was first introduced by Vilman and colleagues[29] in 1992 and is currently the first-line modality for tissue acquisition in patients with pancreatic masses. It involves the passage of a needle through the working channel of a linear-array echoendoscope to obtain samples of the pancreatic mass as well as surrounding lymph nodes, liver masses, and ascites. There are multiple commercially available needles of different sizes (19-G, 22-G, and 25-G) for sampling and multiple techniques have been studied (use of suction, number of needle passes, "fanning" technique, etc), but are beyond the scope of this article and will not be reviewed here.

The pooled sensitivity and specificity of EUS-FNA for diagnosis of pancreatic adenocarcinoma are 85% to 89% and 98% to 99%, respectively.[30,31] In addition to various technical factors, the availability of a cytopathologist on site (for rapid on site evaluation [ROSE]) has been shown to improve the diagnostic yield of EUS-FNA for diagnosis of pancreatic malignancy.[32–35] The beneficial role of ROSE for EUS-FNA of solid pancreatic masses was confirmed by a metaanalysis of 34 studies (3644 patients).[30] However, recent data from a multicenter, randomized, noninferiority trial showed that FNA of solid pancreatic masses with 7 needle passes is noninferior to ROSE but is associated with significant cost reduction.[36]

The role of EUS-FNA is clear in patients with borderline resectable or unresectable pancreatic cancer when tissue diagnosis is required for delivery of chemotherapy and/or radiation therapy. However, when a clearly resectable mass is seen in a patient with high clinical suspicion of pancreatic cancer, there is controversy regarding the need for FNA versus proceeding directly to surgery. In such circumstances, the clinician must balance the value of obtaining a definitive diagnosis and the risk associated with EUS-FNA (discussed elsewhere in this paper). In clinical practice, EUS-FNA is commonly done in patients with resectable pancreatic masses and a high clinical suspicion of cancer. Even though the sensitivity and specificity of EUS-FNA for diagnosis of pancreatic adenocarcinoma is very high, the NPV of EUS-FNA is not very high and ranges from 55% to 65%.[31] This is further decreased by the presence of parenchymal abnormalities seen in patients with chronic pancreatitis.[24,25] In patients with negative cytology but a mass seen on imaging or a high clinical suspicion for pancreatic malignancy, repeat EUS with FNA is a reasonable approach. If still negative, ERCP with brushings and/or intraductal biopsies could be considered (discussed below). EUS guided fine needle core biopsy needles are available, but are usually technically difficult to use owing to the larger needle size and stiffness of these needles. Published data have not shown superiority of fine needle core biopsy needles over the easier to use, more flexible FNA needles for diagnosis of pancreatic adenocarcinoma.[37]

Safety of endoscopic ultrasound imaging

EUS is a safe procedure with a reported overall adverse event rate of 1.1% to 3%.[38] The addition of an ultrasound transducer at the end of the endoscope leads to a rigid distal segment. The endoscopic images are also oblique-view images, making scope manipulation more difficult than with standard forward-viewing endoscopes. The reported risk of perforation with EUS is 0.06%, which is similar to that reported with standard upper endoscopy (0.03%).[38,39] A recent systematic review showed that the incidence of pain, bleeding, fever and infection after EUS-FNA of pancreatic masses were 0.38%, 0.10%, 0.08%, and 0.02%, respectively.[39] Two major possible adverse events of EUS-FNA of solid pancreatic masses include acute pancreatitis and the risk of needle tract seeding. The reported risk of acute pancreatitis after EUS-FNA of solid pancreatic masses is 0.26% to 0.85% and is much lower than what is seen after EUS-FNA of cystic neoplasms of the pancreas.[40–42] This risk can be decreased by minimizing the number of needle passes, minimizing the amount of normal appearing pancreatic parenchyma traversed with each pass, and avoiding needle insertion through the pancreatic duct unless it is absolutely needed. Needle tract seeding is a consideration with biopsy of pancreatic masses, but most of the published data are limited to case reports.[43–45] The reported incidence of needle tract seeding after EUS-FNA is much lower when compared with percutaneous CT or transabdominal ultrasound–guided sampling (2.2% vs 16.3%).[46,47] The majority of the reported cases of EUS-FNA needle tract seeding are for body and tail cancers, which were sampled through the transgastric approach. This is less of an issue for resectable pancreatic head tumors sampled transduodenally, because the site of needle puncture is included in the resection margins of a pancreatoduodenectomy. When available, EUS-FNA is the preferred method for tissue diagnosis of pancreatic masses.

Endoscopic Retrograde Cholangiopancreatography

Owing to the risk of potential adverse effects with ERCP and availability of MR cholangiopancreatography, ERCP rarely has a primary diagnostic role in the management of pancreatic masses. It is mainly used for palliation to relieve biliary obstruction. Pancreatic head tumors commonly present with obstructive jaundice owing to bile duct strictures. The fluoroscopic stricture morphology can give some clues about the etiology of the obstruction, but morphology alone is unreliable for diagnostic purposes. Long, irregular strictures with an abrupt cutoff and shelflike ends are more suggestive of a malignant process compared with smooth tapering strictures, which usually represent a benign inflammatory process, as commonly seen in patients with chronic pancreatitis (**Fig. 3**A). The presence of a double-duct sign (stricture in both bile duct and pancreatic duct with upstream dilatation) is also suggestive of a pancreatic head tumor. In these cases, tissue samples can be obtained either by cytology brushings, intraductal biopsies and cytology from removed stents. ERCP-guided brushings and biopsies have a high specificity for diagnosis of malignancy (approaching 95%), but the sensitivity is very low (23%–56% for biliary brushings and 33%–65% for fluoroscopic biopsies) leading to a low NPV of 58%.[48–51] Combining both brushings and intraductal biopsies can increase the diagnostic yield to 60% to 70%, but still is suboptimal compared with EUS.[52] There are limited published data comparing EUS-FNA with ERCP cytology for diagnosis of solid pancreatic masses, but a recent study showed the superiority of EUS-FNA compared with ERCP alone. In this retrospective analysis of 234 patients with pancreatic neoplasms, it was shown that the sensitivity, specificity, and accuracy for diagnosis of pancreatic

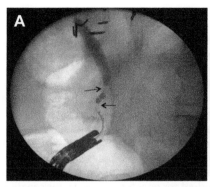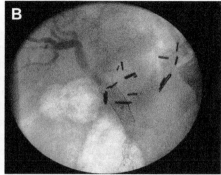

Fig. 3. Patient with metastatic pancreatic head cancer and obstructive jaundice. (*A*) Endoscopic retrograde cholangiopancreatography showed a severe, malignant distal common bile duct stricture (*arrows*). (*B*) An uncovered biliary metal stent was placed with improvement of jaundice followed by initiation of palliative therapy.

neoplasms were 98.9%, 93.3%, and 98.1%, respectively, for EUS-FNA compared with 72.1%, 60%, and 71.4%, respectively, for ERCP alone. The overall adverse events were also significant lower for EUS-FNA compared with ERCP alone (1.9% vs 6.6%).[53]

The main role of ERCP in patients with pancreatic cancer is palliative and involves relief of biliary obstruction. Transpapillary biliary drainage was first introduced in 1980 when only plastic stents were available.[54] These stents range in diameter from 7-Fr to a maximum of 11.5-Fr. These plastic stents have a short average patency of around 3 to 4 months and require scheduled stent exchange every 3 months.[55] Self-expanding uncovered metal biliary stents were developed in 1990s to overcome these issues.[56] The commonly available biliary metal stents have a diameter of 8 or 10 mm. Published data have shown that self-expanding biliary metal stents have a longer patency, have a lower incidence of occlusion and cholangitis, are associated with a shorter duration of hospital stay, and are more cost effective, especially in patients with an expected of survival more than 3 to 6 months without any difference in overall short-term mortality.[55,57–59] The average patency of metal biliary stents approaches 1 year compared with 3 to 4 months for the plastic bile duct stents.[60] The superiority and cost effectiveness of metal stents have been confirmed by metaanalyses as well.[61,62] In a recent metaanalysis comparing use of plastic versus metal stents for inoperable malignant biliary obstruction in 1133 patients (13 studies), it was shown that self-expanding metal stents were associated with lower stent dysfunction (21.6% vs 46.8%; $P<.00001$), lesser need for repeat interventions (21.6% vs 56.6%; $P<.00001$), longer stent patency (250 vs 124 days; $P<.0001$), and longer mean survival (182 vs 150 days; $P<.0001$). However, there was no difference in cost per patient, although a trend toward lower cost was seen in metal stents (€4193.98 vs €4728.65; $P<.0985$).[62]

These data suggest that self-expanding metal stents are superior to plastic stents in patients with unresectable or borderline resectable disease who need neoadjuvant therapy before reevaluation for surgery. However, the debate of metal versus plastic stents is still not resolved in patients with clinically resectable disease who are to undergo surgical resection within a short period of time. In patients with radiologic and endosonographic evidence of resectable disease and biliary obstruction, directly proceeding to surgery without endoscopic biliary drainage is usually the preferred approach. Some investigators propose that preoperative biliary drainage can lead to improved tissue healing.[63,64] Other data suggest that preoperative biliary drainage might increase the risk of complications.[65] Biliary drainage, however, is needed for symptom relief when evaluation for surgery is ongoing, especially in patients with cholangitis or intractable pruritus. There were initial concerns that metal stents could make surgical bile duct anastomosis challenging at the time of resection, but there are no published data to support this claim. Studies have shown that as long as at least 2 cm of nonstrictured common hepatic duct proximal to the stent is available for anastomosis, the surgical outcomes are unaffected.[66,67] Efforts should be made to use the shortest metal stent possible that traverse the stricture. The proximal end of the metal stent should be placed below the line of potential surgical transection of the bile duct leaving adequate length of native, nonstrictured bile duct for anastomosis. It is our practice to place plastic stents in patients who require biliary decompression and are likely to undergo surgery in the near future or when the diagnosis of malignancy has not been confirmed. In patients with metastatic/inoperable disease or borderline resectable disease and who are to receive neoadjuvant therapy, we place self-expanding metal biliary stents (**Fig. 3**B).

Both covered and uncovered metal stents are available. The uncovered stents have a mesh design to allow embedding in the bile duct wall, but it also exposes them to risk of tumor ingrowth and eventual obstruction. The covered metal stents have the mesh covered by silicone, polyurethane, or polytetrafluoroethylene to prevent tissue ingrowth, but this puts them at increased risk of stent migration. There were initial concerns about increased risk of cholecystitis with covered stents owing to blockage of cystic duct drainage, but the data are not conclusive.[68] Although tumor ingrowth is not an issue for covered metal stents, this advantage is offset by the higher incidence of stent migration. In a randomized, nonblinded, multicenter study comparing covered versus uncovered metal stents in patients with malignant distal biliary obstruction, it was shown that there were no differences in stent patency, patient survival, or complications (including cholecystitis) in the 2 groups. Covered stents were associated with a higher migration rate whereas uncovered stents had a higher incidence of tumor ingrowth.[69] These findings have also been confirmed by other groups.[70,71] A metaanalysis involving 1078 patients with malignant biliary obstruction also showed that covered metal biliary stents had higher migration rates compared with uncovered stents without a significant difference in patency.[68] Based on these data, uncovered stents are used more commonly for malignant obstruction and covered stents are usually reserved for benign biliary obstruction.

PRETREATMENT STAGING OF PANCREATIC CANCER

Accurate staging of pancreatic adenocarcinoma is very important to determine operative resectability. The staging includes assessment of local spread and vascular involvement (T stage), nodal involvement (N stage), and metastatic involvement (M stage). The role of EUS in staging pancreatic malignancy is not as well-established; its role in diagnosis and most surgeons rely more on cross-sectional imaging than EUS for determining resectability. MDCT and EUS play a complementary role in the staging of pancreatic cancers and the data about superiority of 1 modality over the other is not conclusive. Although earlier studies showed superiority of EUS over conventional CT for local staging, vascular invasion and nodal staging, subsequent studies have shown that MDCT is either equivalent or superior to EUS for

T and N staging.[7,72–74] In a recent metaanalysis involving 12 studies comparing EUS and CT for staging of pancreatic cancer, EUS was found to have higher sensitivity for nodal staging (58% vs 24%) and vascular involvement (86% vs 58%).[75] The sensitivity for determining resectability was comparable between the 2 modalities (87% vs 90%). There are some data to suggest that CT and MRI can lead to overestimating the T stage compared with EUS and hence exclude potentially resectable tumors from going to the operating room.[74] It should be noted that EUS is user dependent and there are data to indicate that the accuracy of EUS for staging improves with operator experience.[72]

SUMMARY

Endoscopy plays an important role in the diagnosis and management of pancreatic cancer. EUS is the most sensitive modality for diagnosis of pancreatic cancers and should be the preferred modality for obtaining tissue diagnosis with FNA. Both CT and EUS play complementary roles in pancreatic cancer staging and both are comparable in terms of determining resectability. The role of ERCP in the workup of pancreatic cancer is limited to palliative biliary drainage in majority of the cases and uncovered self-expanding metal stents are preferred for biliary drainage in patients who have unresectable disease or need neoadjuvant therapy. The American Society of Gastrointestinal Endoscopy Standards of Practice Committee proposed an algorithm for patients with suspected pancreatic adenocarcinoma, which highlights the role of various diagnostic modalities (**Fig. 4**).[38]

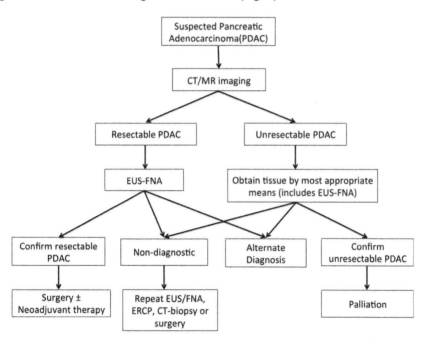

Fig. 4. Proposed algorithm for diagnosis of solid pancreatic neoplasms. CT, computed tomography; ERCP, endoscopic retrograde cholangiopancreatography; EUS-FNA, endoscopic ultrasound imaging–guided fine-needle aspiration. (*Adapted from* ASGE Standards of Practice Committee, Eloubeidi MA, Decker GA, et al. The role of endoscopy in the evaluation and management of patients with solid pancreatic neoplasia. Gastrointest Endosc 2016;83(1):17–28; with permission.)

REFERENCES

1. SEER Stat Fact Sheets: Pancreatic Cancer. NCI Surveillance, Epidemiology, and End Results Program 2005-2011. Bethesda (MD): National Cancer Institute. Available at: http://seer.cancer.gov/statfacts/html/pancreas.html.
2. Rahib L, Smith BD, Aizenberg R, et al. Projecting cancer incidence and deaths to 2030: the unexpected burden of thyroid, liver, and pancreas cancers in the United States. Cancer Res 2014;74(11):2913–21.
3. Partyka K, Maupin KA, Brand RE, et al. Diverse monoclonal antibodies against the CA 19-9 antigen show variation in binding specificity with consequences for clinical interpretation. Proteomics 2012;12(13):2212–20.
4. Winter JM, Yeo CJ, Brody JR. Diagnostic, prognostic, and predictive biomarkers in pancreatic cancer. J Surg Oncol 2013;107(1):15–22.
5. Tamm EP, Balachandran A, Bhosale PR, et al. Imaging of pancreatic adenocarcinoma: update on staging/resectability. Radiol Clin North Am 2012;50(3):407–28.
6. Saini S. Imaging of the hepatobiliary tract. N Engl J Med 1997;336(26):1889–94.
7. Dewitt J, Devereaux B, Chriswell M, et al. Comparison of endoscopic ultrasonography and multidetector computed tomography for detecting and staging pancreatic cancer. Ann Intern Med 2004;141(10):753–63.
8. Dewitt J, Devereaux BM, Lehman GA, et al. Comparison of endoscopic ultrasound and computed tomography for the preoperative evaluation of pancreatic cancer: a systematic review. Clin Gastroenterol Hepatol 2006;4(6):717–25.
9. Shrikhande SV, Barreto SG, Goel M, et al. Multimodality imaging of pancreatic ductal adenocarcinoma: a review of the literature. HPB (Oxford) 2012;14(10):658–68.
10. Bret PM, Nicolet V, Labadie M. Percutaneous fine-needle aspiration biopsy of the pancreas. Diagn Cytopathol 1986;2(3):221–7.
11. Brandt KR, Charboneau JW, Stephens DH, et al. CT- and US-guided biopsy of the pancreas. Radiology 1993;187(1):99–104.
12. Arabul M, Karakus F, Alper E, et al. Comparison of multidetector CT and endoscopic ultrasonography in malignant pancreatic mass lesions. Hepatogastroenterology 2012;59(117):1599–603.
13. Raman SP, Horton KM, Fishman EK. Multimodality imaging of pancreatic cancer-computed tomography, magnetic resonance imaging, and positron emission tomography. Cancer J 2012;18(6):511–22.
14. Canto MI, Hruban RH, Fishman EK, et al. Frequent detection of pancreatic lesions in asymptomatic high-risk individuals. Gastroenterology 2012;142(4):796–804.
15. Lee ES, Lee JM. Imaging diagnosis of pancreatic cancer: a state-of-the-art review. World J Gastroenterol 2014;20(24):7864–77.
16. Rösch T, Lorenz R, Braig C, et al. Endoscopic ultrasound in pancreatic tumor diagnosis. Gastrointest Endosc 1991;37(3):347–52.
17. Palazzo L, Roseau G, Gayet B, et al. Endoscopic ultrasonography in the diagnosis and staging of pancreatic adenocarcinoma. Results of a prospective study with comparison to ultrasonography and CT scan. Endoscopy 1993;25(2):143–50.
18. Agarwal B, Abu-Hamda E, Molke KL, et al. Endoscopic ultrasound-guided fine needle aspiration and multidetector spiral CT in the diagnosis of pancreatic cancer. Am J Gastroenterol 2004;99(5):844–50.
19. Gangi S, Fletcher JG, Nathan MA, et al. Time interval between abnormalities seen on CT and the clinical diagnosis of pancreatic cancer: retrospective review of CT scans obtained before diagnosis. Am J Roentgenol 2004;182(4):897–903.

20. Müller MF, Meyenberger C, Bertschinger P, et al. Pancreatic tumors: evaluation with endoscopic US, CT, and MR imaging. Radiology 1994;190(3):745–51.

21. Wang W, Shpaner A, Krishna SG, et al. Use of EUS-FNA in diagnosing pancreatic neoplasm without a definitive mass on CT. Gastrointest Endosc 2013;78(1): 73–80.

22. Ngamruengphong S, Li F, Zhou Y, et al. EUS and survival in patients with pancreatic cancer: a population-based study. Gastrointest Endosc 2010;72(1):78–83, 83.e1–2.

23. Catanzaro A, Richardson S, Veloso H, et al. Long-term follow-up of patients with clinically indeterminate suspicion of pancreatic cancer and normal EUS. Gastrointest Endosc 2003;58(6):836–40.

24. Fritscher-Ravens A, Brand L, Knöfel WT, et al. Comparison of endoscopic ultrasound-guided fine needle aspiration for focal pancreatic lesions in patients with normal parenchyma and chronic pancreatitis. Am J Gastroenterol 2002; 97(11):2768–75.

25. Varadarajulu S, Tamhane A, Eloubeidi MA. Yield of EUS-guided FNA of pancreatic masses in the presence or the absence of chronic pancreatitis. Gastrointest Endosc 2005;62(5):728–36.

26. Fusaroli P, Spada A, Mancino MG, et al. Contrast harmonic echo-endoscopic ultrasound improves accuracy in diagnosis of solid pancreatic masses. Clin Gastroenterol Hepatol 2010;8(7):629–34.

27. Giovannini M, Thomas B, Erwan B, et al. Endoscopic ultrasound elastography for evaluation of lymph nodes and pancreatic masses: a multicenter study. World J Gastroenterol 2009;15(13):1587–93.

28. Iglesias-Garcia J, Larino-Noia J, Abdulkader I, et al. EUS elastography for the characterization of solid pancreatic masses. Gastrointest Endosc 2009;70(6): 1101–8.

29. Vilmann P, Jacobsen GK, Henriksen FW, et al. Endoscopic ultrasonography with guided fine needle aspiration biopsy in pancreatic disease. Gastrointest Endosc 1992;38(2):172–3.

30. Hébert-Magee S, Bae S, Varadarajulu S, et al. The presence of a cytopathologist increases the diagnostic accuracy of endoscopic ultrasound-guided fine needle aspiration cytology for pancreatic adenocarcinoma: a meta-analysis. Cytopathology 2013;24(3):159–71.

31. Hewitt MJ, McPhail MJ, Possamai L, et al. EUS-guided FNA for diagnosis of solid pancreatic neoplasms: a meta-analysis. Gastrointest Endosc 2012;75(2):319–31.

32. Klapman JB, Logrono R, Dye CE, et al. Clinical impact of on-site cytopathology interpretation on endoscopic ultrasound-guided fine needle aspiration. Am J Gastroenterol 2003;98(6):1289–94.

33. Iglesias-Garcia J, Dominguez-Munoz JE, Abdulkader I, et al. Influence of on-site cytopathology evaluation on the diagnostic accuracy of endoscopic ultrasound-guided fine needle aspiration (EUS-FNA) of solid pancreatic masses. Am J Gastroenterol 2011;106(9):1705–10.

34. Alsohaibani F, Girgis S, Sandha GS. Does onsite cytotechnology evaluation improve the accuracy of endoscopic ultrasound-guided fine-needle aspiration biopsy? Can J Gastroenterol 2009;23(1):26–30.

35. Collins BT, Murad FM, Wang JF, et al. Rapid on-site evaluation for endoscopic ultrasound-guided fine-needle biopsy of the pancreas decreases the incidence of repeat biopsy procedures. Cancer Cytopathol 2013;121(9):518–24.

36. Lee LS, Nieto J, Watson RR, et al. Randomized noninferiority trial comparing diagnostic yield of cytopathologist-guided versus 7 passes for EUS-FNA of pancreatic masses. Dig Endosc 2015. [Epub ahead of print].

37. Bang JY, Hebert-Magee S, Trevino J, et al. Randomized trial comparing the 22-gauge aspiration and 22-gauge biopsy needles for EUS-guided sampling of solid pancreatic mass lesions. Gastrointest Endosc 2012;76(2):321–7.

38. ASGE Standards of Practice Committee, Eloubeidi MA, Decker GA, et al. The role of endoscopy in the evaluation and management of patients with solid pancreatic neoplasia. Gastrointest Endosc 2016;83(1):17–28.

39. Wang KX, Ben QW, Jin ZD, et al. Assessment of morbidity and mortality associated with EUS-guided FNA: a systematic review. Gastrointest Endosc 2011;73(2):283–90.

40. Eloubeidi MA, Gress FG, Savides TJ, et al. Acute pancreatitis after EUS-guided FNA of solid pancreatic masses: a pooled analysis from EUS centers in the United States. Gastrointest Endosc 2004;60(3):385–9.

41. Eloubeidi MA, Tamhane A, Varadarajulu S, et al. Frequency of major complications after EUS-guided FNA of solid pancreatic masses: a prospective evaluation. Gastrointest Endosc 2006;63(4):622–9.

42. Siddiqui AA, Shahid H, Shah A, et al. High risk of acute pancreatitis after endoscopic ultrasound-guided fine needle aspiration of side branch intraductal papillary mucinous neoplasms. Endosc Ultrasound 2015;4(2):109–14.

43. Paquin SC, Gariépy G, Lepanto L, et al. A first report of tumor seeding because of EUS-guided FNA of a pancreatic adenocarcinoma. Gastrointest Endosc 2005;61(4):610–1.

44. Chong A, Venugopal K, Segarajasingam D, et al. Tumor seeding after EUS-guided FNA of pancreatic tail neoplasia. Gastrointest Endosc 2011;74(4):933–5.

45. Ahmed K, Sussman JJ, Wang J, et al. A case of EUS-guided FNA–related pancreatic cancer metastasis to the stomach. Gastrointest Endosc 2011;74(1):231–3.

46. Tomonari A, Katanuma A, Matsumori T, et al. Resected tumor seeding in stomach wall due to endoscopic ultrasonography-guided fine needle aspiration of pancreatic adenocarcinoma. World J Gastroenterol 2015;21(27):8458–61.

47. Micames C, Jowell PS, White R, et al. Lower frequency of peritoneal carcinomatosis in patients with pancreatic cancer diagnosed by EUS-guided FNA vs. percutaneous FNA. Gastrointest Endosc 2003;58(5):690–5.

48. Schoefl R, Haefner M, Wrba F, et al. Forceps biopsy and brush cytology during endoscopic retrograde cholangiopancreatography for the diagnosis of biliary stenoses. Scand J Gastroenterol 1997;32(4):363–8.

49. Ponchon T, Gagnon P, Berger F, et al. Value of endobiliary brush cytology and biopsies for the diagnosis of malignant bile duct stenosis: results of a prospective study. Gastrointest Endosc 1995;42(6):565–72.

50. Pugliese V, Conio M, Nicolò G, et al. Endoscopic retrograde forceps biopsy and brush cytology of biliary strictures: a prospective study. Gastrointest Endosc 1995;42(6):520–6.

51. Burnett AS, Calvert TJ, Chokshi RJ. Sensitivity of endoscopic retrograde cholangiopancreatography standard cytology: 10-y review of the literature. J Surg Res 2013;184(1):304–11.

52. Jailwala J, Fogel EL, Sherman S, et al. Triple-tissue sampling at ERCP in malignant biliary obstruction. Gastrointest Endosc 2000;51:383–90.

53. Malak M, Masuda D, Ogura T, et al. Yield of endoscopic ultrasound-guided fine needle aspiration and endoscopic retrograde cholangiopancreatography for solid pancreatic neoplasms. Scand J Gastroenterol 2016;51(3):360–7.
54. Soehendra N, Reynders-Frederix V. Palliative bile duct drainage - a new endoscopic method of introducing a transpapillary drain. Endoscopy 1980;12(1):8–11.
55. Prat F, Chapat O, Ducot B, et al. A randomized trial of endoscopic drainage methods for inoperable malignant strictures of the common bile duct. Gastrointest Endosc 1998;47(1):1–7.
56. Davids PH, Groen AK, Rauws EA, et al. Randomised trial of self-expanding metal stents versus polyethylene stents for distal malignant biliary obstruction. Lancet 1992;340(8834–8835):1488–92.
57. Knyrim K, Wagner HJ, Pausch J, et al. A prospective, randomized, controlled trial of metal stents for malignant obstruction of the common bile duct. Endoscopy 1993;25(3):207–12.
58. Kaassis M, Boyer J, Dumas R, et al. Plastic or metal stents for malignant stricture of the common bile duct? Results of a randomized prospective study. Gastrointest Endosc 2003;57:178–82.
59. Katsinelos P, Paikos D, Kountouras J, et al. Tannenbaum and metal stents in the palliative treatment of malignant distal bile duct obstruction: a comparative study of patency and cost effectiveness. Surg Endosc 2006;20(10):1587–93.
60. Stern N, Sturgess R. Endoscopic therapy in the management of malignant biliary obstruction. Eur J Surg Oncol 2008;34(3):313–7.
61. Moss AC, Morris E, Leyden J, et al. Do the benefits of metal stents justify the costs? A systematic review and meta-analysis of trials comparing endoscopic stents for malignant biliary obstruction. Eur J Gastroenterol Hepatol 2007; 19(12):1119–24.
62. Zorrón Pu L, de Moura EG, Bernardo WM, et al. Endoscopic stenting for inoperable malignant biliary obstruction: a systematic review and meta-analysis. World J Gastroenterol 2015;21(47):13374–85.
63. Klinkenbijl JH, Jeekel J, Schmitz PI, et al. Carcinoma of the pancreas and periampullary region: palliation versus cure. Br J Surg 1993;80(12):1575–8.
64. van der Gaag NA, Kloek JJ, de Castro SM, et al. Preoperative biliary drainage in patients with obstructive jaundice: history and current status. J Gastrointest Surg 2009;13(4):814–20.
65. van der Gaag NA, Rauws EA, van Eijck CH, et al. Preoperative biliary drainage for cancer of the head of the pancreas. N Engl J Med 2010;362(2):129–37.
66. Wasan SM, Ross WA, Staerkel GA, et al. Use of expandable metallic biliary stents in resectable pancreatic cancer. Am J Gastroenterol 2005;100(9):2056–61.
67. Lawrence C, Howell DA, Conklin DE, et al. Delayed pancreaticoduodenectomy for cancer patients with prior ERCP-placed, nonforeshortening, self-expanding metal stents: a positive outcome. Gastrointest Endosc 2006;63(6):804–7.
68. Almadi MA, Barkun AN, Martel M. No benefit of covered vs uncovered self-expandable metal stents in patients with malignant distal biliary obstruction: a meta-analysis. Clin Gastroenterol Hepatol 2013;11(1):27–37.
69. Kullman E, Frozanpor F, Söderlund C, et al. Covered versus uncovered self-expandable nitinol stents in the palliative treatment of malignant distal biliary obstruction: results from a randomized, multicenter study. Gastrointest Endosc 2010;72(5):915–23.
70. Telford JJ, Carr-Locke DL, Baron TH, et al. A randomized trial comparing uncovered and partially covered self- expandable metal stents in the palliation of distal malignant biliary obstruction. Gastrointest Endosc 2010;72(5):907–14.

71. Lee JH, Krishna SG, Singh A, et al. Comparison of the utility of covered metal stents versus uncovered metal stents in the management of malignant biliary strictures in 749 patients. Gastrointest Endosc 2013;78(2):312–24.

72. Gress FG, Hawes RH, Savides TJ, et al. Role of EUS in the preoperative staging of pancreatic cancer: a large single-center experience. Gastrointest Endosc 1999;50(6):786–91.

73. Harrison JL, Millikan KW, Prinz RA, et al. Endoscopic ultrasound for diagnosis and staging of pancreatic tumors. Am Surg 1999;65(7):659–64 [discussion: 664–5].

74. Soriano A, Castells A, Ayuso C, et al. Preoperative staging and tumor resectability assessment of pancreatic cancer: prospective study comparing endoscopic ultrasonography, helical computed tomography, magnetic resonance imaging, and angiography. Am J Gastroenterol 2004;99(3):492–501.

75. Nawaz H, Yi-Fan C, Kloke J, et al. Performance characteristics of endoscopic ultrasound in the staging of pancreatic cancer: a meta-analysis. JOP 2013;14(5): 484–97.

Surgical Therapy for Pancreatic and Periampullary Cancer

John B. Ammori, MD*, Kevin Choong, MD,
Jeffrey M. Hardacre, MD

KEYWORDS

- Pancreaticoduodenectomy • Pancreatic cancer • Periampullary cancer

KEY POINTS

- Surgery is a key component in the care of pancreatic and periampullary cancers.
- Standard pancreaticoduodenectomy and pyloric-preserving pancreaticoduodenectomy have equivalent outcomes.
- There is no benefit to extended lymphadenectomy.
- There are numerous techniques and maneuvers available to minimize operative complications, particularly those associated with the pancreatic anastomosis.
- Despite the complexities of pancreatic surgery, enhanced recovery after surgery protocols are recommended.

INTRODUCTION

Periampullary cancers encompass cancers arising in the head of pancreas, distal bile duct, ampulla, and periampullary duodenum. The surgical management for these cancers is a pancreaticoduodenectomy or Whipple procedure. Distal pancreatectomy/splenectomy is the surgical procedure for cancers arising in the body and tail of the pancreas. Total pancreatectomy is indicated for tumors in the neck of the gland when a negative margin cannot be achieved with either a proximal or distal pancreatectomy. It is also indicated for patients with diffuse involvement by a main duct intraductal papillary mucinous neoplasm.

Pancreatic cancer is the fourth most common cause of cancer death in the United States, with more than 40,000 estimated deaths yearly and nearly 49,000 new diagnoses. Overall 5-year survival is 7%.[1] Surgical therapy is the only potential curative therapy. Even with surgical therapy as a component of multimodal care, actual 5-year

Division of Surgical Oncology, University Hospitals Cleveland Medical Center, 11100 Euclid Avenue, Cleveland, OH 44106, USA
* Corresponding author.
E-mail address: john.ammori@uhhospitals.org

Surg Clin N Am 96 (2016) 1271–1286
http://dx.doi.org/10.1016/j.suc.2016.07.001
surgical.theclinics.com

survival is approximately 12% to 15% with median survival of approximately 25 months.[2–4] Prognosis is better in other periampullary tumor types, with 5-year survivals of 39% for ampullary cancers, 27% for distal cholangiocarcinomas, and 59% for duodenal cancers.[5]

Because of the poor survival in pancreatic cancer even in surgical candidates, nonoperative therapy with chemoradiation has been studied in a randomized trial against surgery. In this study, 42 patients with locally resectable pancreatic cancer were randomized. With follow-up of at least 5 years, survival at 1 year and 3 years was significantly improved with surgery, 62% versus 35%, $P<.05$ at 1 year and 20% versus 0%, $P<.05$ at 3 years, with no difference in quality-of-life (QOL) measurements.[6] As such, surgery remains the treatment of choice for operable periampullary and pancreatic cancers. This article focuses on data specifically related to the surgical management of periampullary and pancreatic cancers.

PYLORUS-PRESERVING PANCREATICODUODENECTOMY VERSUS STANDARD PANCREATICODUODENECTOMY

To assess whether preservation of the pylorus improves perioperative outcomes and long-term gastrointestinal function, 4 randomized controlled trials (RCTs) have compared pylorus-preserving pancreaticoduodenectomy (PPPD) versus standard pancreaticoduodenectomy (PD) (Table 1).[7–10] No difference was seen in short-term and long-term survival, postoperative morbidity, operating time, blood loss, length of hospital stay (LOS), or QOL. The 2 smaller studies, which included 27 and

Table 1
Studies comparing PPPD with PD

Lead Author	n	Study Groups	Findings
Tran et al,[10] 2004	170	Standard PD n = 83 PPPD n = 87	No difference in overall survival, complications, DGE, blood loss, operative time, and postoperative weight loss.
Seiler et al,[8] 2005	130	Standard PD n = 66 PPPD n = 64	No difference in perioperative morbidity and mortality, overall survival, DGE, QOL, and weight gain. Capacity to work was better in PPPD group at 6 mo (77% vs 56%, $P = .02$).
Lin et al,[7] 2005	36	Standard PD n = 19 PPPD n = 14 Conversion from PPPD standard PD n = 3	No difference in operating time, blood loss, operative mortality, and overall survival. DGE was more frequently encountered in the PPPD group (43% vs 0%, $P<.05$).
Srinarmwong et al,[9] 2008	27	Standard PD n = 13 PPPD n = 14	No difference in operative time, blood loss, operative morbidity and mortality, length of stay, and overall survival. DGE was higher in the PPPD group (64% vs 15%, $P = .02$).

Abbreviations: DGE, delayed gastric emptying; PD, pancreaticoduodenectomy; PPPD, pylorus-preserving pancreaticoduodenectomy; QOL, quality of life.
Data from Refs.[7–10]

36 patients, demonstrated an increased incidence of delayed gastric emptying (DGE) in the PPPD.[7,9] However, the larger studies, which included 170 and 130 patients, did not demonstrate a difference in the incidence of postoperative DGE.[8,10] The authors' practice is to perform PD.

PANCREATICODUODENECTOMY WITH STANDARD VERSUS EXTENDED LYMPHADENECTOMY

To examine whether extended lymphadenectomy (EL) improves oncologic outcomes, 4 RCTs have examined PD with standard lymphadenectomy compared with EL (**Table 2**).[11–14] The conclusion of these studies is that EL does not improve survival from pancreatic or periampullary cancers, but increases operative time, blood loss, and postoperative morbidity. However, in the trial by Yeo and colleagues,[14] there was a trend toward prolonged survival in the EL group, and in the trial by Pedrazzoli and colleagues,[13] there was an improvement in survival in the subgroup of patients with positive lymph nodes who underwent EL. Taken together, these trials suggest that in general there is not a benefit to EL.

PANCREATIC RECONSTRUCTION

Of the 3 anastomoses after PD, the pancreatic anastomosis is the highest risk for leaks and fistulas (12%–33%) and the main driver for overall complications. The International Study Group of Pancreatic Fistula (ISGPF) has defined postoperative pancreatic fistula (POPF) as the output of fluid with amylase level greater than 3 times the upper normal serum value on or after postoperative day 3.[15] There are 3 grades of POPF described. Grade A POPF has no clinical impact, and is treated with the operatively

Table 2
Studies comparing standard PD with PD/EL

Lead Author	n	Study Groups	Findings
Yeo et al,[14] 2002	294	Standard PD n = 146 PD/EL n = 148	No difference in overall survival, blood loss, operative mortality, and node status. PD/EL resulted in increased operative time, postoperative complications, DGE, pancreatic fistula, and LOS.
Jang et al,[12] 2014	167	Standard PD n = 83 PD/EL n = 84	No difference in overall survival. PD/EL resulted in increased operative time, postoperative morbidity, and blood loss.
Pedrazzoli et al,[13] 1998	81	Standard PD n = 40 PD/EL n = 41	No difference in overall survival, operative morbidity and mortality, and operative time. Unplanned subgroup analysis of lymph node positive patients showed longer survival for PD/EL (*P*<.05).
Farnell et al,[11] 2005	79	Standard PD n = 40 PD/EL n = 39	No difference in overall survival, operative morbidity and mortality, and LOS. PD/EL resulted in increased operative time and blood loss, and decreased QOL.

Abbreviations: EL, extended lymphadenectomy; LOS, length of hospital stay; PD, pancreaticoduodenectomy; QOL, quality of life.
Data from Refs.[11–14]

placed drain. Grade B POPF has a clinical impact requiring specific treatment or change in management, such as percutaneous drainage. Grade C POPF has severe clinical impact requiring critical care and possible reoperation. Numerous techniques have been studied in an attempt to improve outcomes and minimize complications related to the pancreatic anastomosis.

Pancreaticogastrostomy Versus Pancreaticojejunostomy

Nine RCTs have compared reconstruction with pancreaticogastrostomy (PG) versus pancreaticojejunostomy (PJ) after PD (**Table 3**), most of which have been done in

Table 3
Studies comparing PG with PJ

Lead Author	n	Study Groups	Findings
Topol et al,[22] 2013	329	PG n = 162 PJ n = 167	Grade B/C POPF lower in PG group, 8.0% vs 19.8%, P = .002.
Keck et al,[21] 2016	320	PG n = 171 PJ n = 149	No difference in grade B/C POPF, PG = 20%, PJ = 22%. PG associated with higher grade A/B bleeding, PG = 10%, PJ = 5%, P = .023.
Bassi et al,[16] 2005	151	PG n = 69 PJ n = 82	No difference in POPF, PG = 13%, PJ = 16%. Lower postoperative collections, DGE, and biliary fistula in PG group.
Duffas et al,[17] 2005	149	PG n = 81 PJ n = 68	No difference in POPF (PG = 16%, PJ = 20%), mortality, reoperations, interventional drainage procedures, and LOS.
Yeo et al,[24] 1995	145	PG n = 73 PJ n = 72	No difference in POPF, PG = 12.3%, PJ = 11.1%. POPF associated with soft texture pancreas.
Figueras et al,[20] 2013	123	PG n = 65 PJ n = 58	POPF lower in PG group, 15% vs 34%, P = .014. Lower readmissions, better exocrine function, and less weight loss in PG group.
Wellner et al,[23] 2012	116	PG n = 59 PJ n = 57	No difference in POPF of any grade, PG = 10%, PJ = 12%. Decreased operative time in PG group.
Fernandez-Cruz et al,[19] 2008	108	PG n = 53 PJ n = 55	POPF of any grade lower in PG group, 4% vs 18%, P<.01. Decreased overall complications with PG, 23% vs 44%, P<.01.
El Nakeeb et al,[18] 2014	90	PG n = 45 PJ n = 45	No difference in grade B/C POPF, PG = 16%, PJ = 9%.

Abbreviations: DGE, delayed gastric emptying; LOS, length of hospital stay; PG, pancreaticogastrostomy; PJ, pancreaticojejunostomy; POPF, postoperative pancreatic fistula.
    Data from Refs.[16–24]

Europe.[16–24] A meta-analysis including 7 of these studies showed no difference in the overall morbidity rate, which was 49% in both groups.[25] Another meta-analysis of 7 studies reported an increased risk of intraluminal bleeding with PG.[26] Overall, the data suggest no overall difference in the rate of complications or POPF between these techniques. The data raise concerns about a higher risk of bleeding after PG. The authors' practice is to perform PJ following PD.

Pancreaticojejunostomy Techniques

PJ is the most common method of reconstruction after PD in the United States. Standard techniques include a 2-layered end-to-side, duct-to-mucosa anastomosis and an invaginating anastomosis.[27] Two RCTs have compared these anastomoses, with one of these studies showing no difference in POPF and the other study showing a lower POPF rate with the invagination technique (12% vs 24%, $P<.05$).[27,28] The most important risk factor for POPF was a soft texture gland.[27] A binding PJ technique demonstrated a lower rate of POPF compared with end-to-end invaginating PJ (0% vs 7%, $P = .01$).[29] Single-institution series have not duplicated a POPF rate near zero for the binding PJ technique, showing no difference to standard techniques at those institutions.[30–32] A comparison of the standard end-to-side duct-to-mucosa PJ to a mattress technique showed no difference in POPF.[33] A multicenter RCT is under way in the United Kingdom to compare 2 methods of duct-to-mucosa PJ, the standard 2-layered end-to-side technique (Cattell-Warren anastomosis) and mattress technique (Blumgart anastomosis).[34] See **Table 4** for a summary of these studies.

Table 4 Studies comparing PJ techniques			
Lead Author	**n**	**Study Groups**	**Findings**
Berger et al,[27] 2009	197	Invagination n = 100 Duct-to-mucosa n = 97	POPF of any grade lower in invagination group, 12% vs 24%, $P<.05$. PF developed in 8% with hard glands, 27% with a soft gland.
Bassi et al,[28] 2003	144	Invagination n = 72 Duct-to-mucosa n = 72	No difference in complications or POPF (invagination = 15%, duct-to-mucosa = 13%).
Peng et al,[29] 2007	217	Binding n = 106 Invagination n = 111	Lower POPF of any grade (0% vs 7%, $P = .014$) and complications (25% vs 37%, $P = .048$) in the binding technique group.
Langrehr et al,[33] 2005	113	Mattress duct-to-mucosa n = 57 Duct-to-mucosa n = 56	No difference in POPF, complications, LOS, or reoperations.
Halloran et al,[34] 2016	506 planned	Mattress duct-to-mucosa Planned n = 253 Duct-to-mucosa Planned n = 253	Trial under way.

Abbreviations: LOS, length of hospital stay; PF, pancreatic fistula; PG, pancreaticogastrostomy; PJ, pancreaticojejunostomy; POPF, postoperative pancreatic fistula.
Data from Refs.[27–29,33,34]

The "best" technique is not defined, and varies based on individual surgeon training and experience. Further, the best method may not be the same in all patients; one type of anastomosis may be better in soft glands with a small duct and another in hard glands with a dilated duct.

Management of the Pancreatic Stump After Distal Pancreatectomy

Pancreatic leak rates after distal pancreatectomy (DP) are approximately 15% to 25%. Numerous methods of addressing the pancreatic stump have been studied in an attempt to improve complication rates. The 2 techniques that are primarily used are to either suture or staple the pancreatic stump. The DISPACT trial addressed this issue with an analysis of 352 randomized patients (177 stapled and 175 hand-sewn closure).[35] There was no difference identified between the 2 techniques in terms of POPF or complications. Stapled transection with mesh reinforcement of the staple line was studied in a single-institution prospective randomized trial of 100 patients. This study demonstrated a significant decrease in POPF with staple line reinforcement compared with nonreinforced staple transection, 2% versus 20%, $P = .0007$.[36] A single-institution experience that compared 18 patients with nonreinforced staple transection with 36 patients with reinforced staple transection showed a significant decrease in POPF with stapler reinforcement, 8% versus 39%, $P = .01$.[37] There also have been a number of prospective RCTs and a meta-analysis examining the use of fibrin glue as an adjunct.[38–42] To summarize these studies, the addition of fibrin glue did not reduce POPF or postoperative complications. Several other randomized trials have assessed numerous additional techniques, such as the use of ultrasonic dissection, pancreaticojejunostomy to the stump, seromuscular patch, a fibrin sealant patch, falciform patch, and prophylactic transpapillary pancreatic duct stent placement.[38,42–47] Although many techniques have been studied, there is no definitively proven best method of dealing with the pancreatic stump after DP. Despite data from only 1 randomized study of 100 patients in addition to retrospective data, the use of a reinforced stapler to transect the pancreas is the preferred approach of the author.

Use and Management of Intraperitoneal Drains After Pancreatectomy

The use of drains after pancreatic resection remains a somewhat controversial topic. Further, if drains are used, there is debate regarding the timing of safe drain removal.

An RCT assessed early versus late removal of operatively placed drains after pancreatic resections.[48] A total of 114 patients with a drain amylase level of less than 5000 U/L on postoperative day 1 were randomized to drain removal on postoperative day 3 or standard drain management with removal on postoperative day 5 or beyond. Early drain removal was associated with a decreased rate of POPF, abdominal and pulmonary complications, LOS, and hospital costs.

There have been 2 prospective RCTs examining whether intraperitoneal drains should be routinely used after pancreatectomy. One study randomized 179 patients (88 drain, 91 no drain), including 139 who underwent PD and 40 who underwent DP.[49] No significant difference in the overall 30-day mortality, number or type of complications, or LOS was identified. However, significant intra-abdominal abscess, collection, or fistula occurred more frequently in patients with a drain, 22% versus 9%, $P = .02$. The second study evaluating drainage after PD was stopped after an interim analysis of 137 evaluable patients (68 drain, 69 no drain) because of increased 90-day mortality in the no-drain group, 12% versus 3%, $P = .097$.[50] In the no-drain group, there was an increase in the use of percutaneous drains (23% vs 9%, $P = .022$), occurrence of intra-abdominal abscess (26% vs 12%, $P = .033$), gastroparesis (42% vs 24%, P = .021), and any complication in grade 2 or higher (68% vs 52%, P = .047). Given the results of this study, routine drainage cannot be abandoned.

Selective use of intraperitoneal drains based on risk stratification has been recommended.[51] In addition to the RCTs evaluating the use of routine drainage, there have been single-institution cohort studies that have shown that the use of drains routinely can be safely avoided.[52–54] These studies have an inherent selection bias, as the patients deemed to be low risk for POPF were less likely to have a drain. A Fistula Risk Score was developed and validated using recognized risk factors for POPF (small duct, soft pancreas, high-risk pathology, excessive blood loss) to stratify patients into 4 categories: negligible risk, low risk, intermediate risk, and high risk.[55,56] The Fistula Risk Score calculator can be found at http://pancreasclub.com/calculators/fistula-risk-score-calculator/. A proposed clinical care path recommends drain placement in intermediate-risk and high-risk patients with omission of drainage in negligible and low-risk patients. Early drain removal is recommended in patients with postoperative day 1 drain amylase less than 5000 U/L.[51]

The authors' practice currently is the routine placement of 2 drains: 1 anterior to the pancreatic and biliary anastomoses and 1 placed posterior to these anastomoses. Drain amylase is checked on postoperative days 3 and 4, and drains are removed if fluid amylase levels are less than 3 times the upper limit of normal for serum amylase.

Pancreatic Duct Stenting

There have been 6 RCTs addressing the use of pancreatic duct stents following PD to reduce POPF (**Table 5**).[57–62] Three studies that compared external stenting to no stents demonstrated a reduction in POPF.[58–60] Two studies that compared internal with external stenting showed no difference between the techniques.[57,61] One study that compared internal stenting with no stents showed no difference between the techniques stratified by texture of pancreas.[62] In the authors' practice, pancreatic duct stenting is not routinely used. When thought to be needed, internal stenting is used.

Use of Somatostatin Analogs

There have been more than 20 RCTs examining the prophylactic use of somatostatin or one of its analogs, most notably octreotide, to reduce complications of pancreatic surgery. The mechanism of action is the reduction of pancreatic fluid production with the theoretic benefit of reduced POPF and pancreatic-associated complications. Three RCTs from Europe with more than 200 patients each published in the 1990s showed lower complication rates with prophylactic octreotide.[63–65] A subsequent French study and 2 studies from the United States showed no difference in outcomes with the use of octreotide.[66–68] Vapreotide, a potent somatostatin analog, was not shown to reduce complications in a multicenter trial.[69] A meta-analysis of 21 RCTs published in 2013 concluded that somatostatin analogs may reduce perioperative complications but do not reduce perioperative mortality.[70] As such, the routine use of octreotide has been abandoned for the most part; however, some still advocate for use in high-risk anastomoses. A subsequent study examining the effects of perioperative treatment with pasireotide, a somatostatin analog with a longer half-life than octreotide, decreased the rate of clinically significant POPF, leak, or abscess.[71] The use of pasireotide has not yet been approved for this indication and comes with a high cost. **Table 6** summarizes these studies.

Table 5
RCTs of pancreatic duct stenting

Lead Author	n	Study Groups	Findings
Pessaux et al,[59] 2011	158	External stent n = 77 No stent n = 81	POPF lower in stent group, 26% vs 42%, $P = .034$. Morbidity lower in stent group, 61.7% vs 41.5%, $P = .01$. DGE lower in stent group, 7.8% vs 27.2%, $P = .001$. No difference in mortality.
Poon et al,[60] 2007	120	External stent n = 60 No stent n = 60	POPF lower in stent group, 6.7% vs 20%, $P = .032$. No difference in overall morbidity and mortality between groups.
Motoi et al,[58] 2012	93	External stent n = 47 No stent n = 46	POPF lower in stent group, 22% vs 61%, $P = .04$.
Tani et al,[61] 2010	100	External stent n = 50 Internal stent n = 50	No difference in POPF, external stent 20% vs internal stent 26%. No difference in other complications.
Kamoda et al,[57] 2008	43	External stent n = 22 Internal stent n = 21	No difference in POPF, external stent 36.4% vs internal stent 33.3%.
Winter et al,[62] 2006	234	Internal stent n = 115 No stent n = 119	Soft pancreas: No difference in POPF, internal stent 21.1% vs no stent 10.7%, $P = .1$. Hard pancreas: No difference in POPF, internal stent 1.7% vs no stent 4.8%, $P = .4$.

Abbreviations: DGE, delayed gastric emptying; POPF, postoperative pancreatic fistula; RCT, randomized controlled trial.
   Data from Refs.[57–62]

SUPERIOR MESENTERIC ARTERY FIRST APPROACH

Local infiltration of the superior mesenteric artery (SMA) is a contraindication for resection. Involvement of the SMA is not frequently obvious on preoperative cross-sectional imaging and must be determined intraoperatively. In the classically described technique for PD, assessment for venous involvement is performed by creating a retropancreatic tunnel before committing to tumor resection, leaving the retroperitoneal and SMA dissection as the final step. Because superior mesenteric vein and portal vein resection/reconstruction can be performed safely with good long-term outcomes, it is sometimes imperative to assess SMA involvement before committing to resection to avoid a positive resection margin and inappropriate surgery. The SMA first approach described by Pessaux and colleagues[72] allows early assessment of the SMA. Briefly, the initial steps of the operation include a wide Kocher maneuver to the point at which the left renal vein crosses the aorta. The SMA is dissected free of connective tissue at its origin and encircled with a vessel loop. Then, the attachments to the uncinate process and superior mesenteric vein and portal vein are dissected, and resectability can be assessed.

MINIMALLY INVASIVE PANCREATECTOMY

Minimally invasive surgery (MIS) approaches to PD include laparoscopic, robotic, and a hybrid approach using laparoscopy for resection and the robot during the

Table 6
RCTs of somatostatin analogues

Lead Author	n	Study Groups	Findings
Buchler et al,[63] 1992	246	Octreotide n = 125 Placebo n = 121	Lower complications with octreotide in patients with cancer, 38% vs 65%, $P<.01$. Lower POPF with octreotide in all patients, 17.6% vs 38%, $P<.05$.
Motorsi et al,[64] 1995	218	Octreotide n = 111 Placebo n = 107	Lower POPF in the octreotide group, 9% vs 19.6%, $P<.05$. Lower morbidity in the octreotide group, 21.6% vs 36.4%, $P<.05$.
Pederzoli et al,[65] 1994	252	Octreotide n = 122 Placebo n = 130	Lower complications in the octreotide group, 15.6% vs 29.2%, $P = .01$. Lower POPF in the octreotide group, 9% vs 18.5%, $P<.05$.
Suc et al,[67] 2004	230	Octreotide n = 122 Placebo n = 108	No difference in intra-abdominal complications, 22% for octreotide and 32% for placebo.
Yeo et al,[68] 2000	211	Octreotide n = 104 Placebo n = 107	No difference in complications (40% octreotide, 34% placebo) or POPF (10.6% octreotide, 9.3% placebo).
Lowy et al,[66] 1997	110	Octreotide n = 57 Placebo n = 53	No difference in POPF (28% octreotide, 21% placebo) or clinically significant POPF (12% octreotide, 6% placebo).
Saar et al,[69] 2003	275	Vapreotide n = 135 Placebo n = 140	No difference in pancreas-related complications (30.4% vapreotide, 26.4% placebo).
Allen et al,[71] 2014	300	Pasireotide n = 152 Placebo n = 148	Lower grade 3 POPF, leak, or abscess in pasireotide group, 9% vs 21%, $P = .006$.

Abbreviations: POPF, postoperative pancreatic fistula; RCT, randomized controlled trial.
 Data from Refs.[63–69,71]

reconstruction phase. Advantages of the robotic approach include full articulation of the instruments, such as a human wrist, elimination of surgeon tremor, and 3-dimensional image. This is a complex procedure predominantly performed in a handful of centers, as it requires expertise in both MIS and pancreatic surgery. There are no RCTs comparing MIS with open PD. Most studies are single-center studies reporting the institutional experience, or comparing MIS with open surgery.[73–80] In general, the studies have shown that MIS is feasible and safe in experienced hands with similar overall morbidity, mortality, and oncologic outcomes to open PD. MIS PD has a significantly increased operative time, but a lower operative blood loss. Using the National Cancer Database, 983 patients with MIS PD were compared with 6078 open procedures.[81] Although there was no difference in the number of lymph nodes retrieved, the rate of positive surgical margins, LOS, or readmissions, the unadjusted 30-day mortality rate was 5.1% for MIS PD versus 3.1% after open PD ($P = .002$). As such, MIS PD remains a complex procedure that should be used only by experienced centers and may not be widely applicable.

MIS DP has become increasingly performed in recent years.[82] This is a less technically demanding procedure than MIS PD. There are no RCTs comparing MIS DP with open DP; however, numerous studies have demonstrated that MIS DP is a safe procedure. In general, the studies indicate that there are lower rates of overall complications, LOS, and operative blood loss without differences in mortality or reoperation rates.[82–85] There is theoretic concern about oncologic outcomes with MIS DP compared with open surgery; however, oncologic outcomes appear similar between approaches.[86,87] Taking these data into consideration, the improved recovery outcomes after MIS DP compared with open DP are not uniform and not as profound as laparoscopic compared with open cholecystectomy. As such, MIS DP for cancer should be done only when the surgeon is confident of his or her ability to perform an oncologically appropriate operation.

ENHANCED RECOVERY AFTER SURGERY FOR PANCREATICODUODENECTOMY

Enhanced recovery after surgery (ERAS) protocols, also known as "fast-track" protocols, have become widely used in postoperative management. These protocols were implemented in patients with postoperative colectomy and reduced resource utilization while improving patient outcomes.[88] Similar findings have been seen with ERAS following PD, with reduced complications and lower hospital costs.[89] The ERAS Society has published guidelines for the perioperative care of patients with PD.[90] Numerous perioperative issues are addressed in the guidelines. One area worth noting is postoperative nutrition. The recommendation is for early oral diet without restriction, with patients cautioned to begin carefully and increase to tolerance over 3 to 4 days. Enteral or parenteral feeding should not be routinely performed. This recommendation contradicts traditional practice of surgeon-controlled slowly advancing diet. Furthermore, routine placement of jejunostomy tubes for enteral feeding has been commonly practiced, predominantly in Europe. An RCT compared postoperative enteral tube feedings with early oral feeding and found no difference in complications.[91] In summary, the use of ERAS protocols is encouraged to benefit both patient outcomes and medical expenditures. ERAS in pancreatic surgery is discussed in detail elsewhere in this volume.

SUMMARY

Pancreatectomy is a complex procedure with numerous perioperative and intraoperative factors that are important to achieving optimal outcomes. There have been several refinements in the care of patients with pancreatic cancer over the past decades. With surgery for pancreatic cancer being a safe procedure, better systemic therapies are clearly needed to improve patient outcomes.

REFERENCES

1. Siegel RL, Miller KD, Jemal A. Cancer statistics, 2015. CA Cancer J Clin 2015; 65(1):5–29.
2. Cleary SP, Gryfe R, Guindi M, et al. Prognostic factors in resected pancreatic adenocarcinoma: analysis of actual 5-year survivors. J Am Coll Surg 2004; 198(5):722–31.
3. Ferrone CR, Brennan MF, Gonen M, et al. Pancreatic adenocarcinoma: the actual 5-year survivors. J Gastrointest Surg 2008;12(4):701–6.
4. Winter JM, Brennan MF, Tang LH, et al. Survival after resection of pancreatic adenocarcinoma: results from a single institution over three decades. Ann Surg Oncol 2012;19(1):169–75.

5. Yeo CJ, Sohn TA, Cameron JL, et al. Periampullary adenocarcinoma: analysis of 5-year survivors. Ann Surg 1998;227(6):821–31.

6. Doi R, Imamura M, Hosotani R, et al. Surgery versus radiochemotherapy for resectable locally invasive pancreatic cancer: final results of a randomized multi-institutional trial. Surg Today 2008;38(11):1021–8.

7. Lin PW, Shan YS, Lin YJ, et al. Pancreaticoduodenectomy for pancreatic head cancer: PPPD versus Whipple procedure. Hepatogastroenterology 2005;52(65): 1601–4.

8. Seiler CA, Wagner M, Bachmann T, et al. Randomized clinical trial of pylorus-preserving duodenopancreatectomy versus classical Whipple resection-long term results. Br J Surg 2005;92(5):547–56.

9. Srinarmwong C, Luechakiettisak P, Prasitvilai W. Standard Whipple's operation versus pylorus preserving pancreaticoduodenectomy: a randomized controlled trial study. J Med Assoc Thai 2008;91(5):693–8.

10. Tran KT, Smeenk HG, van Eijck CH, et al. Pylorus preserving pancreaticoduodenectomy versus standard Whipple procedure: a prospective, randomized, multicenter analysis of 170 patients with pancreatic and periampullary tumors. Ann Surg 2004;240(5):738–45.

11. Farnell MB, Pearson RK, Sarr MG, et al. A prospective randomized trial comparing standard pancreatoduodenectomy with pancreatoduodenectomy with extended lymphadenectomy in resectable pancreatic head adenocarcinoma. Surgery 2005;138(4):618–28 [discussion: 628–30].

12. Jang JY, Kang MJ, Heo JS, et al. A prospective randomized controlled study comparing outcomes of standard resection and extended resection, including dissection of the nerve plexus and various lymph nodes, in patients with pancreatic head cancer. Ann Surg 2014;259(4):656–64.

13. Pedrazzoli S, DiCarlo V, Dionigi R, et al. Standard versus extended lymphadenectomy associated with pancreatoduodenectomy in the surgical treatment of adenocarcinoma of the head of the pancreas: a multicenter, prospective, randomized study. Lymphadenectomy Study Group. Ann Surg 1998;228(4):508–17.

14. Yeo CJ, Cameron JL, Lillemoe KD, et al. Pancreaticoduodenectomy with or without distal gastrectomy and extended retroperitoneal lymphadenectomy for periampullary adenocarcinoma, part 2: randomized controlled trial evaluating survival, morbidity, and mortality. Ann Surg 2002;236(3):355–66 [discussion: 366–8].

15. Bassi C, Dervenis C, Butturini G, et al. Postoperative pancreatic fistula: an international study group (ISGPF) definition. Surgery 2005;138(1):8–13.

16. Bassi C, Falconi M, Molinari E, et al. Reconstruction by pancreaticojejunostomy versus pancreaticogastrostomy following pancreatectomy: results of a comparative study. Ann Surg 2005;242(6):767–71 [discussion: 771–3].

17. Duffas JP, Suc B, Msika S, et al. A controlled randomized multicenter trial of pancreatogastrostomy or pancreatojejunostomy after pancreatoduodenectomy. Am J Surg 2005;189(6):720–9.

18. El Nakeeb A, Hamdy E, Sultan AM, et al. Isolated Roux loop pancreaticojejunostomy versus pancreaticogastrostomy after pancreaticoduodenectomy: a prospective randomized study. HPB 2014;16(8):713–22.

19. Fernandez-Cruz L, Cosa R, Blanco L, et al. Pancreatogastrostomy with gastric partition after pylorus-preserving pancreatoduodenectomy versus conventional pancreatojejunostomy: a prospective randomized study. Ann Surg 2008;248(6): 930–8.

20. Figueras J, Sabater L, Planellas P, et al. Randomized clinical trial of pancreatico-gastrostomy versus pancreaticojejunostomy on the rate and severity of pancreatic fistula after pancreaticoduodenectomy. Br J Surg 2013;100(12):1597–605.

21. Keck T, Wellner UF, Bahra M, et al. Pancreatogastrostomy versus pancreatojejunostomy for RECOnstruction After PANCreatoduodenectomy (RECOPANC, DRKS 00000767): perioperative and long-term results of a multicenter randomized controlled trial. Ann Surg 2016;263(3):440–9.

22. Topal B, Fieuws S, Aerts R, et al. Pancreaticojejunostomy versus pancreaticogastrostomy reconstruction after pancreaticoduodenectomy for pancreatic or periampullary tumours: a multicentre randomised trial. Lancet Oncol 2013;14(7):655–62.

23. Wellner UF, Sick O, Olschewski M, et al. Randomized controlled single-center trial comparing pancreatogastrostomy versus pancreaticojejunostomy after partial pancreatoduodenectomy. J Gastrointest Surg 2012;16(9):1686–95.

24. Yeo CJ, Cameron JL, Maher MM, et al. A prospective randomized trial of pancreaticogastrostomy versus pancreaticojejunostomy after pancreaticoduodenectomy. Ann Surg 1995;222(4):580–8 [discussion: 588–92].

25. Menahem B, Guittet L, Mulliri A, et al. Pancreaticogastrostomy is superior to pancreaticojejunostomy for prevention of pancreatic fistula after pancreaticoduodenectomy: an updated meta-analysis of randomized controlled trials. Ann Surg 2015;261(5):882–7.

26. Clerveus M, Morandeira-Rivas A, Picazo-Yeste J, et al. Pancreaticogastrostomy versus pancreaticojejunostomy after pancreaticoduodenectomy: a systematic review and meta-analysis of randomized controlled trials. J Gastrointest Surg 2014;18(9):1693–704.

27. Berger AC, Howard TJ, Kennedy EP, et al. Does type of pancreaticojejunostomy after pancreaticoduodenectomy decrease rate of pancreatic fistula? A randomized, prospective, dual-institution trial. J Am Coll Surg 2009;208(5):738–47 [discussion: 747–9].

28. Bassi C, Falconi M, Molinari E, et al. Duct-to-mucosa versus end-to-side pancreaticojejunostomy reconstruction after pancreaticoduodenectomy: results of a prospective randomized trial. Surgery 2003;134(5):766–71.

29. Peng SY, Wang JW, Lau WY, et al. Conventional versus binding pancreaticojejunostomy after pancreaticoduodenectomy: a prospective randomized trial. Ann Surg 2007;245(5):692–8.

30. Buc E, Flamein R, Golffier C, et al. Peng's binding pancreaticojejunostomy after pancreaticoduodenectomy: a French prospective study. J Gastrointest Surg 2010;14(4):705–10.

31. Casadei R, Ricci C, Silvestri S, et al. Peng's binding pancreaticojejunostomy after pancreaticoduodenectomy. An Italian, prospective, dual-institution study. Pancreatology 2013;13(3):305–9.

32. Maggiori L, Sauvanet A, Nagarajan G, et al. Binding versus conventional pancreaticojejunostomy after pancreaticoduodenectomy: a case-matched study. J Gastrointest Surg 2010;14(9):1395–400.

33. Langrehr JM, Bahra M, Jacob D, et al. Prospective randomized comparison between a new mattress technique and Cattell (duct-to-mucosa) pancreaticojejunostomy for pancreatic resection. World J Surg 2005;29(9):1111–9 [discussion: 1120–1].

34. Halloran CM, Platt K, Gerard A, et al. PANasta Trial; Cattell Warren versus Blumgart techniques of panreatico-jejunostomy following pancreato-duodenectomy: study protocol for a randomized controlled trial. Trials 2016;17(1):30.

35. Diener MK, Seiler CM, Rossion I, et al. Efficacy of stapler versus hand-sewn closure after distal pancreatectomy (DISPACT): a randomised, controlled multi-centre trial. Lancet 2011;377(9776):1514–22.

36. Hamilton NA, Porembka MR, Johnston FM, et al. Mesh reinforcement of pancreatic transection decreases incidence of pancreatic occlusion failure for left pancreatectomy: a single-blinded, randomized controlled trial. Ann Surg 2012; 255(6):1037–42.

37. Wallace CL, Georgakis GV, Eisenberg DP, et al. Further experience with pancreatic stump closure using a reinforced staple line. Conn Med 2013;77(4):205–10.

38. Carter TI, Fong ZV, Hyslop T, et al. A dual-institution randomized controlled trial of remnant closure after distal pancreatectomy: does the addition of a falciform patch and fibrin glue improve outcomes? J Gastrointest Surg 2013;17(1):102–9.

39. Orci LA, Oldani G, Berney T, et al. Systematic review and meta-analysis of fibrin sealants for patients undergoing pancreatic resection. HPB 2014;16(1):3–11.

40. Suc B, Msika S, Fingerhut A, et al. Temporary fibrin glue occlusion of the main pancreatic duct in the prevention of intra-abdominal complications after pancreatic resection: prospective randomized trial. Ann Surg 2003;237(1):57–65.

41. Suzuki Y, Kuroda Y, Morita A, et al. Fibrin glue sealing for the prevention of pancreatic fistulas following distal pancreatectomy. Arch Surg 1995;130(9): 952–5.

42. Bassi C, Butturini G, Falconi M, et al. Prospective randomised pilot study of management of the pancreatic stump following distal resection. HPB 1999;1(4): 203–8.

43. Frozanpor F, Lundell L, Segersvard R, et al. The effect of prophylactic transpapillary pancreatic stent insertion on clinically significant leak rate following distal pancreatectomy: results of a prospective controlled clinical trial. Ann Surg 2012;255(6):1032–6.

44. Kawai M, Hirono S, Okada KI, et al. Randomized controlled trial of pancreaticojejunostomy versus stapler closure of the pancreatic stump during distal pancreatectomy to reduce pancreatic fistula. Ann Surg 2016;264(1):180–7.

45. Montorsi M, Zerbi A, Bassi C, et al. Efficacy of an absorbable fibrin sealant patch (TachoSil) after distal pancreatectomy: a multicenter, randomized, controlled trial. Ann Surg 2012;256(5):853–9 [discussion: 859–60].

46. Olah A, Issekutz A, Belagyi T, et al. Randomized clinical trial of techniques for closure of the pancreatic remnant following distal pancreatectomy. Br J Surg 2009;96(6):602–7.

47. Suzuki Y, Fujino Y, Tanioka Y, et al. Randomized clinical trial of ultrasonic dissector or conventional division in distal pancreatectomy for non-fibrotic pancreas. Br J Surg 1999;86(5):608–11.

48. Bassi C, Molinari E, Malleo G, et al. Early versus late drain removal after standard pancreatic resections: results of a prospective randomized trial. Ann Surg 2010; 252(2):207–14.

49. Conlon KC, Labow D, Leung D, et al. Prospective randomized clinical trial of the value of intraperitoneal drainage after pancreatic resection. Ann Surg 2001; 234(4):487–93 [discussion: 493–4].

50. Van Buren G 2nd, Bloomston M, Hughes SJ, et al. A randomized prospective multicenter trial of pancreaticoduodenectomy with and without routine intraperitoneal drainage. Ann Surg 2014;259(4):605–12.

51. McMillan MT, Malleo G, Bassi C, et al. Drain management after pancreatoduodenectomy: reappraisal of a prospective randomized trial using risk stratification. J Am Coll Surg 2015;221(4):798–809.

52. Adham M, Chopin-Laly X, Lepilliez V, et al. Pancreatic resection: drain or no drain? Surgery 2013;154(5):1069–77.
53. Correa-Gallego C, Brennan MF, D'Angelica M, et al. Operative drainage following pancreatic resection: analysis of 1122 patients resected over 5 years at a single institution. Ann Surg 2013;258(6):1051–8.
54. Mehta VV, Fisher SB, Maithel SK, et al. Is it time to abandon routine operative drain use? A single institution assessment of 709 consecutive pancreaticoduodenectomies. J Am Coll Surg 2013;216(4):635–42 [discussion: 642–4].
55. Callery MP, Pratt WB, Kent TS, et al. A prospectively validated clinical risk score accurately predicts pancreatic fistula after pancreatoduodenectomy. J Am Coll Surg 2013;216(1):1–14.
56. Miller BC, Christein JD, Behrman SW, et al. A multi-institutional external validation of the fistula risk score for pancreatoduodenectomy. J Gastrointest Surg 2014; 18(1):172–9 [discussion: 179–80].
57. Kamoda Y, Fujino Y, Matsumoto I, et al. Usefulness of performing a pancreaticojejunostomy with an internal stent after a pancreatoduodenectomy. Surg Today 2008;38(6):524–8.
58. Motoi F, Egawa S, Rikiyama T, et al. Randomized clinical trial of external stent drainage of the pancreatic duct to reduce postoperative pancreatic fistula after pancreaticojejunostomy. Br J Surg 2012;99(4):524–31.
59. Pessaux P, Sauvanet A, Mariette C, et al. External pancreatic duct stent decreases pancreatic fistula rate after pancreaticoduodenectomy: prospective multicenter randomized trial. Ann Surg 2011;253(5):879–85.
60. Poon RT, Fan ST, Lo CM, et al. External drainage of pancreatic duct with a stent to reduce leakage rate of pancreaticojejunostomy after pancreaticoduodenectomy: a prospective randomized trial. Ann Surg 2007;246(3):425–33 [discussion: 433–5].
61. Tani M, Kawai M, Hirono S, et al. A prospective randomized controlled trial of internal versus external drainage with pancreaticojejunostomy for pancreaticoduodenectomy. Am J Surg 2010;199(6):759–64.
62. Winter JM, Cameron JL, Campbell KA, et al. Does pancreatic duct stenting decrease the rate of pancreatic fistula following pancreaticoduodenectomy? Results of a prospective randomized trial. J Gastrointest Surg 2006;10(9):1280–90 [discussion: 1290].
63. Buchler M, Friess H, Klempa I, et al. Role of octreotide in the prevention of postoperative complications following pancreatic resection. Am J Surg 1992;163(1): 125–30 [discussion: 130–1].
64. Montorsi M, Zago M, Mosca F, et al. Efficacy of octreotide in the prevention of pancreatic fistula after elective pancreatic resections: a prospective, controlled, randomized clinical trial. Surgery 1995;117(1):26–31.
65. Pederzoli P, Bassi C, Falconi M, et al. Efficacy of octreotide in the prevention of complications of elective pancreatic surgery. Italian Study Group. Br J Surg 1994;81(2):265–9.
66. Lowy AM, Lee JE, Pisters PW, et al. Prospective, randomized trial of octreotide to prevent pancreatic fistula after pancreaticoduodenectomy for malignant disease. Ann Surg 1997;226(5):632–41.
67. Suc B, Msika S, Piccinini M, et al. Octreotide in the prevention of intra-abdominal complications following elective pancreatic resection: a prospective, multicenter randomized controlled trial. Arch Surg 2004;139(3):288–94 [discussion: 295].
68. Yeo CJ, Cameron JL, Lillemoe KD, et al. Does prophylactic octreotide decrease the rates of pancreatic fistula and other complications after

pancreaticoduodenectomy? Results of a prospective randomized placebo-controlled trial. Ann Surg 2000;232(3):419–29.

69. Sarr MG, Pancreatic Surgery Group. The potent somatostatin analogue vapreotide does not decrease pancreas-specific complications after elective pancreatectomy: a prospective, multicenter, double-blinded, randomized, placebo-controlled trial. J Am Coll Surg 2003;196(4):556–64 [discussion: 564–5]; [author reply: 565].

70. Gurusamy KS, Koti R, Fusai G, et al. Somatostatin analogues for pancreatic surgery. Cochrane Database Syst Rev 2013;(4):CD008370.

71. Allen PJ, Gonen M, Brennan MF, et al. Pasireotide for postoperative pancreatic fistula. N Engl J Med 2014;370(21):2014–22.

72. Pessaux P, Varma D, Arnaud JP. Pancreaticoduodenectomy: superior mesenteric artery first approach. J Gastrointest Surg 2006;10(4):607–11.

73. Asbun HJ, Stauffer JA. Laparoscopic vs open pancreaticoduodenectomy: overall outcomes and severity of complications using the Accordion Severity Grading System. J Am Coll Surg 2012;215(6):810–9.

74. Bao PQ, Mazirka PO, Watkins KT. Retrospective comparison of robot-assisted minimally invasive versus open pancreaticoduodenectomy for periampullary neoplasms. J Gastrointest Surg 2014;18(4):682–9.

75. Buchs NC, Addeo P, Bianco FM, et al. Robotic versus open pancreaticoduodenectomy: a comparative study at a single institution. World J Surg 2011;35(12):2739–46.

76. Chalikonda S, Aguilar-Saavedra JR, Walsh RM. Laparoscopic robotic-assisted pancreaticoduodenectomy: a case-matched comparison with open resection. Surg Endosc 2012;26(9):2397–402.

77. Croome KP, Farnell MB, Que FG, et al. Total laparoscopic pancreaticoduodenectomy for pancreatic ductal adenocarcinoma: oncologic advantages over open approaches? Ann Surg 2014;260(4):633–8 [discussion: 638–40].

78. Lai EC, Yang GP, Tang CN. Robot-assisted laparoscopic pancreaticoduodenectomy versus open pancreaticoduodenectomy–a comparative study. Int J Surg 2012;10(9):475–9.

79. Zeh HJ, Zureikat AH, Secrest A, et al. Outcomes after robot-assisted pancreaticoduodenectomy for periampullary lesions. Ann Surg Oncol 2012;19(3):864–70.

80. Zureikat AH, Moser AJ, Boone BA, et al. 250 robotic pancreatic resections: safety and feasibility. Ann Surg 2013;258(4):554–9 [discussion: 559–62].

81. Adam MA, Choudhury K, Dinan MA, et al. Minimally invasive versus open pancreaticoduodenectomy for cancer: practice patterns and short-term outcomes among 7061 patients. Ann Surg 2015;262(2):372–7.

82. Tran Cao HS, Lopez N, Chang DC, et al. Improved perioperative outcomes with minimally invasive distal pancreatectomy: results from a population-based analysis. JAMA Surg 2014;149(3):237–43.

83. Kooby DA, Gillespie T, Bentrem D, et al. Left-sided pancreatectomy: a multicenter comparison of laparoscopic and open approaches. Ann Surg 2008;248(3):438–46.

84. Nigri GR, Rosman AS, Petrucciani N, et al. Metaanalysis of trials comparing minimally invasive and open distal pancreatectomies. Surg Endosc 2011;25(5):1642–51.

85. Venkat R, Edil BH, Schulick RD, et al. Laparoscopic distal pancreatectomy is associated with significantly less overall morbidity compared to the open technique: a systematic review and meta-analysis. Ann Surg 2012;255(6):1048–59.

86. Kooby DA, Hawkins WG, Schmidt CM, et al. A multicenter analysis of distal pancreatectomy for adenocarcinoma: is laparoscopic resection appropriate? J Am Coll Surg 2010;210(5):779–85, 786–7.

87. Magge D, Gooding W, Choudry H, et al. Comparative effectiveness of minimally invasive and open distal pancreatectomy for ductal adenocarcinoma. JAMA Surg 2013;148(6):525–31.

88. Adamina M, Kehlet H, Tomlinson GA, et al. Enhanced recovery pathways optimize health outcomes and resource utilization: a meta-analysis of randomized controlled trials in colorectal surgery. Surgery 2011;149(6):830–40.

89. Coolsen MM, van Dam RM, van der Wilt AA, et al. Systematic review and meta-analysis of enhanced recovery after pancreatic surgery with particular emphasis on pancreaticoduodenectomies. World J Surg 2013;37(8):1909–18.

90. Lassen K, Coolsen MM, Slim K, et al. Guidelines for perioperative care for pancreaticoduodenectomy: enhanced recovery after surgery (ERAS(R)) Society recommendations. Clin Nutr 2012;31(6):817–30.

91. Lassen K, Kjaeve J, Fetveit T, et al. Allowing normal food at will after major upper gastrointestinal surgery does not increase morbidity: a randomized multicenter trial. Ann Surg 2008;247(5):721–9.

Adjuvant and Neoadjuvant Therapy for Resectable Pancreatic and Periampullary Cancer

Stephanie M. Kim, MD[a], Jennifer R. Eads, MD[b],*

KEYWORDS

- Pancreatic cancer - Pancreatic adenocarcinoma - Periampullary cancer - Adjuvant
- Neoadjuvant

KEY POINTS

- Pancreatic cancer is associated with an overall high mortality rate despite the use of curative surgery.
- Adjuvant therapy including chemotherapy with or without radiation improves overall survival rates.
- Neoadjuvant chemotherapy with or without radiation therapy is increasingly being used and studied as a management strategy for pancreatic cancer.
- Periampullary cancers are a rare and heterogeneous group of tumors with many of the treatment recommendations being based on pancreatic cancer studies.

INTRODUCTION

Adjuvant therapy in pancreatic and periampullary adenocarcinoma remains a topic of intense investigation. Initial adjuvant treatment efforts grew out of the recognition that overall survival rates remained low despite curative intent resection for early stage disease. The pool of potentially therapeutic options have largely been derived from the metastatic setting, and numerous regimens have been evaluated. Although chemotherapy offers a significant but modest survival benefit over receipt of no treatment, the use of chemoradiation in the adjuvant setting has not demonstrated a clear survival

Disclosures: J.R. Eads reports research support from Novartis and consulting for Amgen, Oxigene, Portola, and ClearView Healthcare Partners. S.M. Kim reports no disclosures.
[a] Division of Hematology and Oncology, University Hospitals Seidman Cancer Center, Case Comprehensive Cancer Center, Case Western Reserve University, 11100 Euclid Avenue, Lakeside 1200, Cleveland, OH 44106, USA; [b] Division of Hematology and Oncology, University Hospitals Seidman Cancer Center, Case Comprehensive Cancer Center, Case Western Reserve University, 11100 Euclid Avenue, Lakeside 1200, Cleveland, OH 44106, USA
* Corresponding author.
E-mail address: jennifer.eads@uhhospitals.org

benefit among the major studies and, as such, its role is less clear. The rarity of peri-ampullary carcinoma, historically treated similarly to pancreatic adenocarcinoma, limits its evaluation to retrospective studies or subgroup analyses within larger studies. In addition, there have not been many studies demonstrating a clear survival benefit of an adjuvant regimen in this small group, which may be reflective of the histologic heterogeneity that exists among these tumors. This article discusses the data that have led to and support the current standard of care for the adjuvant management of pancreatic adenocarcinoma and periampullary cancers, which in turn illuminates the way forward for more effective adjuvant and potentially neoadjuvant treatment strategies.

PANCREATIC ADENOCARCINOMA
Epidemiology and Rationale for Adjuvant Therapy

Pancreatic adenocarcinoma is the 12th most commonly diagnosed malignancy, but is the 4th leading cause of cancer-related death with 40,560 patients dying from this disease in 2015.[1] Despite curative intent surgical resection of early stage lesions (stages I and II), local and systemic recurrence rates are high and overall survival rates are dismally low. Retrospective surgical studies demonstrate that although perioperative mortality has improved with surgical advances, overall survival continues to be low, with 5-year survival rates of 7% to 25% after a curative intent resection.[2–6] Criteria for resectability relate to the degree of arterial and venous tumor involvement as well as the presence of metastases.[7] Given the high recurrence rates after surgical resection—likely owing to the lingering presence of micrometastatic disease—the role of adjuvant therapy, specifically chemotherapy, radiation therapy or a combination of the 2 modalities, has been evaluated for survival benefit.

Adjuvant Chemotherapy

The efficacy of adjuvant chemotherapy alone has been assessed in several clinical trials with initial studies producing mixed results. An early Norwegian study randomized 61 patients with stages I through III pancreatic cancer to adjuvant chemotherapy with doxorubicin, mitomycin C, and 5-fluorouracil (5-FU) or observation after surgical resection.[8] Median survival in the treatment group was 23 months compared with 11 months in the observation group ($P = .02$); however, there was no significant improvement in 2-year survival ($P = .10$). Similarly, a Japanese group randomized 508 patients with resected stages II through IV pancreaticobiliary cancers to adjuvant mitomycin C and 5-FU. Despite a large overall population, only a fraction of patients with pancreatic cancer underwent curative resection (n = 92). Among this subgroup, no differences were found in 5-year disease-free or 5-year overall survival ($P = .28$ and $P = .45$, respectively).[9] Although neither of these studies was positive for the use of adjuvant chemotherapy, the small number of patients undergoing curative resection in both trials made the results inconclusive.

Historically, 5-FU has been the most extensively studied chemotherapeutic agent of choice for patients with any stage of pancreatic cancer.[10–12] However, the subsequent success of gemcitabine in metastatic disease changed the adjuvant landscape. Burris and colleagues[13] published a randomized phase III trial conducted in patients with advanced pancreatic adenocarcinoma, demonstrating that gemcitabine conferred a superior survival benefit as compared with 5-FU (5.6 vs 4.4 months, respectively; $P = .0025$). Similar efforts to improve adjuvant therapy led to Charite Onkologie's (CONKO) study of gemcitabine in the adjuvant setting. In a randomized controlled phase III trial, 368 patients with T1-4 N0-1 M0 pancreatic adenocarcinoma were randomized to either gemcitabine or observation after resection. Median disease-free survival was significant in favor of adjuvant gemcitabine (13.4 vs 6.9 months; $P<.001$).[14] After long-term analysis, patients in the gemcitabine arm were found to have modest benefit in overall survival as well, with a median overall survival of 22.8 months in the treatment group versus 20.2 months in the observation group ($P = .01$). The 5-year survival rate was reported as 20.7% in the treatment group versus 10.4% in the observation group ($P = .01$).[15] These results thus established gemcitabine as a standard treatment approach for the adjuvant management of pancreatic adenocarcinoma.

With the historical use of 5-FU as a standard adjuvant agent for pancreatic adeno-carcinoma, the objective of ESPAC (European Study Group for Pancreatic Cancer)-3 was to compare gemcitabine with 5-FU in a randomized trial. ESPAC-3 randomized 1088 patients with resected pancreatic cancer to adjuvant gemcitabine or 5-FU for a total of 6 months. This study demonstrated no difference in median overall survival (23.6 vs 23 months; $P = .39$) between gemcitabine and 5-FU. Although gemcitabine was not deemed superior, it is considered to be better tolerated. Gemcitabine did have significantly higher rates of grade 3 and 4 hematologic toxicity, but 5-FU had significantly higher rates of grade 3 and 4 stomatitis and diarrhea.[16] The ability of a patient to complete the entire course of adjuvant therapy also seems to be important. In an ad hoc analysis of the ESPAC-3 data evaluating whether timing or duration of chemotherapy after surgery influenced survival, patients who received chemotherapy within 8 weeks of surgery did not have a survival benefit over those who began therapy after 8 weeks and up to 12 weeks postoperatively. However, completion of all 6 cycles (24 weeks) was an independent prognostic factor, with a median overall survival in this subgroup of 28 months compared with only 14.6 months in patients completing 1 to 5 cycles (hazard ratio [HR], 0.516; $P<.001$).[17]

The finding of nonsuperiority for either gemcitabine or 5-FU was confirmed in RTOG (Radiation Therapy Oncology Group) 9704, where gemcitabine versus 5-FU as part of an adjuvant chemoradiation regimen were compared.[18] Although this study did include a radiation component, the question being studied was which chemothera-peutic backbone was more favorable. In this study, 451 patients with resected pancre-atic cancer were randomized to chemoradiation plus gemcitabine or chemoradiation plus 5-FU. Chemotherapy in both arms was given before and after chemoradiation, and chemotherapeutic radiosensitization with 5-FU was used during radiation in both arms of the study. Of note, the gemcitabine group had a significantly higher num-ber of T3 and T4 tumors than the 5-FU group (81% vs 70%; $P = .01$). As in ESPAC-3, there was no difference in median overall survival between the gemcitabine or 5-FU groups (20.5 vs 16.9 months; $P = .09$). Also similar to ESPAC-3, hematologic toxicities were more commonly seen in the gemcitabine arm. A summary of adjuvant chemo-therapy trials is presented in **Table 1**.

Adjuvant Chemoradiation

Based on promising studies in locally advanced disease, combined modality chemo-radiation has been evaluated in several randomized controlled trials as an alternative adjuvant option for resected pancreatic adenocarcinoma, however with competing results. The Gastrointestinal Study Group (GITSG) was the first to demonstrate a potential survival benefit in favor of adjuvant chemoradiation.[11] In this trial, 43 patients with pancreatic adenocarcinoma were randomized after curative resection to either chemoradiation or observation. In the treatment group, patients underwent a course of concurrent chemoradiation with weekly 5-FU. After a 2-week interval, this was repeated. 5-FU was then continued as maintenance weekly for 2 years or until

Table 1
Major adjuvant randomized trials

	Trial Type	N	Treatment Arms	Primary Endpoint	Result
GITSG[11]	Phase III	43	• ChemoRT with 5-FU • Observation	Median OS	20 vs 11 mo ($P = .03$)
EORTC[a,12]	Phase III	218	• ChemoRT with 5-FU • Observation	Median OS	24.5 vs 19 mo ($P = .2$)
ESPAC-1[19]	Phase III	289	• ChemoRT and chemotherapy • ChemoRT alone • Chemotherapy alone • Observation	Median OS	*Chemo vs no chemo:* 20.1 vs 15.5 mo ($P = .009$) *ChemoRT vs no chemoRT:* 15.9 vs 17.9 mo ($P = .05$)
CONKO-001[15]	Phase III	368	• Gemcitabine • Observation	DFS	13.4 vs 6.9 mo ($P<.001$)
RTOG 9704[18]	Phase III	451	• Gemcitabine before and after chemoRT • 5-FU before and after chemoRT	Median OS	20.5 vs 16.9 mo ($P = .09$)
ESPAC-3[a,16]	Phase III	1088	• Gemcitabine • 5-FU	Median OS	23.6 vs 23 mo ($P = .39$)
JASPAC[23]	Phase III	385	• S1 • Gemcitabine	2-year OS	70% vs 53% ($P<.0001$)

Abbreviations: 5-FU, 5-fluorouracil; ChemoRT, chemoradiation; CONKO, Charité Onkologie trial; DFS, disease-free survival; EORTC, European Organisation for Research and Treatment of Cancer; ESPAC, European Study Group for Pancreatic Cancer; GITSG, Gastrointestinal Tumor Study Group; JASPAC, Japan Adjuvant Study Group of Pancreatic Cancer[22]; OS, overall survival; RTOG, Radiation Therapy Oncology Group.
[a] Denotes studies including both pancreatic adenocarcinoma and ampullary cancers.
Data from Refs.[11,12,15,16,18,19,23]

recurrence. Median overall survival was 20 months in the treatment arm compared with 11 months in the observation arm ($P = .3$). Median disease-free survival was 11 versus 9 months, respectively ($P = .1$). The study was terminated prematurely owing to low accrual, and statistical conclusions could not be made; however, it did suggest an underlying survival benefit, which resulted in the use of adjuvant 5-FU and radiation therapy as a standard adjuvant therapy option.

A subsequent study conducted by the European Organization of Research and Treatment of Cancer (EORTC) reported results of a larger prospective trial that did not show survival benefit for the use of adjuvant chemoradiation.[12] This study randomized 218 patients with resectable head of the pancreas or periampullary adenocarcinoma postoperatively in a similar fashion as the GITSG study. The treatment arm consisted of radiation given over 2 weeks to a total of 40 Gy, in combination with 24-hour continuous 5-FU (given as a bolus in the GITSG study) given on the first day of radiation. This regimen was given again after a 2-week hiatus, and 5-FU was continued weekly for 2 years until recurrence. The control arm consisted of observation only. Median survival was 24.5 months in the treatment group compared with 19.0 months in the observation group ($P = .208$). When further stratified by tumor type, patients with pancreatic adenocarcinoma had a median survival of 17.1 months in the treatment arm compared with 12.6 months in the observation arm ($P = .099$). Of note, the sample size was too small to make a separate conclusion in this subset of patients. This study concluded that adjuvant chemoradiation did not confer a significant survival benefit over observation alone. When taken into consideration alongside results from the GITSG study, the role of chemoradiation in the adjuvant pancreatic cancer setting remains unclear. A summary of trials assessing adjuvant chemoradiation is included in **Table 1**.

Adjuvant Chemotherapy Versus Adjuvant Chemoradiation

Given the inconclusive data regarding the role for a component of chemoradiation in the adjuvant treatment setting, ESPAC sought to investigate this question in a large randomized controlled trial, ESPAC-1.[19] One of their reported aims was to evaluate whether chemoradiation or chemotherapy alone resulted in an improved survival benefit. A second objective was to determine if chemoradiation followed by chemotherapy (as in GITSG) improved survival. A total of 289 patients were randomized after surgery in a 2 × 2 design; 73 patients were assigned to chemoradiation alone, 75 to chemotherapy alone, 72 to chemoradiation followed by chemotherapy, and 69 to observation. The trial was not powered to compare these 4 groups directly. Survival estimates were based on 145 patients receiving chemoradiation (one-half of the patients also receiving chemotherapy) compared with 144 patients not receiving chemoradiation. Median survival was 15.9 months in patients receiving chemoradiation compared with 17.9 months in those not receiving chemoradiation ($P = .05$). Similarly, 147 patients received chemotherapy (one-half of them also receiving chemoradiation) and 142 patients did not receive chemotherapy. Median survival was 20.1 months in patients receiving chemotherapy compared with 15.5 months in those not receiving chemotherapy ($P = .009$). From these results, ESPAC-1 concluded that standard of care should consist of adjuvant chemotherapy, and that adjuvant chemoradiation could actually be detrimental to patient survival, even in patients receiving a component of chemotherapy alone. It should be noted, however, that in this trial the dose of radiation administered was well below the standard of care today—20 Gy in 10 fractions over a 2-week period in EPCAC-1 versus current standard of care consisting of 45 to 46 Gy in 1.8 to 2 Gy fractions over 5 weeks with a possible additional 5 to 9 Gy if clinically appropriate.[20] The fact that the chemoradiation arm was deemed detrimental may be secondary to patients receiving suboptimal radiation dosing in combination with an associated delay in administration of single agent chemotherapy.

To clarify the conflicting results of the major adjuvant trials to date, Stocken and colleagues[21] published a metaanalysis to evaluate the efficacy of adjuvant chemoradiation and chemotherapy, especially because some of the studies and subgroup analyses were inadequately powered. This metaanalysis reviewed the data from GITSG,[11] EORTC,[12] Bakkevold and colleagues,[8] Takada and colleagues,[9] and ESPAC-1.[19] Data from an additional group of patients in the ESPAC trial outside of the 2 × 2 factorial design were also included.[22] To evaluate the question of benefit from adjuvant chemoradiation, the trial data from EORTC and ESPAC-1 were reanalyzed. The HR indicated no reduction in the risk of death (HR, 1.09), and no difference in median survival (15.8 vs 15.2 months), 2-year survival (30% vs 34%) or 5-year survival (12% vs 17%) with or without chemoradiation, respectively. To evaluate the question of benefit from adjuvant chemotherapy, a pooled analysis of trial data from Bakkevold and colleagues, Takada and colleagues, and ESPAC-1 was conducted and reported an estimated HR of 0.75, indicating a 25% reduction in the risk of death with chemotherapy compared with no chemotherapy. Within subgroups, chemoradiation seemed to have a benefit in patients with positive resection margins, whereas chemotherapy seemed less beneficial in these situations; however, this was not powered to be statistically conclusive. The authors noted that their data were dominated by the ESPAC trial data, and came to the similar conclusion that adjuvant chemotherapy should be the standard of care for resected pancreatic cancer. Studies comparing chemotherapy and chemoradiation in the adjuvant pancreatic cancer setting are summarized in **Table 1**.

Ongoing Adjuvant Therapy Studies

With gemcitabine as the adjuvant standard, ongoing studies are evaluating gemcitabine in combination with additional agents. Two active trials, RTOG 0848 and CONKO-005, are evaluating the addition of erlotinib to gemcitabine in the adjuvant setting. Both of these studies draw on the approval of erlotinib, a tyrosine kinase inhibitor, that has a demonstrated survival benefit in advanced pancreatic cancer when given in combination with gemcitabine as compared with gemcitabine alone.[24] Combination adjuvant gemcitabine and metformin is also being evaluated. RTOG 0848 also hopes to further define the role of adjuvant chemoradiation. More recently, Nab-paclitaxel was found to have a survival benefit in combination with gemcitabine in advanced pancreatic cancers as compared with gemcitabine alone.[25] As such, the role for combination therapy with Nab-paclitaxel and gemcitabine in the adjuvant setting is being addressed in the APACT (Nab-paclitaxel and Gemcitabine vs Gemcitabine Alone as Adjuvant Therapy for Patients With Resected Pancreatic Cancer) trial, which has completed accrual but has pending results. Finally, the role for immunotherapy in pancreatic adenocarcinoma is also under intense investigation with studies assessing vaccine therapies, immune checkpoint inhibitors, and other immunotherapeutic agents. Combination therapy with low dose cyclophosphamide, GVAX (a vaccine composed of a granulocyte-macrophage colony-stimulating factor secreting pancreatic cancer cell line), gemcitabine, and chemoradiation (5-FU based) with or without nivolumab (an immune checkpoint inhibitor) is being assessed based on promising results demonstrated with GVAX in the metastatic pancreatic adenocarcinoma setting.[26] The largest completed immunotherapy study conducted in the adjuvant setting (with results still pending) was IMPRESS (Immunotherapy Study for Surgically Resected Pancreatic Cancer), which evaluated the role of algenpantucel-L, a vaccine composed of human pancreatic adenocarcinoma cell lines expressing a murine enzyme that is theorized to mount an immune response against cancer cells. This study was founded on results demonstrated in a phase II trial showing 1-year disease-free survival and 1-year overall survival rates of 62% and 86%, respectively.[27] In the pending phase III trial, patients received standard adjuvant therapy with gemcitabine alone or gemcitabine and 5-FU–based chemoradiation then were randomized to receive either vaccine or no vaccine. **Table 2** summarizes selected ongoing clinical trials in the adjuvant setting.

Neoadjuvant Management

More recently, the question of whether or not there may be a benefit from administration of neoadjuvant chemotherapy with or without neoadjuvant chemoradiation has been increasingly asked. This is likely owing to the fact that the large majority of patients undergoing what is an intended curative surgical resection develop disease recurrence in a relatively short period of time. As such, administration of neoadjuvant treatment may aid in identifying which patients are more likely to benefit from surgery and which patients may be spared undergoing an unnecessary surgery owing to the rapid development of metastatic disease. By virtue of their questionably resectable status, neoadjuvant therapy has been evaluated most extensively in patients with borderline resectable disease (see Jason W. Denbo and Jason B. Fleming

Table 2
Selected active adjuvant and neoadjuvant trials

Study	Type of Trial	N	Planned Enrollment Dates	Treatment Arms	Primary Endpoint
RTOG 0848 NCT01013649	Phase II/III	950	2009–2020	• Adjuvant gemcitabine for 5 cycles • Adjuvant gemcitabine + erlotinib hydrochloride for 5 cycles then Patients without disease progression are randomized again • One more cycle of previous regimen • One more cycle of previous regimen followed by chemoRT	OS
NEOPAC NCT01314027	Phase III	350	2009–2014	• Neoadjuvant gemcitabine/oxaliplatin + adjuvant gemcitabine • Adjuvant gemcitabine	PFS
NCT01526135	Phase III	490	2012–2018	• Adjuvant gemcitabine • Adjuvant mFOLFIRINOX	DFS
APACT NCT01964430	Phase III	846	2014–2020	• Adjuvant Nab-paclitaxel followed by gemcitabine • Adjuvant gemcitabine	DFS
NCT02172976	Phase II/III	126	2014–2019	• Neoadjuvant and adjuvant FOLFIRINOX • Adjuvant gemcitabine	OS
NEONAX NCT02047513	Phase II	166	2015–2019	• Neoadjuvant and adjuvant Nab-paclitaxel and gemcitabine • Adjuvant Nab-paclitaxel and gemcitabine	DFS
NCT02005419	Phase II	300	2013–2017	• Adjuvant gemcitabine • Adjuvant gemcitabine plus metformin	RFS
SWOG 1505 NCT02562716	Phase II	112	2015–2019	• Neoadjuvant and adjuvant mFOLFIRINOX • Neoadjuvant and adjuvant Nab-paclitaxel and gemcitabine	OS
NCT02451982	Phase I/II	50	2016–2020	• Neoadjuvant and adjuvant cyclophosphamide/GVAX, gemcitabine and radiation • Neoadjuvant and adjuvant cyclophosphamide/GVAX and nivolumab, gemcitabine and radiation	IL-17A expression in resected tumors
IMPRESS NCT01072981	Phase III	722	2010–2016	• Adjuvant gemcitabine with or without 5-FU chemoradiation • Adjuvant gemcitabine with or without 5-FU chemoradiation plus HyperAcute immunotherapy (Algenpantucel-L)	OS

Abbreviations: 5-FU, 5-fluorouracil; APACT, Nab-paclitaxel and Gemcitabine for Patients With Resected Pancreatic Cancer; chemoRT, chemoradiation; DFS, disease-free survival; ESPAC, European Study Group for Pancreatic Cancer; GVAX, a vaccine composed of a granulocyte-macrophage colony-stimulating factor secreting pancreatic cancer cell line; IMPRESS, Immunotherapy Study for Surgically Resected Pancreatic Cancer; mFOLFIRINOX, modified 5-fluorouracil irinotecan and oxaliplatin; NEONAX, Neoadjuvant Plus Adjuvant or Only Adjuvant Nab- Paclitaxel Plus Gemcitabine for Resectable Pancreatic Cancer; NEOPAC, Adjuvant Versus Neoadjuvant Plus Adjuvant Chemotherapy in Resectable Pancreatic Cancer; OS, overall survival; PFS, progression free survival; RFS, recurrence free survival; RTOG, Radiation Therapy Oncology Group; SWOG, Southwest Oncology Group.

article, "Definition and Management of Borderline Resectable Pancreatic Cancer", in this issue). This is in an effort to both convert these patients to a resectable status and to identify patients who are unlikely to be surgical candidates. For this patient population, despite the lack of category 1 evidence, it is the current recommendation of the National Comprehensive Cancer Center[20] Pancreatic Adenocarcinoma Clinical Practice Guidelines in Oncology panel that this patient population receive neoadjuvant treatment with either of the 2 most standardly used metastatic regimens—FOLFIRINOX (folinic acid, 5-FU, irinotecan, and oxaliplatin) or gemcitabine and abraxane.[28] This further begs the question as to whether these same regimens should be used in a resectable patient population. In a retrospective review of 69 patients with resectable pancreatic adenocarcinoma who received neoadjuvant treatment (chemotherapy, radiation, or both) followed by surgical resection, 60 of the initial 69 patients were able to undergo surgical resection and achieved a median overall survival of 44.9 months; the median overall survival for all 69 patients was 32 months.[29] This reported median overall survival is superior to what has been reported previously for stage IA and IIB pancreatic cancer patients, which ranges from 12.7 to 24.1 months.[30] In light of this, active neoadjuvant trials are evaluating similar regimens to those being investigated in the adjuvant setting. NEOPAC (Adjuvant Versus Neoadjuvant Plus Adjuvant Chemotherapy in Resectable Pancreatic Cancer) is studying neoadjuvant gemcitabine and oxaliplatin plus adjuvant gemcitabine in comparison with adjuvant gemcitabine alone. Neoadjuvant plus adjuvant Nab-paclitaxel and gemcitabine will be compared with adjuvant only Nab-paclitaxel and gemcitabine in the NEONAX (Neoadjuvant Plus Adjuvant or Only Adjuvant Nab- Paclitaxel Plus Gemcitabine for Resectable Pancreatic Cancer) trial. Neoadjuvant plus adjuvant FOLFIRINOX is being compared with current standard adjuvant gemcitabine. Finally, SWOG 1505 is comparing neoadjuvant plus adjuvant FOLFIRINOX with neoadjuvant plus adjuvant Nab-paclitaxel and gemcitabine. Full trial details of ongoing neoadjuvant trials are summarized in **Table 2**.

Surveillance

There is not good evidence for surveillance after the completion of adjuvant therapy. Given the high incidence of relapse and poor prognosis, the National Comprehensive Cancer Network panel recommends symptom assessment, CA 19-9, and computed tomography scans every 3 to 6 months for the first 2 years, then annually.[20] However, the data do not show that routine surveillance computed tomography scans offers any survival benefit.[31]

PERIAMPULLARY CARCINOMA
Epidemiology and Histologic Classification

Periampullary carcinomas comprise a rare and heterogeneous group, making them challenging to evaluate for effective therapy. Any neoplasm in the vicinity of the ampulla of Vater is considered periampullary, and can arise from pancreatic, duodenal, biliary, or ampullary epithelia. Pancreatic cancers account for the majority of periampullary cancers, which has resulted in many of the treatment recommendations for these tumors arising from the pancreatic cancer trials. From a series of 242 resected periampullary cancers from Johns Hopkins, 62% were pancreatic, 19% were ampullary, 12% arose from the distal bile duct, and 7% were duodenal.[32] True ampullary cancers have an incidence of 4 to 6 cases per million and account for 0.2% of all gastrointestinal cancers.[33,34] Ampullary cancers themselves have 2 distinct histologic subtypes—pancreaticobiliary and nonpancreaticobiliary (also known as intestinal). The distinction among the subtypes comprising periampullary carcinomas carries prognostic significance with implications for different therapeutic strategies.

Survival and Prognostic Factors

Patients with periampullary cancers have a better prognosis compared with those with pancreatic cancer. Among the periampullary cancers, tumor origin carries prognostic significance, with pancreatic cancers not surprisingly conferring the poorest outcomes.[35,36] From a Johns Hopkins series of 890 periampullary patients with long-term follow-up, the 5-year survival of the entire cohort was 23%. Duodenal cancers carried the best prognosis with a 5-year survival rate of 51% (n = 47). True ampullary cancers had the next best 5-year survival rate of 37% (n = 135), followed by distal bile duct cancers at 23% (n = 144), and pancreatic cancers at 17% (n = 564).[37]

Similarly, among the true ampullary cancers, the pancreaticobiliary histologic subtype confers a worse prognosis than the intestinal subtype. In retrospective studies, histologic subtypes were found to be independent predictors of survival.[38,39] Chang and colleagues[40] further delineated these subtypes with histopathologic and molecular criteria, using immunostains for MUC1 to identify pancreaticobiliary cancers, and CDX2 to identify nonpancreaticobiliary cancers. Using this stratification, the pancreaticobiliary histomolecular phenotype was found to be an independent adverse prognostic variable compared with the intestinal histomolecular phenotype (median survival, 16 vs 115 months; $P<.001$). Despite these findings, tumor histology is still not used as a standard to drive treatment decisions.

Other factors predicting survival and outcomes after resection of periampullary cancers include nodal metastases as well as neural and lymphovascular invasion.[41] Negative margins and tumor size do not seem to be independent prognostic variables. Predictive factors did, however, vary among cancers of different tumor origins. Prognostically, this has clinical implications for more tailored therapeutic strategies based on the stratification of periampullary cancers into types of tumor origin and histologic phenotype; however, this is not included as part of any treatment guideline.

Adjuvant Therapy

Owing to the rarity of periampullary cancers, current standards of adjuvant therapy are based on retrospective studies and subgroup analyses of larger prospective studies that included both pancreatic cancer and periampullary cancers. As a result, adjuvant chemoradiation and/or chemotherapy alone have not been shown definitively to provide significant survival benefit in this specific group of patients. The use of chemoradiation is largely extrapolated from the adjuvant pancreatic trials.[8,12] After the EORTC group published its prospective study on chemoradiation with 5-FU in pancreatic and periampullary cancers,[12] several groups retrospectively examined the efficacy of similar chemoradiation regimens in ampullary cancers. Bhatia and colleagues[42] published one of the largest series from the Mayo Clinic, suggesting a benefit for chemoradiation in high-risk patients, defined as locally advanced T3 and T4 disease, positive lymph nodes, or high-grade tumor. There was no difference in median overall survival between patients receiving adjuvant chemoradiation (n = 29) and those being observed (n = 96; 5.6 vs 3.5 years; $P = .64$). The presence of positive lymph nodes, however, was found to be a negative prognostic factor, and adjuvant chemoradiation was found to confer a survival benefit in this subgroup (median overall survival of 3.4 years in the chemoradiation group vs 1.6 years in the observation group; $P = .01$). Despite these findings, this study is inconclusive because it is limited by its retrospective nature and small number of patients in each of the subgroups.

Table 3
Periampullary trials

Author	Type of Trial	Types of Cancer	N	Treatment Arms	Results
Klinkenbijl et al,[12] 1999 EORTC	Prospective Phase III	Pancreas, periampullary	93	• ChemoRT with 5-FU • Observation	No difference in median OS (P = .208)
Chakravarthy et al,[50] 2000	Prospective Phase II	Pancreas, periampullary	16	ChemoRT with 5-FU /DPM/MMC[a]	Trend toward survival benefit
Lee et al,[43] 2000	Retrospective	Ampullary	39	• ChemoRT with 5-FU • Observation	No difference in 3-y OS rate (P = .132), suggestive of benefit in high-risk patients (P = .032)
Sikora et al,[44] 2005	Retrospective	Ampullary	113	• ChemoRT with 5-FU • Observation	No difference in median survival (P = .3)
Bhatia et al,[42] 2006	Retrospective	Ampullary	125	• ChemoRT with 5-FU • Observation	No difference in median OS (P = .64), suggestive of benefit in patients with positive LNs (P = .01)
Krishnan et al,[45] 2008	Retrospective	Ampullary	96	• ChemoRT with 5-FU or capecitabine • Observation	No difference in 5-y OS rate (P = .53), trend toward benefit in T3/T4 tumors (P = .06)
Kim et al,[46] 2009	Retrospective	Ampullary	118	• ChemoRT with 5-FU • Observation	No difference in 5-y OS rate (P = .22)
Zhou et al,[47] 2009	Retrospective	Ampullary	111	• ChemoRT with 5-FU or capecitabine • Observation	No difference in median OS (P = .969)
Palta et al,[48] 2012	Retrospective	Ampullary	137	• ChemoRT • Observation	No difference in median OS (P = .074)
Neoptolemos et al,[49] 2012 ESPAC-3	Prospective Phase III	Periampullary	434	• 5-FU • Gemcitabine • Observation	No difference in median OS (P = .25) between chemotherapy groups and observation; statistically significant benefit after adjusting for prognostic variables (P = .03)

Abbreviations: 5-FU, 5-fluoracil; DPM, dipyridamole; EORTC, European Organization of Research and Treatment of Cancer; ESPAC, European Study Group for Pancreatic Cancer; LNs, lymph nodes; MMC, mitomycin C; OS, overall survival.

[a] As compared with historical control.

Data from Refs.[12,42–50]

Several other retrospective studies were similarly inconclusive in regard to a survival benefit derived from adjuvant chemoradiation in periampullary cancers.[43–48]

The data on adjuvant chemotherapy in periampullary cancers are also mixed. The largest prospective trial to date, ESPAC-3, compared adjuvant gemcitabine versus 5-FU versus observation in 434 patients after surgical resection.[49] Investigators found there was no difference in overall survival between chemotherapy and observation. Only after the data were adjusted for prognostic variables including age, bile duct cancer, poor tumor differentiation, and positive lymph nodes, was there a survival benefit in favor of chemotherapy (as compared with observation; HR, 0.75; $P = .03$). Subgroup analysis was only hypothesis generating given the small number of patients in each subset. Interestingly, the authors distinguished only between ampullary and bile duct tumor origins, with 35 remaining patients described as "other." They also noted no significant survival benefit of chemotherapy when ampullary cancers were further stratified to pancreaticobiliary and intestinal subtypes; however, the number of patients in these subgroups was very small. **Table 3** provides a summary of prospective and retrospective studies assessing chemotherapy and/or chemoradiation in periampullary cancers.

Given the data from the pancreatic trials, and the added toxicity of radiation without proven benefit, the standard of care for periampullary cancers remains adjuvant chemotherapy. The difficulty in achieving survival benefit with adjuvant regimens is likely owing to their underlying histologic heterogeneity. There are no data to guide therapy based on histologic subtype (intestinal type vs pancreaticobiliary type). However, given the activity of 5-FU in the management of both pancreatic adenocarcinoma as well as intestinal cancers, it may be reasonable to use a fluoropyrimidine-based regimen for tumors with an intestinal histology and a gemcitabine-based regimen for tumors with a pancreaticobiliary histology. Therapy for this malignancy should be discussed in a multidisciplinary setting.

SUMMARY

- The rationale for adjuvant therapy in resectable pancreatic cancer is based on high local and systemic recurrence rates and poor overall survival despite curative-intent surgical resection.
- Data regarding the role of adjuvant chemoradiation in resectable disease are conflicting.
- Adjuvant chemotherapy results in a survival benefit after surgical resection with the current standard being administration of adjuvant gemcitabine for 6 cycles (months), beginning up to 12 weeks after surgery.
- Ongoing studies are evaluating new adjuvant regimens, as well as the role for neoadjuvant therapy for resectable disease.
- There are no convincing data for surveillance after resection; however, current guidelines suggest measurement of the CA 19-9 tumor marker every 3 to 6 months for the first 2 years, then annually for up to 5 years. Computed tomography imaging may also be included, but there is no definitive recommendation.
- Periampullary cancers are a rare and heterogeneous group of tumors in terms of site of origin and histologic subtype with an overall better survival rate compared with pancreatic adenocarcinomas; however, the pancreaticobiliary histology among these cancers carries the worst prognosis.
- Data for adjuvant therapy, and hence current treatment standards, for periampullary cancers are derived from subgroup analyses within prospective trials for pancreatic cancer

REFERENCES

1. Siegel RL, Miller KD, Jemal A. Cancer statistics, 2015. CA Cancer J Clin 2015;65:5–29.
2. Trede M, Schwall G, Saeger HD. Survival after pancreaticoduodenectomy. Ann Surg 1990;211:447–58.
3. Cameron JL, Crist DW, Sitzmann JV. Factors influencing survival after pancreaticoduodenectomy for pancreatic cancer. Am J Surg 1991;161:120–5.
4. Geer RJ, Brennan MF. Prognostic indicators for survival after resection of pancreatic adenocarcinoma. Am J Surg 1993;165:68–73.
5. Nitecki SS, Sarr MG, Colby TV, et al. Long-term survival after resection for ductal adenocarcinoma of the pancreas. Is it really improving? Ann Surg 1995;221: 59–66.
6. Sperti C, Pasquali C, Piccoli A, et al. Survival after resection for ductal adenocarcinoma of the pancreas. Br J Surg 1996;83:625–31.
7. Al-Hawary MM, Francis IR, Chari ST, et al. Pancreatic ductal adenocarcinoma radiology reporting template: consensus statement of the Society of Abdominal Radiology and the American Pancreatic Association. Radiology 2014;270: 248–60.
8. Bakkevold KE, Arnesjø B, Dahl O, et al. Adjuvant combination chemotherapy (AMF) following radical resection of carcinoma of the pancreas and papilla of Vater—results of a controlled, prospective, randomised multicentre study. Eur J Cancer 1993;29:698–703.
9. Takada T, Amano H, Yasuda H, et al. Is postoperative adjuvant chemotherapy useful for gallbladder carcinoma? Cancer 2002;95:1685–95.
10. Van Rijswijk RE, Jeziorski K, Wagener DT, et al. Weekly high-dose 5-fluorouracil and folinic acid in metastatic pancreatic carcinoma: a phase II study of the EORTC GastroIntestinal Tract Cancer Cooperative Group. Eur J Cancer 2004; 40:2077–81.
11. Kalser MH, Ellenberg SS. Pancreatic cancer: adjuvant combined radiation and chemotherapy following curative resection. Arch Surg 1985;120:899–903.
12. Klinkenbijl JH, Jeekel J, Sahmoud T, et al. Adjuvant radiotherapy and 5-fluorouracil after curative resection of cancer of the pancreas and periampullary region: phase III trial of the EORTC gastrointestinal tract cancer cooperative group. Ann Surg 1999;230:776–82 [discussion: 782–4].
13. Burris HA, Moore MJ, Andersen J, et al. Improvements in survival and clinical benefit with gemcitabine as first-line therapy for patients with advanced pancreas cancer: a randomized trial. J Clin Oncol 1997;15:2403–13.
14. Oettle H, Post S, Neuhaus P, et al. Adjuvant chemotherapy with gemcitabine vs observation in patients undergoing curative-intent resection of pancreatic cancer: a randomized controlled trial. JAMA 2007;297:267–77.
15. Oettle H, Neuhaus P, Hochhaus A, et al. Adjuvant chemotherapy with gemcitabine and long-term outcomes among patients with resected pancreatic cancer: the CONKO-001 randomized trial. JAMA 2013;310:1473–81.
16. Neoptolemos JP, Stocken DD, Bassi C, et al. Adjuvant chemotherapy with fluorouracil plus folinic acid vs gemcitabine following pancreatic cancer resection: a randomized controlled trial. JAMA 2010;304:1073–81.
17. Valle JW, Palmer D, Jackson R, et al. Optimal duration and timing of adjuvant chemotherapy after definitive surgery for ductal adenocarcinoma of the pancreas: ongoing lessons from the ESPAC-3 study. J Clin Oncol 2014;32:504–12.
18. Regine WF, Winter KA, Abrams RA, et al. Fluorouracil vs gemcitabine chemotherapy before and after fluorouracil-based chemoradiation following resection

of pancreatic adenocarcinoma: a randomized controlled trial. JAMA 2008;299: 1019–26.

19. Neoptolemos JP, Stocken DD, Friess H, et al. A randomized trial of chemoradiotherapy and chemotherapy after resection of pancreatic cancer. N Engl J Med 2004;350:1200–10.

20. National Comprehensive Cancer Network (NCCN). NCCN clinical practice guidelines in oncology. Pancreatic Cancer Version 2.2015. National Comprehensive Cancer Network. Available at: http://www.nccn.org/professionals/physician_gls/pdf/pancreatic.pdf. Accessed April 2, 2016.

21. Stocken D, Büchler M, Dervenis C, et al. Meta-analysis of randomised adjuvant therapy trials for pancreatic cancer. Br J Cancer 2005;92:1372–81.

22. Neoptolemos J, Dunn J, Stocken D, et al. Adjuvant chemoradiotherapy and chemotherapy in resectable pancreatic cancer: a randomised controlled trial. Lancet 2001;358:1576–85.

23. Uesaka K, Boku N, Fukutomi A, et al. Adjuvant chemotherapy of S-1 versus gemcitabine for resected pancreatic cancer: a phase 3, open-label, randomized, non-inferiority trial (JASPAC 01). Lancet 2016;388:248–57.

24. Moore MJ, Goldstein D, Hamm J, et al. Erlotinib plus gemcitabine compared with gemcitabine alone in patients with advanced pancreatic cancer: a phase III trial of the National Cancer Institute of Canada Clinical Trials Group. J Clin Oncol 2007;25:1960–6.

25. Von Hoff DD, Ervin T, Arena FP, et al. Increased survival in pancreatic cancer with nab-paclitaxel plus gemcitabine. N Engl J Med 2013;369:1691–703.

26. Le D, Wang-Gillam A, Picozzi V, et al. Safety and survival with GVAX pancreas prime and Listeria Monocytogenes-expressing mesothelin (CRS-207) boost vaccines for metastatic pancreatic cancer. J Clin Oncol 2015;33:1325–33.

27. Hardacre JM, Mulcahy M, Small W, et al. Addition of algenpantucel-L immunotherapy to standard adjuvant therapy for pancreatic cancer: a phase 2 study. J Gastrointest Surg 2013;17:94–100.

28. Conroy T, Desseigne F, Ychou M, et al. FOLFIRINOX versus gemcitabine for metastatic pancreatic cancer. N Engl J Med 2011;364:1817–25.

29. Christians KK, Heimler JW, George B, et al. Survival of patients with resectable pancreatic cancer who received neoadjuvant therapy. Surgery 2016;159: 893–900.

30. Compton CC, Byrd DR, Garcia-Aguilar J, et al. American joint committee on cancer (AJCC) Cancer staging manual. 7th edition. New York: Springer; 2010.

31. Witkowski ER, Smith JK, Ragulin-Coyne E, et al. Is it worth looking? Abdominal imaging after pancreatic cancer resection: a national study. J Gastrointest Surg 2012;16:121–8.

32. Yeo CJ, Sohn TA, Cameron JL, et al. Periampullary adenocarcinoma: analysis of 5-year survivors. Ann Surg 1998;227:821–31.

33. Goodman M, Yamamoto J. Descriptive study of gallbladder, extrahepatic bile duct, and ampullary cancers in the United States, 1997-2002. Cancer Causes Control 2007;18:415–22.

34. Albores-Saavedra J, Schwartz AM, Batich K, et al. Cancers of the ampulla of Vater: demographics, morphology, and survival based on 5,625 cases from the SEER program. J Surg Oncol 2009;100:598–605.

35. Yeo CJ, Cameron JL, Sohn TA, et al. Six hundred fifty consecutive pancreaticoduodenectomies in the 1990s: pathology, complications, and outcomes. Ann Surg 1997;226:248–57.

36. Talamini MA, Moesinger RC, Pitt HA, et al. Adenocarcinoma of the ampulla of Vater. A 28-year experience. Ann Surg 1997;225:590–9 [discussion: 599–600].
37. Riall TS, Cameron JL, Lillemoe KD, et al. Resected periampullary adenocarcinoma: 5-year survivors and their 6-to 10-year follow-up. Surgery 2006;140: 764–72.
38. Carter JT, Grenert JP, Rubenstein L, et al. Tumors of the ampulla of Vater: histopathologic classification and predictors of survival. J Am Coll Surg 2008;207: 210–8.
39. Westgaard A, Tafjord S, Farstad IN, et al. Pancreaticobiliary versus intestinal histologic type of differentiation is an independent prognostic factor in resected periampullary adenocarcinoma. BMC Cancer 2008;8:1.
40. Chang DK, Jamieson NB, Johns AL, et al. Histomolecular phenotypes and outcome in adenocarcinoma of the ampulla of Vater. J Clin Oncol 2013;31: 1348–56.
41. Hatzaras I, George N, Muscarella P, et al. Predictors of survival in periampullary cancers following pancreaticoduodenectomy. Ann Surg Oncol 2010;17:991–7.
42. Bhatia S, Miller RC, Haddock MG, et al. Adjuvant therapy for ampullary carcinomas: the Mayo Clinic experience. Int J Radiat Oncol Biol Phys 2006;66:514–9.
43. Lee JH, Whittington R, Williams NN, et al. Outcome of pancreaticoduodenectomy and impact of adjuvant therapy for ampullary carcinomas. Int J Radiat Oncol Biol Phys 2000;47:945–53.
44. Sikora SS, Balachandran P, Dimri K, et al. Adjuvant chemo-radiotherapy in ampullary cancers. Eur J Surg Oncol 2005;31:158–63.
45. Krishnan S, Rana V, Evans DB, et al. Role of adjuvant chemoradiation therapy in adenocarcinomas of the ampulla of Vater. Int J Radiat Oncol Biol Phys 2008;70: 735–43.
46. Kim K, Chie EK, Jang JY, et al. Role of adjuvant chemoradiotherapy for ampulla of Vater cancer. Int J Radiat Oncol Biol Phys 2009;75:436–41.
47. Zhou J, Hsu CC, Winter JM, et al. Adjuvant chemoradiation versus surgery alone for adenocarcinoma of the ampulla of Vater. Radiother Oncol 2009;92:244–8.
48. Palta M, Patel P, Broadwater G, et al. Carcinoma of the ampulla of Vater: patterns of failure following resection and benefit of chemoradiotherapy. Ann Surg Oncol 2012;19:1535–40.
49. Neoptolemos JP, Moore MJ, Cox TF, et al. Effect of adjuvant chemotherapy with fluorouracil plus folinic acid or gemcitabine vs observation on survival in patients with resected periampullary adenocarcinoma: the ESPAC-3 periampullary cancer randomized trial. JAMA 2012;308:147–56.
50. Chakravarthy A, Abrams RA, Yeo CJ, et al. Intensified adjuvant combined modality therapy for resected periampullary adenocarcinoma: acceptable toxicity and suggestion of improved 1-year disease-free survival. Int J Radiat Oncol Biol Phys 2000;48:1089–96.

Enhanced Recovery Pathways in Pancreatic Surgery

Joshua G. Barton, MD

KEYWORDS

- Enhanced recovery after surgery • ERAS • Fast-track • Pancreatoduodenectomy
- Distal pancreatectomy

KEY POINTS

- Enhanced recovery after surgery (ERAS) protocols, or fast-track pathways, use evidence-based medicine to improve recovery from surgery via institutional guidelines, nursing protocols, and order templates.
- ERAS protocols address factors in preoperative, intraoperative, and postoperative settings.
- ERAS protocols in pancreatic surgery focus on early mobilization, early oral intake, neutral fluid balance, optimal analgesia, drain management, and antibiotic selection.

INTRODUCTION

Mortality following pancreatic surgery, particularly pancreatoduodenectomy (PD), has improved dramatically over the past 4 decades. Mortality in the 1970s was as high as 25% and is now commonly lower than 2% in high-volume centers.[1] Morbidity, however, often remains in excess of 40%, despite advances in surgical technique, anesthesia, preoperative imaging, and antimicrobials. In fact, the complications most particular to pancreatic surgery, postoperative pancreatic fistula (POPF) and delayed gastric emptying (DGE), have not improved.[1]

Enhanced recovery after surgery (ERAS), or fast-track protocols, were first introduced in the 1990s to help recovery following colorectal surgery.[2] The purpose of such pathways is to use evidence-based medicine in a multidisciplinary fashion to optimize recovery from surgery and potentially decrease postoperative pain, improve complications, and shorten hospital stay. Enhanced recovery protocols focus on the entire range of surgical care, including preoperative assessment, intraoperative technique, postoperative care, and outpatient follow-up. There is significant evidence

No disclosures.

Center for Pancreatic and Liver Diseases, St. Luke's Mountain States Tumor Institute, 100 E Idaho St, STE 301, Boise, ID 83712, USA

E-mail address: bartonjo@slhs.org

http://dx.doi.org/10.1016/j.suc.2016.07.003
surgical.theclinics.com

supporting the utility of enhanced recovery protocols following colorectal surgery with few dissenting studies.[3] Studies have shown earlier resolution of postoperative ileus, shorter hospital stay, and fewer complications.[4,5] ERAS protocols have since been studied in a variety of other general surgery specialties and even orthopedics with similarly promising results.[6–9]

STUDIES ON ENHANCED RECOVERY AFTER SURGERY PROTOCOLS IN PANCREATIC SURGERY

Enhanced recovery protocols following pancreatic surgery have been studied since the early 2000s.[10–20] Each study, however, used different institutional-based protocols, which makes comparisons difficult. Furthermore, not all studies share the details of the protocol used. To address the difficulty of comparing studies and implementing protocols in institutions interested in ERAS, the ERAS Society, European Society for Clinical Nutrition and Metabolism (ESPEN), and the International Association for Surgical Metabolism (IASMEN) recently published a framework to guide future ERAS programs and studies in pancreatic surgery based on best-practices and clinical evidence.[21]

None of the available studies on ERAS in pancreatic surgery contain high levels of evidence.[22] Studies covering ERAS protocols are limited to retrospective case series or comparative case-control studies using historical controls. No completely prospective, randomized studies have been published. Despite the limited strengths of studies covering ERAS protocols in pancreatic surgery, several important findings have been made. Of 8 studies assessing length of stay (LOS), 7 found that their ERAS protocols decreased LOS by 6 to 10 days with no increase in readmission rates.[10,11,13–15,17,18,20] All the studies found that their protocols were safe with none finding an increase in morbidity or mortality. Only 1 study found a reduction in morbidity from 59% to 47% and was the largest study to date.[10] Two of 4 studies assessing hospital costs found a reduction when using ERAS protocols[11,14,15,18] (**Table 1**).

Table 1
Enhanced recovery after surgery (ERAS) protocols in pancreatic surgery

Authors, Year of Publication	Length of Stay, Days		Readmissions Rate n (%)		Morbidity, n (%)	
	Control	ERAS	Control	ERAS	Control	ERAS
Porter et al,[18] 2000	15	12[a]	10 (15)	9 (11)	20 (29)	24 (30)
Vanounou et al,[11] 2007	8	8	4 (6)	13 (9)	40 (62)	77 (54)
Kennedy et al,[15] 2007	13	7[a]	3 (7)	7 (8)	19 (44)	34 (37)
Berberat et al,[16] 2007	—	10	—	9 (4)	—	105 (41)
Balzano et al,[10] 2008	15	13[a]	16 (6)	18 (7)	148 (59)	119 (47)[a]
Kennedy et al,[14] 2009	10	7[a]	10 (25)	5 (7)[a]	15 (38)	11 (16)
di Sebastiano et al,[12] 2011	—	10	—	9 (6)	—	56 (39)
Robertson et al,[19] 2012	—	10	—	2 (4)	—	23 (46)
Nikfarjam et al,[17] 2013	14	8[a]	0 (0)	3 (15)	—	—
Abu Hilal et al,[13] 2013	13	8[a]	2 (10)	1 (4)	16 (67)	8 (40)
Coolsen et al,[20] 2014	20	14[a]	14 (14)	11 (12.8)	19 (20)	29 (34)

[a] Significant difference: $P > .05$.
Data from Refs.[10–20]

There are several systematic reviews covering ERAS protocols in pancreatic surgery and 1 meta-analysis.[23–27] The meta-analysis by Coolsen and colleagues[24] included 8 studies that met final inclusion criteria with a total of 1558 patients. Despite no overwhelming evidence within the individual studies reviewed, Coolsen and colleagues[24] found a significant risk reduction in postoperative complications by 8.2% with no increase in mortality or readmission rates when the data were assessed from a meta-analysis perspective.

FACETS OF ENHANCED RECOVERY AFTER SURGERY PROTOCOLS IN PANCREATIC SURGERY

ERAS protocols cover a variety of preoperative, intraoperative, and postoperative factors that are implemented through a variety of institutional guidelines, nursing protocols, and order templates (**Box 1**). Some facets within ERAS protocols include measures commonly accepted or previously controlled by governing bodies.[28] These facets include the following:

1. Preoperative hair removal
2. Venous thromboembolism prophylaxis
3. Neutral fluid balance
4. Early mobilization
5. Normothermia

Other facets of ERAS protocols in pancreatic surgery are not commonly accepted or controlled by governing bodies. These facets are detailed in the following sections.

Perioperative Antibiotics

The Centers for Medicare and Medicaid Services and the Centers for Disease Control and Prevention implemented the Surgical Infection Prevention Project and Surgical Care Improvement Project (SCIP) to decrease the morbidity and mortality associated

---

Box 1
Facets of enhanced recovery after surgery (ERAS) protocols

1. Preoperative
   a. Preoperative counseling (operation expectations, smoking cessation, alcohol consumption, nutrition optimization, mobility)
   b. Biliary drainage
   c. Mechanical bowel preparation
   d. Deep venous thrombosis prophylaxis
   e. Preoperative carbohydrate loading

2. Intraoperative
   a. Perioperative antibiotics
   b. Hypothermia management
   c. Pain management
   d. Fluid management

3. Postoperative
   a. Nutrition management
   b. Nasogastric tube management
   c. Urinary catheter management
   d. Pain management
   e. Medication management (somatostatin analogues)
   f. Drain management

with surgical site infections (SSI) in 2003.[29,30] SCIP measures addressing SSIs include the following:

1. Administration of antibiotics within 1 hour of incision time
2. Selection of appropriate antibiotic therapy
3. Discontinuation of antibiotics within 24 hours of surgery end time

SCIP measures do not specifically address antibiotic selection for pancreatic operations. For patients who are not allergic to penicillin, SCIP measures recommend cefotetan, cefoxitin, ampicillin-sulbactam, ertapenem, or cefazolin/cefuroxime with metronidazole for colonic surgery.[31] SCIP antibiotic selection for colonic surgery is often used in pancreatic surgery. Interestingly, guidelines published by the American Society of Health-System Pharmacists (ASHP), the Infectious Disease Society of America, the Surgical Infection Society, and the Society for Healthcare Epidemiology of America specify antibiotic selection for pancreatoduodenectomy, and this recommendation is limited to cefazolin.[32]

Several studies have found that antibiotics recommended by SCIP and ASHP do not address SSI concerns in pancreatic surgery adequately.[33–35] This is likely due to the prevalence of *Enterococcus* and *Enterobacter* species in SSIs following pancreatic operations. As such, piperacillin-tazobactam is considered a more appropriate choice for antibiotic prophylaxis in pancreatic surgery, particularly pancreatoduodenectomy[34] in patients who have had preoperative biliary stenting.

Preoperative Biliary Drainage

Obstructive jaundice is the most common presenting symptom of peri-ampullary carcinomas. Preoperative biliary drainage (PBD) is commonly done in the setting of obstructive jaundice to alleviate symptoms and prevent complications, namely vitamin K–associated coagulopathy. Several studies have supported the role of PBD and have indicated it is associated with a decrease in morbidity and mortality.[36–38] Other studies, including 2 meta-analyses, however, failed to show positive or negative effects of PBD.[39–41] In fact, a multicenter, randomized trial comparing routine plastic endoscopic biliary stenting with surgery alone showed that routine PBD increases the rate of complications following PD.[42] A follow-up study on that trial assessing fully covered self-expanding metal stents (FCSEMS) reaffirmed that surgery alone was associated with fewer complications, but indicated that FCSEMS were superior to plastic stents with regard to stent-related complications (but not surgery-related complications).[43] The preponderance of evidence indicates that PBD should be done only when surgery cannot be scheduled within a reasonable time frame (eg, neoadjuvant therapy) or if prolonged prothrombin time indicates that there is a risk of vitamin K–deficient coagulopathy.[44]

Oral Bowel Preparation

Historically, oral bowel preparation was used in a vast majority of gastrointestinal operations, not only as means of decreasing intracolonic bacterial counts and, hence, decreasing SSIs, but also to aid in the manipulation of bowel and conducting operations in general.[45] The negative physiologic effect of bowel preparation is not insignificant.[46] Dehydration associated with oral bowel preparation can lead to adverse effects, particularly in the elderly. Multiple clinical and animal studies fail to reveal any benefit of oral bowel preparations in colon surgery.[47,48] As a result, current recommendations by the ERAS Society recommend against oral bowel preparation for colon operations.[49]

Oral bowel preparation in pancreatic surgery has not been well studied. Retrospective studies have not found a benefit with oral bowel preparation in pancreatic surgery.[50] Therefore, oral bowel preparation is not recommended in pancreatic surgery.

Intra-Abdominal Drainage

Intra-abdominal drainage following pancreatic surgery has been an intensely debated and studied topic. In 2001, a single-institution randomized trial indicated that intra-abdominal drainage failed to reduce the morbidity and mortality following PD. Additionally, this study indicated that patients with drains were more likely to develop intra-abdominal abscesses and various fistulae, including POPF.[51] Subsequent studies, including meta-analyses, supported the findings that intra-abdominal drainage following pancreatic surgery may not offer any benefit and might increase complications, particularly in patients undergoing PD.[52–54]

In 2005, the International Study Group on Pancreatic Fistula (ISGPF) proposed a unifying definition of POPF.[55] Using a modern definition of POPF, a recent multicenter, randomized trial found that the elimination of drainage in PD was associated with a fourfold increase in mortality.[56] The findings were so profound that the trial was stopped early despite the study group hypothesizing that routine intra-abdominal drainage was unnecessary. Additionally, 2 prospective randomized trials found that early drain removal was not only safe, but actually improved postoperative morbidity, even when they were removed aggressively. Accordingly, intra-abdominal drains are recommended following pancreatic surgery with early removal on postoperative day 3 when the drain amylase content is less than 3 times the normal serum amylase (ISGPF definition of POPF).[57,58]

Preoperative Fasting and Carbohydrate Loading

Current guidelines from the American Academy of Anesthesiologists recommend the cessation of liquids and solids 2 and 6 hours before the induction of anesthesia, respectively. Although the ingestion of a carbohydrate-rich liquid approximately 2 hours before the induction of anesthesia may not result in decreased postoperative morbidity, it does decrease patient discomfort, and it may improve insulin sensitivity and skeletal muscle preservation without increasing aspiration or complications. Because it may offer some benefit and does not violate the recommended fasting guidelines, the ingestion of a carbohydrate liquid 2 hours before induction of anesthesia is recommended before pancreatic surgery.[59–61]

Gastric Decompression

Gastric decompression via nasogastric (NG) intubation is likely one of the more dogmatically adhered to principles in gastrointestinal surgery with little substantive evidence supporting its usage. Although NG tubes are commonly thought to prevent pulmonary complications, decrease the length of ileus, and decrease the risk of anastomotic dehiscence and fistula, routine usage has been long shown to be unwarranted and possibly not necessary at all,[62–65] even following pancreatoduodenectomy.[66] One of the most common facets of studies assessing ERAS protocols in pancreatic surgery is either the removal of NG tubes at the end of operation[12,16,20] or on postoperative day 1,[10,14,15,19] with no increase in overall complications. Although DGE is not an insignificant complication following pancreatic surgery,[1,67] gastric decompression does not appear to be preventive, and NG tube insertion should be used if it develops. Therefore, it is recommended that NG tubes be removed ideally at the end of pancreatic operations or on postoperative day 1 with usage only for the treatment of DGE.

Postoperative Nutrition

In a manner similar to the placement of NG tubes, maintaining a nil per os (NPO) status until bowel function returns has been adhered to particularly after upper gastrointestinal surgery, including pancreatic surgery, despite a lack of supporting evidence. A multicenter, randomized controlled trial indicated that withholding oral nutrition does not offer any benefit.[68] Along those lines, feeding jejunostomy tubes are not beneficial and possibly harmful following pancreatic surgery.[69,70] The early resumption of oral intake on postoperative day 1 is a common feature of published studies assessing ERAS protocols after pancreatic surgery and has not been associated with increased morbidity.[12–16,20]

Somatostatin Analogues

The use of somatostatin analogues in the postoperative setting to decrease the incidence of POPF is not entirely agreed on. Randomized trials have shown both that it is effective[71–73] and ineffective.[74,75] A meta-analysis involving 17 trials and 2143 patients found that although somatostatin analogues appear to decrease postoperative complications and overall POPF, they do not decrease LOS, mortality, or clinically significant POPF (ISGPF Grades B and C).[76] It is theorized that the utility of somatostatin analogues may be found in using it only for high-risk glands (soft texture and/or small duct diameter), but even this usage has dissenting evidence.[75] Until further subset studies are conducted, the routine use of somatostatin analogues cannot be recommended.

Postoperative Analgesia

The management of postoperative pain can be difficult. Although patient-controlled analgesia (PCA) with intravenous opioids can control pain, midthoracic continuous epidural analgesia (CEA) appears to provide better pain relief[77] with fewer postoperative complications.[78,79] CEA catheter malfunction, however, can occur frequently and is associated with complications and increased workload.[80]

Continuous wound infusion (CWI) with local anesthetics (OnQ Pain Relief System; Halyard Health, Inc, Alpharetta, GA) in conjunction with PCA appears to be superior to PCA alone[81] and provides pain relief equal to CEA[82] following colorectal surgery. Few studies other than case series have been conducted following pancreatic surgery, but CWI with PCA appears to at least decrease opioid consumption compared with PCA alone.[83] Alternatively, transversus abdominis plane (TAP) blocks may be equivalent to CEA in relief of pain.[84] If an institution's CEA malfunction rate can be optimized, CEA should be considered. Otherwise, CWI plus PCA or TAP block can be used.

SUMMARY

ERAS protocols were designed to optimize postoperative management in several surgical specialties. An example of an ERAS protocol used at the St. Luke's Center for Pancreatic and Liver Diseases in Boise, Idaho, is provided (**Box 2**). ERAS protocols in colorectal surgery have been shown to be effective at improving several patient outcomes, including LOS and, perhaps, morbidity. Although outcomes specific to pancreatic surgery have not been completely studied, they appear to be similar to outcomes in colorectal surgery.

Box 2
St. Luke's Center for Pancreatic and Liver Diseases ERAS protocol in pancreatic surgery

Daily pathway

Preoperative evaluation
    <30-day-old imaging
    Counseling (nutrition, hand hygiene, mobility exercises)
    Informed consent

Day before operation
    Normal oral intake until 6 hours before anesthesia
    Chlorhexidine shower PM before or AM of operation

Day of operation
    Carbohydrate drink 2 hours before anesthesia
    Hair clipping in preoperative holding
    SCD placement in preoperative holding
    Heparin 5000 IU subcutaneously in preoperative holding
    Preoperative piperacillin-tazobactam within 1 hour of incision
    Removal of nasogastric tube at end of operation
    Usage of wound protector
    Closing instruments separated from main instruments
    Gloves changed for closing
    OnQ catheters + patient-controlled analgesia (PCA)[a]

POD 1
    Up and out of bed in AM and then > 4 times a day (QID)
    Clear liquids limited 60–100 mL/h
    Acetaminophen intravenously (IV) and ketorolac[b] adjunct to analgesia
    IV fluids decreased for neutral fluid balance
    Incision cleaned with chlorhexidine wipes

POD 2
    Ambulating in hallways > QID
    Unlimited full liquids if clear liquids tolerated
    IV fluids reduced to keep vein open if oral intake >500 mL on POD 1
    Remove urinary catheter
    Incision cleaned with chlorhexidine wipes

POD 3
    Continue ambulation
    Regular diet
    Discontinue IV fluids if liquids tolerated >1000 mL
    Discontinue PCA and start oral analgesics

POD 4+
    See discharge criteria

Drain management

Check daily drain amylase

Remove on POD 3 regardless of volume if
    Drain amylase <3× normal serum value
    No sinister appearance of fluid

Discharge criteria[c]

Ambulating independently

Pain controlled with oral analgesia

Bowel function resumed
    Tolerating >67% of kcal needs orally
    Capable of self-care
    Patient consenting to discharge

> *Abbreviations*: POD, post-operative day; SCD, sequential compression device.
> [a] We have abandoned epidural usage at our institution due to a high malfunction rate.
> [b] If not contraindicated due to renal function or bleeding risk.
> [c] Evaluate daily (especially beyond POD 5). If ambulation or self-care criteria are not met while all other criteria are met, then consider referral to rehabilitation center.

REFERENCES

1. Cameron JL, He J. Two thousand consecutive pancreaticoduodenectomies. J Am Coll Surg 2015;220(4):530–6.
2. Kehlet H. Fast-track colorectal surgery. Lancet 2008;371(9615):791–3.
3. Dy SM, Garg P, Nyberg D, et al. Critical pathway effectiveness: assessing the impact of patient, hospital care, and pathway characteristics using qualitative comparative analysis. Health Serv Res 2005;40(2):499–516.
4. Chestovich PJ, Lin AY, Yoo J. Fast-track pathways in colorectal surgery. Surg Clin North Am 2013;93(1):21–32.
5. Kehlet H, Wilmore DW. Evidence-based surgical care and the evolution of fast-track surgery. Ann Surg 2008;248(2):189–98.
6. Kehlet H. Fast-track hip and knee arthroplasty. Lancet 2013;381(9878):1600–2.
7. Kehlet H, Thienpont E. Fast-track knee arthroplasty–status and future challenges. Knee 2013;20(Suppl 1):S29–33.
8. Mertz BG, Kroman N, Williams H, et al. Fast-track surgery for breast cancer is possible. Dan Med J 2013;60(5):A4615.
9. Schultz NA, Larsen PN, Klarskov B, et al. Evaluation of a fast-track programme for patients undergoing liver resection. Br J Surg 2013;100(1):138–43.
10. Balzano G, Zerbi A, Braga M, et al. Fast-track recovery programme after pancreatico-duodenectomy reduces delayed gastric emptying. Br J Surg 2008; 95(11):1387–93.
11. Vanounou T, Pratt W, Fischer JE, et al. Deviation-based cost modeling: a novel model to evaluate the clinical and economic impact of clinical pathways. J Am Coll Surg 2007;204(4):570–9.
12. di Sebastiano P, Festa L, De Bonis A, et al. A modified fast-track program for pancreatic surgery: a prospective single-center experience. Langenbecks Arch Surg 2011;396(3):345–51.
13. Abu Hilal M, Di Fabio F, Badran A, et al. Implementation of enhanced recovery programme after pancreatoduodenectomy: a single-centre UK pilot study. Pancreatology 2013;13(1):58–62.
14. Kennedy EP, Grenda TR, Sauter PK, et al. Implementation of a critical pathway for distal pancreatectomy at an academic institution. J Gastrointest Surg 2009;13(5): 938–44.
15. Kennedy EP, Rosato EL, Sauter PK, et al. Initiation of a critical pathway for pancreaticoduodenectomy at an academic institution–the first step in multidisciplinary team building. J Am Coll Surg 2007;204(5):917–23 [discussion: 923–4].
16. Berberat PO, Ingold H, Gulbinas A, et al. Fast track–different implications in pancreatic surgery. J Gastrointest Surg 2007;11(7):880–7.
17. Nikfarjam M, Weinberg L, Low N, et al. A fast track recovery program significantly reduces hospital length of stay following uncomplicated pancreaticoduodenectomy. JOP 2013;14(1):63–70.

18. Porter GA, Pisters PW, Mansyur C, et al. Cost and utilization impact of a clinical pathway for patients undergoing pancreaticoduodenectomy. Ann Surg Oncol 2000;7(7):484–9.

19. Robertson N, Gallacher PJ, Peel N, et al. Implementation of an enhanced recovery programme following pancreaticoduodenectomy. HPB (Oxford) 2012;14(10): 700–8.

20. Coolsen MM, van Dam RM, Chigharoe A, et al. Improving outcome after pancreaticoduodenectomy: experiences with implementing an enhanced recovery after surgery (ERAS) program. Dig Surg 2014;31(3):177–84.

21. Lassen K, Coolsen MM, Slim K, et al. Guidelines for perioperative care for pancreaticoduodenectomy: Enhanced Recovery After Surgery (ERAS(R)) Society recommendations. Clin Nutr 2012;31(6):817–30.

22. Balshem H, Helfand M, Schunemann HJ, et al. GRADE guidelines: 3. Rating the quality of evidence. J Clin Epidemiol 2011;64(4):401–6.

23. Ypsilantis E, Praseedom RK. Current status of fast-track recovery pathways in pancreatic surgery. JOP 2009;10:646–50.

24. Coolsen MM, van Dam RM, van der Wilt AA, et al. Systematic review and meta-analysis of enhanced recovery after pancreatic surgery with particular emphasis on pancreaticoduodenectomies. World J Surg 2013;37(8):1909–18.

25. Darido EF, Farrell TM. Fast-track concepts in major open upper abdominal and thoracoabdominal surgery: a review. World J Surg 2011;35(12):2594–5.

26. Kagedan DJ, Ahmed M, Devitt KS, et al. Enhanced recovery after pancreatic surgery: a systematic review of the evidence. HPB (Oxford) 2015;17(1):11–6.

27. Spelt L, Ansari D, Sturesson C, et al. Fast-track programmes for hepatopancreatic resections: where do we stand? HPB (Oxford) 2011;13(12):833–8.

28. Measures JCNQC. Specifications Manual for Joint Commission National Quality Core Measures (2010A1). 2010; Available at: https://manual.jointcommission. org/releases/archive/TJC2010B/SurgicalCareImprovementProject.html.   Accessed January 31, 2016.

29. Bratzler DW, Hunt DR. The surgical infection prevention and surgical care improvement projects: national initiatives to improve outcomes for patients having surgery. Clin Infect Dis 2006;43(3):322–30.

30. Jones RS, Brown C, Opelka F. Surgeon compensation: "Pay for performance," the American College of Surgeons National Surgical Quality Improvement Program, the Surgical Care Improvement Program, and other considerations. Surgery 2005;138(5):829–36.

31. Measures JCNQC. Prophylactic antibiotic regimen selection for surgery. Available at: https://manual.jointcommission.org/releases/archive/TJC2010B/ ProphylacticAntibioticRegimenSelectionForSurgery.html.   Accessed   January 31, 2016.

32. Bratzler DW, Dellinger EP, Olsen KM, et al. Clinical practice guidelines for antimicrobial prophylaxis in surgery. Surg Infect (Larchmt) 2013;14(1):73–156.

33. Ceppa EP, Pitt HA, House MG, et al. Reducing surgical site infections in hepatopancreatobiliary surgery. HPB (Oxford) 2013;15(5):384–91.

34. Donald GW, Sunjaya D, Lu X, et al. Perioperative antibiotics for surgical site infection in pancreaticoduodenectomy: does the SCIP-approved regimen provide adequate coverage? Surgery 2013;154(2):190–6.

35. Fong ZV, McMillan MT, Marchegiani G, et al. Discordance between perioperative antibiotic prophylaxis and wound infection cultures in patients undergoing pancreaticoduodenectomy. JAMA Surg 2016;151(5):432–9.

36. Kimmings AN, van Deventer SJ, Obertop H, et al. Endotoxin, cytokines, and endotoxin binding proteins in obstructive jaundice and after preoperative biliary drainage. Gut 2000;46(5):725–31.

37. Klinkenbijl JH, Jeekel J, Schmitz PI, et al. Carcinoma of the pancreas and periampullary region: palliation versus cure. Br J Surg 1993;80(12):1575–8.

38. van der Gaag NA, Kloek JJ, de Castro SM, et al. Preoperative biliary drainage in patients with obstructive jaundice: history and current status. J Gastrointest Surg 2009;13(4):814–20.

39. Mumtaz K, Hamid S, Jafri W. Endoscopic retrograde cholangiopancreaticography with or without stenting in patients with pancreaticobiliary malignancy, prior to surgery. Cochrane Database Syst Rev 2007;(3):CD006001.

40. Salem AI, Alfi M, Winslow E, et al. Has survival following pancreaticoduodenectomy for pancreas adenocarcinoma improved over time? J Surg Oncol 2015; 112(6):643–9.

41. Sewnath ME, Karsten TM, Prins MH, et al. A meta-analysis on the efficacy of preoperative biliary drainage for tumors causing obstructive jaundice. Ann Surg 2002;236(1):17–27.

42. van der Gaag NA, Rauws EA, van Eijck CH, et al. Preoperative biliary drainage for cancer of the head of the pancreas. N Engl J Med 2010;362(2):129–37.

43. Tol JA, van Hooft JE, Timmer R, et al. Metal or plastic stents for preoperative biliary drainage in resectable pancreatic cancer. Gut 2015. [Epub ahead of print].

44. Boulay BR, Parepally M. Managing malignant biliary obstruction in pancreas cancer: choosing the appropriate strategy. World J Gastroenterol 2014;20(28): 9345–53.

45. Fry DE. Colon preparation and surgical site infection. Am J Surg 2011;202(2): 225–32.

46. Holte K, Nielsen KG, Madsen JL, et al. Physiologic effects of bowel preparation. Dis Colon Rectum 2004;47(8):1397–402.

47. Guenaga KF, Matos D, Wille-Jorgensen P. Mechanical bowel preparation for elective colorectal surgery. Cochrane Database Syst Rev 2011;(9):CD001544.

48. Piroglu I, Tulgar S, Thomas DT, et al. Mechanical bowel preparation does not affect anastomosis healing in an experimental rat model. Med Sci Monit 2016; 22:26–30.

49. Gustafsson UO, Scott MJ, Schwenk W, et al. Guidelines for perioperative care in elective colonic surgery: Enhanced Recovery After Surgery (ERAS((R))) Society recommendations. World J Surg 2013;37(2):259–84.

50. Lavu H, Kennedy EP, Mazo R, et al. Preoperative mechanical bowel preparation does not offer a benefit for patients who undergo pancreaticoduodenectomy. Surgery 2010;148(2):278–84.

51. Conlon KC, Labow D, Leung D, et al. Prospective randomized clinical trial of the value of intraperitoneal drainage after pancreatic resection. Ann Surg 2001; 234(4):487–93 [discussion: 493–4].

52. Mehta VV, Fisher SB, Maithel SK, et al. Is it time to abandon routine operative drain use? A single institution assessment of 709 consecutive pancreaticoduodenectomies. J Am Coll Surg 2013;216(4):635–42 [discussion: 642–4].

53. Peng S, Cheng Y, Yang C, et al. Prophylactic abdominal drainage for pancreatic surgery. Cochrane Database Syst Rev 2015;(8):CD010583.

54. van der Wilt AA, Coolsen MM, de Hingh IH, et al. To drain or not to drain: a cumulative meta-analysis of the use of routine abdominal drains after pancreatic resection. HPB (Oxford) 2013;15(5):337–44.

55. Bassi C, Dervenis C, Butturini G, et al. Postoperative pancreatic fistula: an international study group (ISGPF) definition. Surgery 2005;138(1):8–13.
56. Van Buren G 2nd, Bloomston M, Hughes SJ, et al. A randomized prospective multicenter trial of pancreaticoduodenectomy with and without routine intraperitoneal drainage. Ann Surg 2014;259(4):605–12.
57. Bassi C, Molinari E, Malleo G, et al. Early versus late drain removal after standard pancreatic resections: results of a prospective randomized trial. Ann Surg 2010; 252(2):207–14.
58. Kawai M, Tani M, Terasawa H, et al. Early removal of prophylactic drains reduces the risk of intra-abdominal infections in patients with pancreatic head resection: prospective study for 104 consecutive patients. Ann Surg 2006;244(1):1–7.
59. Ljunggren S, Hahn RG, Nystrom T. Insulin sensitivity and beta-cell function after carbohydrate oral loading in hip replacement surgery: a double-blind, randomised controlled clinical trial. Clin Nutr 2014;33(3):392–8.
60. Smith MD, McCall J, Plank L, et al. Preoperative carbohydrate treatment for enhancing recovery after elective surgery. Cochrane Database Syst Rev 2014;(8):CD009161.
61. Yuill KA, Richardson RA, Davidson HI, et al. The administration of an oral carbohydrate-containing fluid prior to major elective upper-gastrointestinal surgery preserves skeletal muscle mass postoperatively–a randomised clinical trial. Clin Nutr 2005;24(1):32–7.
62. Bauer JJ, Gelernt IM, Salky BA, et al. Is routine postoperative nasogastric decompression really necessary? Ann Surg 1985;201(2):233–6.
63. Cheatham ML, Chapman WC, Key SP, et al. A meta-analysis of selective versus routine nasogastric decompression after elective laparotomy. Ann Surg 1995; 221(5):469–76 [discussion: 476–8].
64. Nelson R, Edwards S, Tse B. Prophylactic nasogastric decompression after abdominal surgery. Cochrane Database Syst Rev 2007;(3):CD004929.
65. Nelson R, Tse B, Edwards S. Systematic review of prophylactic nasogastric decompression after abdominal operations. Br J Surg 2005;92(6):673–80.
66. Fisher WE, Hodges SE, Cruz G, et al. Routine nasogastric suction may be unnecessary after a pancreatic resection. HPB (Oxford) 2011;13(11):792–6.
67. Traverso LW, Shinchi H, Low DE. Useful benchmarks to evaluate outcomes after esophagectomy and pancreaticoduodenectomy. Am J Surg 2004;187(5):604–8.
68. Lassen K, Kjaeve J, Fetveit T, et al. Allowing normal food at will after major upper gastrointestinal surgery does not increase morbidity: a randomized multicenter trial. Ann Surg 2008;247(5):721–9.
69. Gerritsen A, Besselink MG, Gouma DJ, et al. Systematic review of five feeding routes after pancreatoduodenectomy. Br J Surg 2013;100(5):589–98 [discussion: 599].
70. Nussbaum DP, Zani S, Penne K, et al. Feeding jejunostomy tube placement in patients undergoing pancreaticoduodenectomy: an ongoing dilemma. J Gastrointest Surg 2014;18(10):1752–9.
71. Friess H, Beger HG, Sulkowski U, et al. Randomized controlled multicentre study of the prevention of complications by octreotide in patients undergoing surgery for chronic pancreatitis. Br J Surg 1995;82(9):1270–3.
72. Suc B, Msika S, Piccinini M, et al. Octreotide in the prevention of intra-abdominal complications following elective pancreatic resection: a prospective, multicenter randomized controlled trial. Arch Surg 2004;139(3):288–94 [discussion: 295].
73. Allen PJ, Gonen M, Brennan MF, et al. Pasireotide for postoperative pancreatic fistula. N Engl J Med 2014;370(21):2014–22.

74. Sarr MG. The potent somatostatin analogue vapreotide does not decrease pancreas-specific complications after elective pancreatectomy: a prospective, multicenter, double-blinded, randomized, placebo-controlled trial. J Am Coll Surg 2003;196(4):556–64 [discussion: 564–5; author reply: 565].

75. Yeo CJ, Cameron JL, Lillemoe KD, et al. Does prophylactic octreotide decrease the rates of pancreatic fistula and other complications after pancreaticoduodenectomy? Results of a prospective randomized placebo-controlled trial. Ann Surg 2000;232(3):419–29.

76. Koti RS, Gurusamy KS, Fusai G, et al. Meta-analysis of randomized controlled trials on the effectiveness of somatostatin analogues for pancreatic surgery: a Cochrane review. HPB (Oxford) 2010;12(3):155–65.

77. Werawatganon T, Charuluxanun S. Patient controlled intravenous opioid analgesia versus continuous epidural analgesia for pain after intra-abdominal surgery. Cochrane Database Syst Rev 2005;(1):CD004088.

78. Popping DM, Elia N, Marret E, et al. Protective effects of epidural analgesia on pulmonary complications after abdominal and thoracic surgery: a meta-analysis. Arch Surg 2008;143(10):990–9 [discussion: 1000].

79. Jorgensen H, Wetterslev J, Moiniche S, et al. Epidural local anaesthetics versus opioid-based analgesic regimens on postoperative gastrointestinal paralysis, PONV and pain after abdominal surgery. Cochrane Database Syst Rev 2000;(4):CD001893.

80. Sugimoto M, Nesbit L, Barton JG, et al. Epidural anesthesia dysfunction is associated with postoperative complications after pancreatectomy. J Hepatobiliary Pancreat Sci 2016;23(2):102–9.

81. Beaussier M, El'Ayoubi H, Schiffer E, et al. Continuous preperitoneal infusion of ropivacaine provides effective analgesia and accelerates recovery after colorectal surgery: a randomized, double-blind, placebo-controlled study. Anesthesiology 2007;107(3):461–8.

82. Bertoglio S, Fabiani F, Negri PD, et al. The postoperative analgesic efficacy of preperitoneal continuous wound infusion compared to epidural continuous infusion with local anesthetics after colorectal cancer surgery: a randomized controlled multicenter study. Anesth Analg 2012;115(6):1442–50.

83. Thompson TK, Hutchison RW, Wegmann DJ, et al. Pancreatic resection pain management: is combining PCA therapy and a continuous local infusion of 0.5% ropivacaine beneficial? Pancreas 2008;37:103–4.

84. Ayad S, Babazade R, Elsharkawy H, et al. Comparison of transversus abdominis plane infiltration with liposomal bupivacaine versus continuous epidural analgesia versus intravenous opioid analgesia. PLoS One 2016;11(4):e0153675.

Postpancreatectomy Complications and Management

Giuseppe Malleo, MD, PhD[a], Charles M. Vollmer Jr, MD[b],*

KEYWORDS

- Pancreatic resection • Postoperative complications • Pancreatic fistula
- Delayed gastric emptying • Postpancreatectomy hemorrhage

KEY POINTS

- The incidence of postoperative complications after pancreatectomy remains high, in the range of 30% to 60%.
- The International Study Group of Pancreatic Surgery (ISGPS) derived consensus definitions of major complications, allowing a reliable comparison among different experiences.
- Advances in perioperative care have ushered a paradigm shift from operative to nonoperative complication management, with a reduction of associated mortality rates.

INTRODUCTION

An early surgical tenet used to be, "eat when you can, sleep when you can, and don't operate on the pancreas." For decades, postoperative complications after pancreatic resection have been feared events that spelled disaster, thus hampering the dissemination of what were called "formidable" (high-acuity) procedures. More recently, mortality has decreased to less than 5%, such that indications for pancreatic resections have broadened from pancreatic cancer to now include cystic, neuroendocrine, and other uncommon neoplasms. Yet, these procedures remain associated with substantial postoperative morbidity, ranging from 30% to 60%.[1] The management of complications after pancreatic resection has shifted from an operative to a conservative approach, thanks to the establishment of multidisciplinary teams with high degrees of expertise. In general, the development of high-volume, specialist pancreatic centers has been credited with the dramatic improvement of outcomes after pancreatic

The authors have nothing to disclose.
[a] Unit of General and Pancreatic Surgery, Department of Surgery and Oncology, The Pancreas Institute, University of Verona Hospital Trust, P.Le L.A. Scuro 10, Verona 37134, Italy; [b] Department of Surgery, University of Pennsylvania Perelman School of Medicine, 3400 Spruce Street, Philadelphia, PA 19104, USA
* Corresponding author.
E-mail address: Charles.Vollmer@uphs.upenn.edu

Surg Clin N Am 96 (2016) 1313–1336
http://dx.doi.org/10.1016/j.suc.2016.07.013
0039-6109/16/© 2016 Elsevier Inc. All rights reserved.

surgical.theclinics.com

resection.[2] Nevertheless, postoperative complications often have a profound impact on patient recovery and length of hospital stay and are associated with increased utilization of resources as well as with increased hospital costs.[3] The ISGPS established standardized definitions and clinical grading systems for the most common complications, including pancreatic fistula, postpancreatectomy hemorrhage (PPH), and delayed gastric emptying (DGE).[4–6] In addition to improving the quality of comparative research, these classification systems have enabled unbiased comparisons of intraoperative techniques and management decisions. They have also ushered in risk-assessment and risk-adjustment models. This review focuses on postoperative pancreatic fistula (POPF), DGE, and PPH, with the aim of providing practicing physicians state-of-the art concepts regarding diagnosis and management.

PANCREATIC FISTULA
Definition and Risk Assessment

POPF is the most common complication after pancreatic resection. The 2005 consensus definition of POPF by the International Study Group of Pancreatic Fistula (**Table 1**) has since been used in most of the studies investigating outcome measures in pancreatic surgery.[4,7–9] A recent pooled analysis of these studies showed that the incidence of POPF after pancreaticoduodenectomy (PD) was between 22% and 26%, whereas in distal pancreatectomy it was in excess of 30%.[10] Although POPF occurs more frequently after distal pancreatectomy, it is associated with a lesser average complication burden compared with PD.[11,12] The highest rate of POPF follows middle-segment pancreatectomy, which ranges from 20% to 60%, because of the creation of 2 pancreatic remnants and, thus, 2 potential sites for fistula development.[13] The ISGPF clinical grading system (grades A, B, and C), which was originally developed qualitatively around the concept of clinical severity, was validated in different articles and has been shown to correlate with hospital expenditure.[3] The POPF grading system suffered from the inability to be compared quantitatively.[14] In a North American study, the utilization of a postoperative morbidity index, based on the Modified

Table 1			
International Study Group of Pancreatic Fistula definition and grading system			
Definition			
Output via an operatively placed drain (or a subsequently placed percutaneous drain) of any measurable volume of drain fluid on or after POD 3, with an amylase content greater than 3 times the upper normal serum value.			
Grading system			
Grade	*A*	*B*	*C*
Clinical condition	Well	Often well	Ill appearing/bad
Specific treatment	No	Yes/no	Yes
Ultrasound/CT scan	Negative	Negative/positive	Positive
Persistent drainage (after 3 wk)	No	Usually yes	Yes
Reoperation	No	No	Yes
POPF-related death	No	No	Possibly yes
Signs of infection	No	Yes	Yes
Sepsis	No	No	Yes
Readmission	No	Yes/No	Yes/No

Data from Refs.[4,7–9]

Accordion Severity Grading System, showed that each grade of POPF segregated into discrete Accordion profiles. Clinically relevant fistulae (grades B–C) usually reflect a patient's highest Accordion score, whereas biochemical fistulas are often superseded by more severe, nonfistulous complications.[15] Pancreatic fistula contributes significantly to mortality after pancreatic resections.[16]

Since the advent of the ISGPF and standardization of fistula nomenclature, there has been a systematic investigation of risk factors, in an attempt to improve outcomes. Numerous articles showed that fistula risk encompasses endogenous, perioperative, and intraoperative factors, including age, gender, body mass index (BMI), diabetes mellitus, cardiovascular comorbidities, disease pathology, neoadjuvant therapy, use of prophylactic somatostatin analogs, pancreatic duct caliber, pancreatic remnant texture, anastomotic technique, use of transanastomotic stent, intraoperative blood loss, operative time, and routine drain placement.[1] Because factors analyzed in isolation might not reflect thoroughly individual patient risk, investigators have instead assessed composite metrics based on the aggregate of weighted risk factors. Many of the resulting scoring systems were developed and validated for pancreatic head resection (**Table 2**),[17–26] whereas such a system is missing for distal pancreatectomy – largely due to the lack of reproducible risk factors in isolation. In the authors' practice, it is believed that risk should be better evaluated using variables that are evident up to, and including, the point of execution of the operation. Variables evident thereafter (in the postoperative period), although possibly contributing to the ultimate severity of the fistula, should be considered a reflection of the consequences of fistula occurrence. Accordingly, the Fistula Risk Score (FRS) is the preferred method of individual fistula risk assessment at the authors' institutions, because it has been the most rigorously scrutinized and applied system thus far in the literature.

The FRS is a system for the prediction of clinically relevant POPF (CR-POPF) after PD that was developed using an extensive multivariate analysis of all known endogenous, perioperative, and operative risk factors for fistula (54 variables in total). After the regression analysis, the following significant risk factors were weighted and assigned quantitative values: soft gland parenchyma, high-risk pathology (anything other than pancreatic adenocarcinoma or pancreatitis), small duct diameter (<5 mm), and elevated intraoperative blood loss (>400 mL) (**Table 3**). The aggregate sum tabulated from these values creates a simple score on a scale from 0 to 10, which could be further segregated into 4 risk zones: negligible (0), low (1–2), moderate (3–6), and high (7–10).[20] CR-POPF risk has been shown to escalate linearly across individual FRS scores as well as risk zones. For instance, the predicted CR-POPF rates for negligible risk, low risk, moderate risk, and high risk are 0%, 6.6%, 12.9%, and 28.1%, respectively. This scoring system has been recently validated externally.[21–23]

In addition, the FRS provides a risk adjustment process that has the potential to conduct assessments of surgeon and institutional performance. In this regard, a recent multi-institutional study of more than 4000 PDs performed by 55 surgeons at 15 institutions sought to identify variability between surgeons and institutions in terms of CR-POPF risk, CR-POPF occurrence, and risk-adjusted performance (based largely on FRS but with other variables) with PD. The results demonstrated there is significant variability in both the risk and occurrence of CR-POPF between surgeons and institutions. Much of the variability in the rate of CR-POPF could be explained not only by patients' inherent fistula risk (through the FRS, odds ratio [OR] 1.49 per point) but also by surgical management decisions, including the use of prophylactic octreotide (OR 3.30) and pancreaticogastrostomy (OR 2.05).[27] As a consequence, comparisons of CR-POPF rates between surgeons and institutions in a non–risk-adjusted setting could be misleading. Surgical management decisions differ substantially across the

Table 2
Scoring systems for postoperative pancreatic fistula prediction after pancreaticoduodenectomy

Reference (Study Period)	Outcome of Interest	Incidence (%)	Type of Score	Variables Included in the Score (Risk Factors, *Protective Factors*)	Proposed Score Scale	Risk Groups	Predictive Accuracy	Internal Validation	External Validation
Gaujoux et al,[17] 2010 (2004–2005)	POPF (A–C) CR-POPF (B–C)	31/100 (31%) 27/100 (27%)	Postoperative	BMI >25 kg/m² Fatty pancreas *Absence of fibrosis*	0–3	4	AUC 0.78 (A–C) AUC 0.81(B–C)	Not done	Not done
Wellner et al,[18] 2010 (2006–2008)	POPF (A–C)	19/62 (31%)	Preoperative	Age >66 y Preoperative diagnosis other than PDAC or pancreatitis *History of weight loss* *History of smoking* *History of acute pancreatitis*	–3–2	3	Correlation coefficient = 0.47 P<.001	Correlation coefficient = 0.35 P<.001	No
Yamamoto et al,[19] 2011 (2004–2009)	CR-POPF (B–C)	103/279 (37%)	Preoperative	MPD index <0.25 Away from portal vein on CT Male gender Intra-abdominal fat thickness >65 mm Preoperative diagnosis other than PDAC	0–7	7	AUC = 0.808	AUC = 0.834	No

Callery et al,[20] 2013 (2002–2007)	CR-POPF (B–C)	58/233 (25%)	Intraoperative	Soft pancreatic parenchyma Preoperative diagnosis other than PDAC or pancreatitis Pancreatic duct diameter Intraoperative blood loss	0–10	3	—	AUC = 0.942	Miller et al,[21] 2014 Kunstman et al,[22] 2014 Shubert et al,[23] 2015
Graham et al,[24] 2013 (2007–2012)	Drain amylase >3× normal serum amylase on or after POD 4	50/146 (34%)	Postoperative	Age BMI Pancreatic duct diameter POD 2 drain amylase	Continuous 0%–100%	—	Hosmer and Lemeshow test P = .452	Not done	Not done
Roberts et al,[25] 2014 (2007–2012)	POPF (A–C)	48/217 (22%)	Preoperative	BMI Pancreatic duct diameter	Continuous 0%–100%	—	AUC = 0.832	AUC = 0.751	No
Chen et al,[26] 2015 (2008–2013)	—	—	—	BMI ≥28 Pancreatic duct <3 mm Soft pancreatic parenchyma (intraoperative blood loss –intraoperative transfusions) ≥800 mL	0–6	2	AUC = 0.812	Not done	Not done

Abbreviations: AUC, area under the curve; PDAC, pancreatic ductal adenocarcinoma.
Data from Refs.[17–20,24–26]

Table 3
Fistula Risk Score for prediction of clinically relevant pancreatic fistula after pancreatoduodenectomy

Risk Factor	Parameter	Points
Gland texture	Firm	0
	Soft	2
Pathology	Pancreatic adenocarcinoma or pancreatitis	0
	Ampullary, duodenal, cystic, islet cell	1
Pancreatic duct diameter, mm	≥5	0
	4	1
	3	2
	2	3
	≤1	4
Intraoperative blood loss, mL	≤400	0
	401–700	1
	701–1000	2
	>1000	3

Fistula Risk Zones	Points
Negligible	0
Low	1–2
Intermediate	3–6
High	7–10

Adapted from Callery MP, Pratt WB, Kent TS, et al. A prospectively validated clinical risk score accurately predicts pancreatic fistula after pancreatoduodenectomy. J Am Coll Surg 2013;216:6; with permission.

world, as recently demonstrated by a survey on the variability in the practice of PD distributed to 897 members of 22 international gastrointestinal (GI) surgical societies. Surprisingly, many of the management choices were in contrast with the established randomized evidence.[28]

Furthermore, risk adjustment through the FRS has been used in assessing the value of various mitigation strategies; for instance, guidelines for selective drainage based on CR-POPF risk have been developed (**Fig. 1**).[29] Patients with drain fluid amylase less than 5000 U/L on postoperative day (POD) 1 enrolled in a previously reported randomized controlled trial on early versus late drain removal after PD[30] were assessed using a risk-adjusted process. Based on the trial reanalysis, a clinical care protocol was proposed whereby drains are recommended for moderate/high-risk FRS patients but may be omitted in patients with negligible/low risk. Drain fluid amylase values in moderate/high-risk patients can then be evaluated on POD 1 to determine the optimal timing for drain removal.[31] The protocol has subsequently been applied prospectively in 260 PDs from the Authors' Institutions,[32] and this has led to a reduction of CR-POPF in excess of 40% compared with an historic cohort. In particular, no POPF developed in the low/negligible-risk patients, in whom drains had been omitted.[32]

Management

Along with the effluent appearance and the measurement of drain fluid amylase, the suspicion of POPF begins whenever there is a deviation in the normal clinical course of a patient who has just undergone partial pancreatic resection.[2] Contrast-enhanced

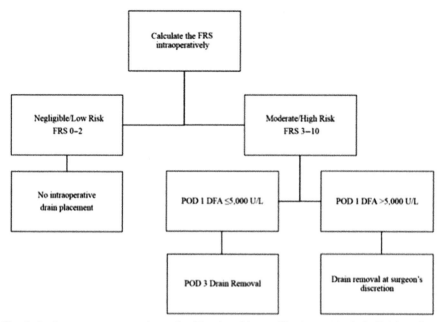

Fig. 1. Drain management pathway for PD using risk stratification. DFA, drain fluid amylase. (*Adapted from* McMillan MT, Malleo G, Bassi C, et al. Drain management after pancreatoduodenectomy: reappraisal of a prospective randomized trial using risk stratification. J Am Coll Surg 2015;221:798–809.)

CT, or transabdominal ultrasound, can show collections in contiguity with the pancreatic remnant and the possible disruption of pancreatic anastomosis, if any.[33]

Nutritional support has been regarded as a key element of conservative therapy, because most POPF patients are in a hypercatabolic state. Furthermore, high-output fistulae (those producing >200 mL of exocrine secretion daily) are associated with fluid/electrolyte imbalances and nutritional depletion.[34] In patients with POPF, enteral nutrition (EN) therapy seems to offer important benefits over total parenteral nutrition (TPN). Klek and colleagues[35] demonstrated, by an open-label, randomized controlled clinical trial of EN versus TPN, that the former increased by more than 2-fold the probability of fistula closure, shortened the time to closure, and was associated with faster recovery, lower rates of nutrition-related complications, and lower cost than TPN. Another mainstay of conservative therapy has been the administration of somatostatin analogs, the anticipated effects of which are to reduce the volume of the fistula output and to potentially mitigate its natural course. A recent systematic review and meta-analysis of somatostatin analogs for the treatment of fistula of the GI tract, including POPF, analyzed 7 randomized clinical trials published between 1990 and 2009. No significant advantage of the use of somatostatin analogs in terms of the fistula closure rate was shown.[36] Because most studies were published before the ISGPF definition, substantial differences existed with regard to the criteria applied for a proved POPF. Nevertheless, there is no solid evidence that somatostatin analogs result in a higher or faster closure rate of POPF compared with other treatments. Accordingly, these drugs should not be considered standard treatment.

In cases of clinical deterioration and/or signs of infection, including abdominal pain and distension with impaired bowel function, DGE, fever (>38°C), high serum leukocyte count, increased C-reactive protein, and purulent drain effluent, antibiotic therapy is required. Selection of empiric antibiotic therapy should be based on institution-specific bacterial growth spectrum and resistance; subsequently, therapies should be tailored according to drain effluent cultures, if needed.

Image-guided percutaneous drainage of peripancreatic fluid collections/abscesses subsequent to a POPF is the most common indication for interventional radiology after pancreatic resection.[37] Peripancreatic collections can be approached percutaneously as long as a patient is hemodynamically stable and has an acceptable coagulation panel and there is a safe access route for a needle. Multiple studies have shown that more than 85% of patients were managed successfully with percutaneous drainages without the need for reoperation.[38,39] The use of endoscopic ultrasound–guided transmural drainage, initially applied for management of pseudocysts, has grown in frequency to drain collections associated with POPF, after both PD and distal pancreatectomy.[40,41] Although most POPFs can be managed nonoperatively, some require reoperative surgical intervention and are thus classified as ISGPF grade C. Indications for relaparotomy are not uniform across different studies and depend on institutional expertise and patient conditions. In general, an operative intervention has to be considered in cases of clinical deterioration despite maximal supporting care, infected intra-abdominal collections inaccessible to percutaneous or endoscopic drainage, suspected peritonitis due to visceral perforation, and drainage limb necrosis.[42,43] Because serious bleeding from pseudoaneurysms can further complicate POPF, ongoing bleeding after failure or contraindication of radiologic endovascular procedures mandates emergency relaparotomy and operative bleeding control.[6] Unfortunately, this is usually a morbid, if not mortal, endeavor.

Pancreatic stump management at relaparotomy encompasses multiple surgical options, including débridement and wide drainage of the peripancreatic region (with or without bridge stenting of the main pancreatic duct), attempted repair of the site of leakage, construction of a new pancreatic-enteric anastomosis (usually ill advised), resection of the pancreatic-enteric anastomosis with remnant closure, and completion pancreatectomy, The choice is often dictated by intraoperative findings and a patient's physiology. Whatever the surgical approach, it has been shown that subsequent operations were required in approximately 50% of patients with redo-operations.[2] A majority of these were necessary in patients with septic complications and the need for open abdominal lavage with secondary abdominal wall closure.[44]

A comprehensive analysis of clinical presentations and risk factors for the highly morbid grade C POPF has been recently carried out by McMillan and colleagues.[45] The incidence of grade C POPF among the multi-institutional database, including more than 4000 PDs, was only 1.8% but incurred a 90-day mortality rate of 35%. Adjuvant chemotherapy might have benefited 56% of grade C POPF patients, yet it was delayed in 26% and never delivered in 67% of these patients. On multivariate analysis, both preoperative factors (alcohol consumption, previous cardiac events, and pathologies other than ductal adenocarcinoma/pancreatitis) and intraoperative factors (operative time) were associated with grade C POPF. Although not applicable in the preoperative setting, it could potentially assist surgeons in identifying patients who may require heightened surveillance and preventative care after their surgery.

DELAYED GASTRIC EMPTYING

Despite being self-limiting in most cases, DGE is a potentially serious event that may lead to patient discomfort, further interventions, prolonged hospitalization, higher readmission rates, and increased hospital costs.[46–51] Yet, among all the complications in pancreatic surgery, DGE is that endowed with the highest degree of subjectivity. This lack of objective evidence, along with the confounding influence of clinical masquerades, leads to misclassification, leaving clinicians to a large extent confused about the true nature of this phenomenon.

The pathogenesis of DGE still represents a medical conundrum. Most research in the field has been focused on PD. Decreased plasma motilin levels as a consequence of duodenal resection and pylorospasm secondary to operative devascularization and/or denervation have traditionally been considered possible triggers of postoperative gastroparesis after PD.[5] Furthermore, the performance of standard Whipple versus pylorus-preserving PD,[52] antecolic versus retrocolic gastric/duodenal reconstruction,[53] hand-sewn versus stapled duodenojejunostomy, Billroth I versus II reconstruction, pancreaticogastrostomy versus pancreaticojejunostomy, and other operative details, such as use of pancreatic stent, length of the gastrojejunostomy, performance of a Braun enteroenterostomy, portal vein resection, operative time, and blood loss, have been investigated as putative risk factors.[54–63] In addition, patient characteristics (ie, female gender, preoperative heart failure, high BMI, pulmonary comorbidities, and smoking history) have also been proposed to influence the occurrence of DGE.[64,65] Unfortunately, none of these has been rigorously studied or accepted.

On the other hand, there is general agreement that perturbation of the operative bed by localized inflammation from a second complication might be a key contributor to the development of DGE. DGE is associated with POPF, intra-abdominal abscesses, and postoperative sepsis.[46–48,63–66] The 2007 ISGPS classification and grading system (**Table 4**)[5] has been validated by several studies demonstrating its feasibility and correlation with clinical course (**Table 5**).[48–51] Many criticisms have been raised, however, regarding the applicability of DGE definition. Unlike POPF, the diagnosis of which relies on an objective biochemical measurement (drain amylase content), DGE remains a nebulous concept, with no test that clearly defines the physiologic function of GI tract. DGE assessment is solely based on how it is treated and, therefore, is more arbitrary and open to interpretation. The placement of a nasogastric tube (NGT) as well as the decision to progress to solid diet is a subjective choice made by the treating surgeon according to institutional policies. The influence of institution-specific clinical pathways has led to a great variability in the reported DGE incidence, ranging from 13.8% to more than 40%,[48–51,63–67] even when the ISGPS definition is

Table 4
International Study Group of Pancreatic Surgery consensus definition and grading system of delayed gastric emptying

Delayed Gastric Emptying Grade	Nasogastric Tube Required	Unable to Tolerate Solid Diet by Postoperative Day	Vomiting/ Gastric Distension	Use of Prokinetics
A	4–7 d or reinsertion > POD 3	7	±	±
B	8–14 d or reinsertion > POD 7	14	+	+
C	>14 d or reinsertion > POD 14	21	+	+

Adapted from Wente MN, Bassi C, Dervenis C, et al. Delayed gastric emptying (DGE) after pancreatic surgery: a suggested definition by the International Study Group of Pancreatic Surgery (ISGPS). Surgery 2007;142:764; with permission.

Table 5
Main literature reports on delayed gastric emptying

Reference (Study Period)	Type of Surgery, n (%)	Incidence (%)	Association with Postoperative Pancreatic Fistula (%)	Isolated Delayed Gastric Emptying	Risk Factors
Park et al,[50] 2009 (2002–2007)	ppPD 76 (58.9) Whipple 53 (41.1)	Overall 43/129 (33.3) Grade A 16 (12.4) Grade B 14 (10.9) Grade C 13 (10.1)	POPF 19 (44.2) CR-POPF 14 (32.6)	21 (48.9)	DGE (grades A–C) CR-POPF Benign pathology
Akizuki et al,[66] 2009 (2003–2007)	ppPD 49 (57.7) ssPD 36 (42.3)	Overall 36/85 (42.4) Grade A 17 (20.0) Grade B 9 (10.6) Grade C 10 (11.8)	POPF[a] 3 (8.3)	Not reported	No significant factors at multivariate analysis
Welsch et al,[49] 2010 (2001–2008)	ppPD 648 (84.8) Whipple 107 (14.0) Total pancreatectomy 9 (1.2)	Overall 340/764 (44.5) Grade A 209 (27.4) Grade B 63 (8.2) Grade C 68 (8.9)	Not reported	168/209 (80.4) of grade DGE A patients had no or only minor complications	DGE (grade A) Female gender Preoperative heart failure Major complications
Malleo et al,[48] 2010 (2007–2009)	ppPD 260 (100)	Overall 36/260 (13.8) Grade A 16 (6.1) Grade B 18 (6.9) Grade C 2 (0.8)	CR-POPF 16 (44.4)	12 (33.3)	DGE (grades A–C) CR-POPF Sepsis
Tan et al,[67] 2011 (2005–2009)	ppPD 46 (59.7) Whipple 31 (40.3)	Overall 16/77 (20.8)	Not reported	Not reported	Not reported
Kunstman et al,[63] 2012 (2003–2011)	ppPD 158 (67.2) Whipple 77 (32.8)	Overall 42/235 (17.9) Grade A 16 (6.8) Grade B 11 (4.7) Grade C 15 (6.4)	POPF[a] 9 (21.4)	Not reported	DGE (grades A–C) Intra-abdominal abscess POPF Pulmonary comorbidity Intraoperative blood loss

Study (study period)	Procedure (n, %)	POPF (n, %)	CR-POPF (n, %)	DGE (n, %)	Risk factors
Sakamoto et al,[54] 2011 (2004–2009)	ppPD 302 (78.0) Whipple/ssPD 85 (22.0)	Overall 188/387 (48.6) Grade A 118 (30.5) Grade B 38 (9.8) Grade C 32 (8.3)	CR-POPF 40 (21.3)	Not reported	DGE (grades B–C) Male gender CR-POPF Hand-sewn reconstruction
Parmar et al,[65] 2013 (2011–2012)	ppPD 304 (42.8) Whipple 387 (54.4) Total pancreatectomy 20 (2.8)	Overall 143/711 (20.1) (Not using ISGPS definition)[b]	POPF[c] 44 (31.2)	52 (36.4)	DGE POPF Postoperative sepsis Need for reoperation
Eisenberg et al,[64] 2015 (2006–2012)	ppPD 618 (85.7) Whipple 103 (14.3)	Overall 140/721 (19.4) Grade A 78 (10.8) Grade B 36 (5.0) Grade C 26 (3.6)	POPF 47 (33.6) CR-POPF 33 (23.6)	88 (12.2)	DGE (grades A–C) Abdominal infection Male gender Smoking history Periampullary carcinoma
Robinson et al,[51] 2015 (2000–2012)	ppPD 259 (62.3) Whipple 157 (37.7)	Overall 153/416 (36.8) Grade A 55 (13.2) Grade B 55 (13.2) Grade C 43 (10.4)	POPF 58 (59)[d] CR-POPF 51 (52)[d]	Not reported	DGE (grades B–C) Operating length >5.5 h BMI ≥35 Prophylactic octreotide use
Healy et al,[70] 2015 (2003–2013)	ppPD 219 (61.3) Whipple 138 (38.7)	Overall 52/357 (14.6) Grade A 22 (6.2) Grade B 13 (3.6) Grade C 17 (4.8)	CR-POPF 15 (28.8)	Not reported	Not reported

Abbreviations: ppPD, pylorus-preserving PD; ssPD, subtotal stomach-preserving PD.

[a] Unclear POPF definition.
[b] DGE defined as the need for gastric decompression for 7 days postoperatively or the absence of oral intake by POD 14.
[c] POPF defined as following: persistent drainage of amylase-rich fluid from an intraoperative drain or a clinical diagnosis; also require 1 of 3 following criteria: (1) drain in place longer than 7 days, (2) percutaneous drainage performed, and (3) reoperation performed.
[d] Only patients with DGE grades B–C are considered.

Data from Refs.[48–51,63–67,70]

applied. In line with these considerations, Reber suggested that "the diagnosis of DGE should require in every case the demonstration by a radiographic contrast study that the stomach is emptying at a slower rate than normal, and that there is no mechanical cause for the problem."[68] The addition of endoscopy or radiologic examination, however, as an absolute requirement to the ISGPS definition might limit its applicability according to some authorities.[69]

At the authors' institution, DGE is diagnosed through a triple-approach strategy, including CT, upper GI Gastrografin series, and endoscopy (**Fig. 2**).

Furthermore, several investigators expressed concern that the actual incidence of DGE is overestimated by the prolonged use of NGT in some clinical scenarios that are not directly correlated to a gastroparesis (ie, ileus). Welsch and colleagues[49] observed that a majority of patients with prolonged stay in the ICU received a diagnosis of DGE. This may more reasonably reflect the widespread use of NGT in the treatment of critically ill ICU patients, however, rather than the presence of true DGE. Other severe complications, such as relaparotomy and high-output pancreatic fistula as well as medical conditions (ie, postoperative pneumonia or pharyngeal dysfunction) may require prolonged fasting, leading to an incorrect diagnosis of DGE. An ongoing problem with the ISGPS definition is also its inability to differentiate true DGE from postoperative ileus[48] and technical problems at the anastomosis (stenosis and edema). To overcome these issues, Kunstman and colleagues[63] proposed a Yale modification to the ISGPS definition of DGE, excluding patients who required NGT replacement due to relaparotomy or reintubation or prolonged fasting for an objectively diagnosed non-DGE cause. A later work by the same group on an implemented cohort of patients further refined the criteria, including the evaluation of available radiological data. Although radiological assessment was not required for the diagnosis of DGE, patients without either gastric distention and/or normal passage of contrast into the small bowel were not considered as having DGE.[70] Yet, this proposal also leaves room for subjective interpretation. The recourse to imaging was not standardized and, because no standard definition of gastric distention after PD exists, it is assessed subjectively. Similarly, Eisenberg and colleagues[64] recently reclassified DGE as either primary (when primary gastric dismotility was strongly suspected) or

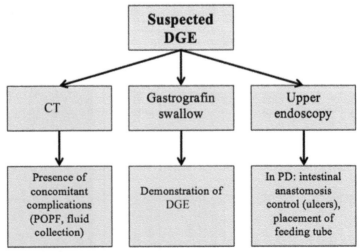

Fig. 2. Triple-approach diagnostic strategy for DGE.

secondary to a concomitant abdominal complication. The decision of whether DGE should be classified as primary or secondary was arbitrary, however, and was mainly based on the temporal association with the onset of the second complication.

A recent study based on the American College of Surgeons National Surgical Quality Improvement Program, analyzed 711 patients undergoing PD at 33 different institutions and considered both ISGPS-DGE and isolated DGE (in the absence of any other complication) as outcomes.[65] The incidence of grade B/C DGE was 20.1%, whereas isolated DGE occurred in only 53 patients (7.5%). At multivariate analysis, POPF, sepsis, and relaparotomy were related with ISGPS-DGE. When considering isolated DGE as an outcome measure, no significant association was found – again, underscoring its confounding origins.

In the absence of a clear understanding of the pathologic mechanisms responsible for DGE development, treatment remains mainly symptomatic, based on nasogastric decompression and fasting. Erythromycin has been proposed to augment gastric motility by binding to motilin receptors and triggering phase III of the gastric migratory motor complex. This action seems to be exerted at lower doses than those used for antibiotic effect.[71] Studies in patients undergoing PD revealed a 37% to 75% decrease in DGE incidence and an increased gastric motility when erythromycin was preventively administered.[72,73] Literature on the topic is scarce and dated, however, mainly extrapolated from gastroparesis studies, and indications to erythromycin administration (prophylactic vs therapeutic) and dosages remain undefined. Otherwise, the prophylactic use of somatostatin analogs has been studied prospectively in a randomized placebo-controlled trial and was shown to have no beneficial effect on DGE.[74]

Although the benefits of early EN over TPN after major abdominal surgery are well established, the specific impact of enteral feeding in DGE management is still largely undefined. Some studies supported the positive effects of EN on DGE prevention and treatment[75–77] whereas others have not shown any major advantages.[78,79] A recent retrospective study by the Indiana group compared outcomes between patients without DGE, those with DGE who received supplemental nutrition (EN and/or TPN) within 10 days after PD (early intervention), and those treated after 10 days (late intervention). The early intervention group resumed a regular diet sooner and were readmitted less than those in the late intervention group.[47] Given the observed strong association between DGE and other complications, especially POPF, many investigators claimed that POPF preventing strategies may be the key to mitigate DGE.[51]

In the authors' experience, in the setting of a defined clinical recovery pathway and a low average length of stay (7–8 days), clinically relevant DGE rates of approximately 10% have been observed. A vast majority of DGE are self-limiting and generally have minor effects on postoperative recovery. For instance, most patients manifest postoperative vomiting after initial tolerance of oral intake for a few days' duration. This is handled conservatively in approximately 75% of patients who require a downshift to nothing-by-mouth status with or without NGT decompression. After another few days, the resumption of oral intake can resume and more often than not it is adequately tolerated. The cost to the patient is an additional 3 to 5 days of hospital stay in most cases. A fraction of patients fail this original strategy and require resumption of this approach again. Only a rare group of patients with DGE (1%–5%) requires a long course of hospitalization (weeks) with extended parenteral feeding (TPN) and/or interventional measures (endoscopy and percutaneous endoscopic gastrostomy/jejunostomy tube placement). Chronic sequelae of DGE are exceedingly rare.

POSTPANCREATECTOMY HEMORRHAGE

With reported rates between 3% and 10% in most series,[80–87] PPH constitutes an uncommon but potentially devastating complication, accounting for a substantial proportion of mortality after pancreatic resection.[16] The ISGPS classification grading system (grades A, B, and C) is based on the time of onset (early or late), site of bleeding (intraluminal or extraluminal), and severity (mild or severe)[6] (**Table 6**).

Early hemorrhage, within 24 hours from the index operation, generally derives from a technical failure or an underlying coagulopathy and, if severe, is best managed with reexploration, because a surgically correctable source of bleeding is likely to be found.[82,83] Endoscopic approaches to early intraluminal PPH – especially in patients with pancreaticogastrostomy – have also been proposed, but are not favored by

Table 6
International Study Group of Pancreatic Surgery definition and grading system of postpancreatectomy hemorrhage

Grade	Time of Onset and Severity — Early (≤24 h)	Late (>24 h)	Clinical Condition	Therapeutic Consequences
A	Mild, intraluminal or extraluminal		Well	No
B	Severe, intraluminal, or extraluminal	Mild, intraluminal, or extraluminal	Often well/ intermediate, rarely life-threatening	Transfusion of fluid/ blood, intermediate/ICU, therapeutic endoscopy, embolization, and relaparotomy for early PPH
C		Severe, intraluminal, or extraluminal	Severely impaired and life threatening	Localization of bleeding, angiography and embolization, (endoscopy) or relaparotomy, and ICU

Severity of Postpancreatectomy Hemorrhage	Mild	Severe
Blood loss	Decrease in hemoglobin concentration by <3 g/dL	Decrease in hemoglobin concentration by ≥3 g/dL
Volume resuscitation/ blood transfusions	Volume resuscitation or blood transfusions (2–3 units packed cells within 24 h of end of operation or 1–3 units if later than 24 h after operation)	Clinically significant impairment (eg, tachycardia, hypotension, oliguria, and hypovolemic shock) and need for blood transfusion (>3 units packed cells)
Need for invasive (interventional or operative) treatment	No (endoscopic treatment of anastomotic bleeding may occur provided the other conditions apply)	Yes

Adapted from Wente MN, Veit JA, Bassi C, et al. Postpancreatectomy hemorrhage (PPH): an International Study Group of Pancreatic Surgery (ISGPS) definition. Surgery 2007;142:23; with permission.

most investigators due to the possible anastomotic damage consequent to GI insuf-flation.[81,84,85] After definitive reintervention, the subsequent postoperative course is, in most cases, uneventful. Late PPH is a highly threatening complication (mortality is up to 41% in some series)[79] and can occur many days or even weeks after the oper-ation, often after patients' discharge.[82,88] Late PPH has a complex pathogenesis, which includes surgical trauma (including vascular skeletonization during lymphade-nectomy), vascular erosion secondary to anastomotic leakage or intra-abdominal ab-scess, pseudoaneurysm formation, and intraluminal ulcerations. In the setting of a delayed hemorrhage, surgical access to the bleeding vessel is often difficult because of the overlying anastomosis as well as the presence of postsurgical adhesions.[89] The operative field can be made even more hostile when a second complication is present. For these reasons, interventional procedures (angiography or endoscopy depending on the location of the bleeding, intraluminal or extraluminal) are emerging as first-line treatment options for late PPH.[82,83,88] Open surgery is generally reserved for hemodynamically unstable patients or when an associated septic complication is pre-sent. In particular, interventional angiography has been associated with a high rate of control of arterial bleeding, up to 50% to 80% in different series.[83,90–92] In a recent large analysis, however, failure of nonoperative management occurred in 36% of pa-tients with late hemorrhage. This ultimately led to undesired emergency laparotomy,

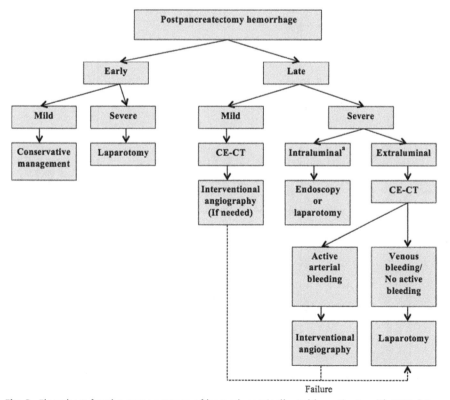

Fig. 3. Flowchart for the management of hemodynamically stable patients with PPH. [a] Per-formance of endoscopy versus relaparotomy in the first PODs is at surgeon's discretion. CE-CT, contrast-enhanced CT.

Table 7
Main literature reports of postpancreatectomy hemorrhage as defined by the International Study Group of Pancreatic Surgery

Reference (Study Period)	Type of Surgery	Incidence	Mortality	Association with Postoperative Pancreatic Fistula (%)	Differences in Postoperative Course Between International Study Group of Pancreatic Surgery Grades	Risk Factors for Postpancreatectomy Hemorrhage
Rajarathinam et al,[86] 2008 (1998–2007)	PD	Overall 14/458 (3.1) Grade A not reported Grade B 7 (1.6) Grade C 7 (1.6)	Overall 4 (29)[a]	Overall 8 (57)[a]		Not reported
Welsch et al,[81] 2011 (2001–2008)	PD	Overall 232/796 (29.1) Grade A 38 (4.8) Grade B 121 (15.2) Grade C 73 (9.2)	Overall 17 (7.2) Grade A 1 (2.6) Grade B 4 (3.3) Grade C 12 (16.4)	Overall 22 (9.3) Grade A 0 Grade B 4 (3.2) Grade C 18 (24.7)	A/B vs C	Early PPH Preoperative Hb <11 g/dL Multivisceral resection Late PPH Age ≥70 CRI Blood loss ≥1500 Operative time ≥420
Grützmann et al,[80] 2012 (1993–2009)	All pancreatic resections	Overall 54/945 (5.7) Grade A not reported Grade B 16 (1.7) Grade C 38 (4.0)	Overall 14 (25.9) Grade A not reported Grade B 1 (6.2) Grade C 13 (34.2)	Overall 28 (51.9) Grade A not reported Grade B 6 (37.5) Grade C 22 (57.9)	B vs C	Not reported

Study	Resection					Risk factors
Correa-Gallego et al,[82] 2012 (2006–2011)	All pancreatic resections	Overall 33/1122 (2.9) Grade A 0 Grade B 19 (1.7) Grade C 14 (1.2)	Overall 1 (3.0) — Grade B 0 (0) Grade C 1 (7.1)	Not reported	No difference between grades	Not reported
Wellner et al,[83] 2014 (1994–2012)	All pancreatic resections	Overall 78/1082 (7.2) Grades A/B 49 (4.5) Grade C 29 (2.7)	Overall 11 (14.1) Grades A/B 2 (4.1) Grade C 9 (31.0)	Overall 40 (51.3) Grades A/B 18 (36.7) Grade C 22 (75.9)	A/B vs C (mortality)	Grade C PPH Age BMI Male gender Intraoperative transfusion Portal venous resection Multivisceralresection POPF Learning Effect Preoperative biliary drainage (protective)
Ansari et al,[87] 2016 (2000–2015)	Whipple, distal pancreatectomy	Overall 68/500 (13.6) Grade A 34 (6.8) Grade B 15 (3.0) Grade C 19 (3.8)	Overall 2 (10.5) — — Grade C 2 (10.5)	Not reported	Not reported	Grade B/C PPH POPF grades B/C Biliary leakage

Abbreviations: CRI, chronic renal insufficiency; Hb, haemoglobin.

[a] PPH grades B/C.

Data from Refs.[80–83,86,87]

with a considerably increased mortality risk.[93] Delayed massive arterial hemorrhages may be preceded by mild, self-limiting bleeds (the so-called herald bleed) in approximately one-third of cases.[94] Despite not being immediately life-threatening to the patient, sentinel bleeds prompt the employment of an abdominal CT scan to exclude the presence of vascular lesions, such as arterial pseudoaneurysms. Given their harmful potential, immediate angiography has also been proposed as the initial tool for management of every detected sentinel bleed after PD,[91] but this is currently not a common practice. A current flowchart for the management of hemodynamically stable patients at the authors' institutions is depicted in **Fig. 3**.

Several studies have evaluated the validity and applicability of the ISGPS definition, with mixed results (**Table 7**). Grützmann and colleagues,[80] in their analysis of 54 patients with grade B/C PPH, described a good correlation between PPH grades and other complications (especially grade C POPF and DGE), mortality, and postoperative stay. Similarly, Welsch and colleagues[81] reported a significant increase in postoperative transfusion events, prevalence of POPF, duration of postoperative ICU stay, and rates of PPH-associated relaparotomy and mortality between grades A/B and grade C. The differences between grades A and B, however, were not significant.[81] On the contrary, in a recent work from the Memorial Sloan Kettering group, the ISGPS definition seemed unable to stratify patients in terms of outcome.[82] This inconsistency might be explained by the inherent limitations of the ISGPS definition. First, it is affected by oversensitivity in defining mild hemorrhage. A decrease in hemoglobin levels is frequently observed in the early perioperative period as a result of fluid management, especially in the ICU, and does not necessarily indicate the presence of bleeding. Moreover, indications for blood transfusion may vary among institutions, thus resulting in a certain rate of arbitrariness in the diagnosis. In the work by Welsch and colleagues,[81] a strict application of the ISGPS criteria revealed a very high incidence of PPH (29%); however, 97% of the patients with mild PPH had no clinical sign of bleeding. Due to its poor impact on clinical course, grade A PPH is not reported in some series[80,82,83] and probably underestimated by many others.

Moreover, the 24-hour limit used to define early bleeding might be overly stringent because the pathophysiology and management of bleeding within the first 72 postoperative hours are unlikely to differ. A final problematic issue concerns the definition of grade B PPH, which includes both early severe and late mild bleeding. These conditions might be too heterogeneous, however, in terms of pathogenesis, treatment, and impact on clinical course to be considered a single entity. In this context, a 4-grade classification, addressing separately early and late PPH according to their degree of severity, might be more appropriate and should be taken into account in any proposed future revision of the ISGPS definition.

SUMMARY

The introduction of common and worldwide-accepted definitions of postoperative complications by the ISGPS has allowed standardized reporting of surgical results. Despite significant improvements in surgical techniques and postoperative care, the overall morbidity rate has not diminished, presumably because indications for pancreatic resections have broadened to include high-risk diseases, such as cystic and neuroendocrine neoplasms. In addition, a growing number of adenocarcinomas are now resected after neoadjuvant therapy. This often requires complex procedures with vascular resections that may increase the risk of morbidity. The variability in the incidence of complications and the reported outcomes could be explained by patients' risk (ie, fistula risk through the FRS) and institutional practices regarding anastomotic techniques and fistula mitigation strategies. The management policies of these complications are most often driven by a patient's condition and local surgical expertise and is not always based on the available high-level, randomized evidence. Accordingly, comparisons of complication rates (especially of CR-POPF) between surgeons and institutions in a non–risk-adjusted setting could be disingenuous. The development of high-volume, specialized units with appropriate resources and multidisciplinary experience in complication management might further improve the evidence and the outcomes. This will likely be augmented by surgeon and institution performance assessment feedback practices.

REFERENCES

1. McMillan MT, Vollmer CM. Predictive factors for pancreatic fistula following pancreatectomy. Langenbecks Arch Surg 2014;399:811–24.
2. Malleo G, Pulvirenti A, Marchegiani G, et al. Diagnosis and management of postoperative pancreatic fistula. Langenbecks Arch Surg 2014;399:801–10.
3. Pratt WB, Maithel SK, Vanounou T, et al. Clinical and economic validation of the International Study Group of Pancreatic Fistula (ISGPF) classification scheme. Ann Surg 2007;245:443–51.
4. Bassi C, Dervenis C, Butturini G, et al. Postoperative pancreatic fistula: an international study group (ISGPF) definition. Surgery 2005;138:8–13.
5. Wente MN, Bassi C, Dervenis C, et al. Delayed gastric emptying (DGE) after pancreatic surgery: a suggested definition by the International Study Group of Pancreatic Surgery (ISGPS). Surgery 2007;142:761–8.
6. Wente MN, Veit JA, Bassi C, et al. Postpancreatectomy hemorrhage (PPH): an International Study Group of Pancreatic Surgery (ISGPS) definition. Surgery 2007; 142:20–5.
7. Daskalaki D, Butturini G, Molinari E, et al. A grading system can predict clinical and economic outcomes of pancreatic fistula after pancreaticoduodenectomy: results in 755 consecutive patients. Langenbecks Arch Surg 2011;396:91–8.
8. Dong X, Zhang B, Kang MX, et al. Analysis of pancreatic fistula according to the International Study Group on Pancreatic Fistula classification scheme for 294 patients who underwent pancreaticoduodenectomy in a single center. Pancreas 2011;40:222–8.
9. Liang TB, Bai XL, Zheng SS. Pancreatic fistula after pancreaticoduodenectomy: diagnosed according to International Study Group Pancreatic Fistula (ISGPF) definition. Pancreatology 2007;7:325–31.
10. Harnoss JC, Ulrich AB, Harnoss JM, et al. Use and results of consensus definitions in pancreatic surgery: a systematic review. Surgery 2014;155:47–57.
11. Pratt W, Maithel SK, Vanounou T, et al. Postoperative pancreatic fistulas are not equivalent after proximal, distal, and central pancreatectomy. J Gastrointest Surg 2006;10:1264–78.
12. McMillan MT, Christein JD, Callery MP, et al. Comparing the burden of pancreatic fistulas after pancreatoduodenectomy and distal pancreatectomy. Surgery 2015; 159:1–10.
13. Goudard Y, Gaujoux S, Dockmak S, et al. Reappraisal of central pancreatectomy: a 12-year single-center experience. JAMA Surg 2014;149:1–8.
14. Strasberg SM, Hall BL. Postoperative morbidity index: a quantitative measure of severity of postoperative complications. J Am Coll Surg 2011;213:616–26.

15. Miller BC, Christein JD, Behrman SW, et al. Assessing the impact of a fistula after a pancreaticoduodenectomy using the post-operative morbidity index. HPB (Oxford) 2013;15:781–8.

16. Vollmer CM Jr, Sanchez N, Gondek S, et al. A root-cause analysis of mortality following major pancreatectomy. J Gastrointest Surg 2012;16:89–102.

17. Gaujoux S, Cortes A, Couvelard A, et al. Fatty pancreas and increased body mass index are risk factors of pancreatic fistula after pancreaticoduodenectomy. Surgery 2010;148:15–23.

18. Wellner UF, Kayser G, Lapshyn H, et al. A simple scoring system based on clinical factors related to pancreatic texture predicts postoperative pancreatic fistula preoperatively. HPB (Oxford) 2010;12:696–702.

19. Yamamoto Y, Sakamoto Y, Nara S, et al. A preoperative predictive scoring system for postoperative pancreatic fistula after pancreaticoduodenectomy. World J Surg 2011;35:2747–55.

20. Callery MP, Pratt WB, Kent TS, et al. A prospectively validated clinical risk score accurately predicts pancreatic fistula after pancreatoduodenectomy. J Am Coll Surg 2013;216:1–14.

21. Miller BC, Christein JD, Behrman SW, et al. A multi-institutional external validation of the fistula risk score for pancreatoduodenectomy. J Gastrointest Surg 2014;18: 172–80.

22. Kunstman JW, Kuo E, Fonseca AL, et al. Evaluation of a recently described risk classification scheme for pancreatic fistulae development after pancreaticoduodenectomy without routine post-operative drainage. HPB (Oxford) 2014;16: 987–93.

23. Shubert CR, Wagie AE, Farnell MB, et al. Clinical risk score to predict pancreatic fistula after pancreatoduodenectomy: independent external validation for open and laparoscopic approaches. J Am Coll Surg 2015;221:689–98.

24. Graham JA, Kayser R, Smirniotopoulos J, et al. Probability prediction of a postoperative pancreatic fistula after a pancreaticoduodenectomy allows for more transparency with patients and can facilitate management of expectations. J Surg Oncol 2013;108:137–8.

25. Roberts KJ, Hodson J, Mehrzad H, et al. A preoperative predictive score of pancreatic fistula following pancreatoduodenectomy. HPB (Oxford) 2014;16: 620–8.

26. Chen JY, Feng J, Wang XQ, et al. Risk scoring system and predictor for clinically relevant pancreatic fistula after pancreaticoduodenectomy. World J Gastroenterol 2015;21:5926–33.

27. McMillan MT, Soi S, Asbun HJ, et al. Risk-adjusted outcomes of clinically relevant pancreatic fistula following pancreatoduodenectomy: a model for performance evaluation. Ann Surg 2016;264(2):344–52.

28. McMillan MT, Malleo G, Bassi C, et al. Defining the practice of pancreatoduodenectomy around the world. HPB (Oxford) 2015;17:1145–54.

29. McMillan MT, Fisher WE, Van Buren G, et al. The value of drains as a fistula mitigation strategy for pancreatoduodenectomy: something for everyone? Results of a randomized prospective multi-institutional study. J Gastrointest Surg 2014;19: 21–31.

30. Bassi C, Molinari E, Malleo G, et al. Early versus late drain removal after standard pancreatic resections: results of a prospective randomized trial. Ann Surg 2010; 252:207–14.

31. McMillan MT, Malleo G, Bassi C, et al. Drain management after pancreatoduodenectomy: reappraisal of a prospective randomized trial using risk stratification. J Am Coll Surg 2015;221:798–809.
32. McMillan MT, Malleo G, Bassi C, et al. A multicenter, prospective trial of drain management for pancreatoduodenectomy using risk stratification. Ann Surg 2016. [Epub ahead of print].
33. Raman SP, Horton KM, Cameron JL, et al. CT after pancreaticoduodenectomy: spectrum of normal findings and complications. AJR Am J Roentgenol 2013; 201:2–13.
34. Meier R, Ockenga J, Pertkiewicz M, et al. ESPEN guidelines on enteral nutrition: pancreas. Clin Nutr 2006;25:275–84.
35. Klek S, Sierzega M, Turczynowski L, et al. Enteral and parenteral nutrition in the conservative treatment of pancreatic fistula: a randomized clinical trial. Gastroenterology 2011;141:157–63.
36. Gans SL, van Westreenen HL, Kiewiet JJS, et al. Systematic review and meta-analysis of somatostatin analogues for the treatment of pancreatic fistula. Br J Surg 2012;99:754–60.
37. Sohn TA, Yeo CJ, Cameron JL, et al. Pancreaticoduodenectomy: role of interventional radiologists in managing patients and complications. J Gastrointest Surg 2003;7:209–19.
38. Sanjay P, Kellner M, Tait IS. The role of interventional radiology in the management of surgical complications after pancreatoduodenectomy. HPB (Oxford) 2012;14:812–7.
39. Munoz-Bongrand N, Sauvanet A, Denys A, et al. Conservative management of pancreatic fistula after pancreaticoduodenectomy with pancreaticogastrostomy. J Am Coll Surg 2004;199:198–203.
40. Reddymasu SC, Pakseresht K, Moloney B, et al. Incidence of pancreatic fistula after distal pancreatectomy and efficacy of endoscopic therapy for its management: results from a tertiary care center. Case Rep Gastroenterol 2013;7:332–9.
41. Bartoli E, Rebibo L, Robert B, et al. Efficacy of the double-pigtail stent as a conservative treatment for grade B pancreatic fistula after pancreatoduodenectomy with pancreatogastric anastomosis. Surg Endosc 2013;28:1528–34.
42. Fuks D, Piessen G, Huet E, et al. Life-threatening postoperative pancreatic fistula (grade C) after pancreaticoduodenectomy: incidence, prognosis, and risk factors. Am J Surg 2009;197:702–9.
43. Balzano G, Pecorelli N, Piemonti L, et al. Relaparotomy for a pancreatic fistula after a pancreaticoduodenectomy: a comparison of different surgical strategies. HPB (Oxford) 2014;16:40–5.
44. Standop J, Glowka T, Schmitz V, et al. Operative re-intervention following pancreatic head resection: indications and outcome. J Gastrointest Surg 2009;13: 1503–9.
45. McMillan MT, Vollmer CM, Asbun HJ, et al. The characterization and prediction of ISGPF grade C fistulas following pancreatoduodenectomy. J Gastrointest Surg 2016;20:262–76.
46. Glowka TR, von Websky M, Pantelis D, et al. Risk factors for delayed gastric emptying following distal pancreatectomy. Langenbecks Arch Surg 2016;401: 161–7.
47. Beane JD, House MG, Miller A, et al. Optimal management of delayed gastric emptying after pancreatectomy: an analysis of 1,089 patients. Surgery 2014; 156:939–48.

48. Malleo G, Crippa S, Butturini G, et al. Delayed gastric emptying after pylorus-preserving pancreaticoduodenectomy: validation of International Study Group of Pancreatic Surgery classification and analysis of risk factors. HPB (Oxford) 2010;12:610–8.

49. Welsch T, Bonn M, Degrate L, et al. Evaluation of the International Study Group of Pancreatic Surgery definition of delayed gastric emptying after pancreatoduodenectomy in a high-volume centre. Br J Surg 2010;97:1043–50.

50. Park JS, Hwang HK, Kim JK, et al. Clinical validation and risk factors for delayed gastric emptying based on the International Study Group of Pancreatic Surgery (ISGPS) classification. Surgery 2009;146:882–7.

51. Robinson JR, Marincola P, Shelton J, et al. Peri-operative risk factors for delayed gastric emptying after a pancreaticoduodenectomy. HPB (Oxford) 2015;17: 495–501.

52. Hüttner FJ, Fitzmaurice C, Schwarzer G, et al. Pylorus-preserving pancreaticoduodenectomy (pp Whipple) versus pancreaticoduodenectomy (classic Whipple) for surgical treatment of periampullary and pancreatic carcinoma. Cochrane Database Syst Rev 2016;(2):CD006053.

53. Joliat GR, Labgaa I, Demartines N, et al. Effect of antecolic versus retrocolic gastroenteric reconstruction after pancreaticoduodenectomy on delayed gastric emptying: a meta-analysis of six randomized controlled trials. Dig Surg 2016; 33:15–25.

54. Sakamoto Y, Yamamoto Y, Hata S, et al. Analysis of risk factors for delayed gastric emptying (DGE) after 387 pancreaticoduodenectomies with usage of 70 stapled reconstructions. J Gastrointest Surg 2011;15:1789–97.

55. Goei TH, van Berge Henegouwen MI, Slooff MJ, et al. Pylorus-preserving pancreatoduodenectomy: influence of a Billroth I versus a Billroth II type of reconstruction on gastric emptying. Dig Surg 2001;18:376–80.

56. Bassi C, Falconi M, Molinari E, et al. Reconstruction by pancreaticojejunostomy versus pancreaticogastrostomy following pancreatectomy: results of a comparative study. Ann Surg 2005;242:767–71.

57. Fernández-Cruz L, Cosa R, Blanco L, et al. Pancreatogastrostomy with gastric partition after pylorus-preserving pancreatoduodenectomy versus conventional pancreatojejunostomy: a prospective randomized study. Ann Surg 2008;248: 930–8.

58. Keck T, Wellner UF, Bahra M, et al. Pancreatogastrostomy versus pancreatojejunostomy for RECOnstruction after PANCreatoduodenectomy (RECOPANC, DRKS 00000767): Perioperative and Long-term Results of a Multicenter Randomized Controlled Trial. Ann Surg 2016;263:440–9.

59. Pessaux P, Sauvanet A, Mariette C, et al. External pancreatic duct stent decreases pancreatic fistula rate after pancreaticoduodenectomy. Ann Surg 2011; 253:879–85.

60. Walters DM, Shada AL, LaPar DJ, et al. A long gastrojejunostomy is associated with decreased incidence and severity of delayed gastric emptying after pancreaticoduodenectomy. Pancreas 2015;44:1273–9.

61. Watanabe Y, Ohtsuka T, Kimura H, et al. Braun enteroenterostomy reduces delayed gastric emptying after pylorus-preserving pancreatoduodenectomy: a retrospective review. Am J Surg 2015;209:369–77.

62. Ravikumar R, Sabin C, Hilal MA, et al. Portal vein resection in borderline resectable pancreatic cancer: a United Kingdom multicenter study. J Am Coll Surg 2014;218:401–11.

63. Kunstman JW, Fonseca AL, Ciarleglio MM, et al. Comprehensive analysis of variables affecting delayed gastric emptying following pancreaticoduodenectomy. J Gastrointest Surg 2012;16:1354–61.
64. Eisenberg JD, Rosato EL, Lavu H, et al. Delayed gastric emptying after pancreaticoduodenectomy: an analysis of risk factors and cost. J Gastrointest Surg 2015; 19:1572–80.
65. Parmar AD, Sheffield KM, Vargas GM, et al. Factors associated with delayed gastric emptying after pancreaticoduodenectomy. HPB (Oxford) 2013;15: 763–72.
66. Akizuki E, Kimura Y, Nobuoka T, et al. Reconsideration of postoperative oral intake tolerance after pancreaticoduodenectomy: prospective consecutive analysis of delayed gastric emptying according to the ISGPS definition and the amount of dietary intake. Ann Surg 2009;249:986–94.
67. Tan WJ, Kow AWC, Liau KH. Moving towards the New International Study Group for Pancreatic Surgery (ISGPS) definitions in pancreaticoduodenectomy: a comparison between the old and new. HPB (Oxford) 2011;13:566–72.
68. Reber HA. Delayed gastric emptying–what should be required for diagnosis? Surgery 2007;142:769–70.
69. Castillo CF. Consensus defining postpancreatectomy complications: an opportunity we cannot ignore. Surgery 2007;142:771–2.
70. Healy JM, Kunstman JW, Salem RR. Proposal and critical appraisal of exclusion criteria to the international study group for pancreatic surgery definition of delayed gastric emptying. J Am Coll Surg 2015;220:1036–43.
71. Lytras D, Paraskevas KI, Avgerinos C, et al. Therapeutic strategies for the management of delayed gastric emptying after pancreatic resection. Langenbecks Arch Surg 2007;392:1–12.
72. Ohwada S, Satoh Y, Kawate S, et al. Low-dose erythromycin reduces delayed gastric emptying and improves gastric motility after Billroth I pylorus-preserving pancreaticoduodenectomy. Ann Surg 2001;234:668–74.
73. Matsunaga H, Tanaka M, Takahata S, et al. Manometric evidence of improved early gastric stasis by erythromycin after pylorus-preserving pancreatoduodenectomy. World J Surg 2000;24:1236–41.
74. Kollmar O, Moussavian MR, Richter S, et al. Prophylactic octreotide and delayed gastric emptying after pancreaticoduodenectomy: results of a prospective randomized double-blinded placebo-controlled trial. Eur J Surg Oncol 2008;34: 868–75.
75. van Berge Henegouwen MI, Akkermans LM, van Gulik TM, et al. Prospective, randomized trial on the effect of cyclic versus continuous enteral nutrition on postoperative gastric function after pylorus-preserving pancreatoduodenectomy. Ann Surg 1997;226:677–85.
76. Rayar M, Sulpice L, Meunier B, et al. Enteral nutrition reduces delayed gastric emptying after standard pancreaticoduodenectomy with child reconstruction. J Gastrointest Surg 2012;16:1004–11.
77. Mack LA, Kaklamanos IG, Livingstone AS, et al. Gastric decompression and enteral feeding through a double-lumen gastrojejunostomy tube improves outcomes after pancreaticoduodenectomy. Ann Surg 2004;240:845–51.
78. Martignoni ME, Friess H, Sell F, et al. Enteral nutrition prolongs delayed gastric emptying in patients after Whipple resection. Am J Surg 2000;180:18–23.
79. Lermite E, Pessaux P, Brehant O, et al. Risk factors of pancreatic fistula and delayed gastric emptying after pancreaticoduodenectomy with pancreaticogastrostomy. J Am Coll Surg 2007;204:588–96.

80. Grützmann R, Rückert F, Hippe-Davies N, et al. Evaluation of the International Study Group of Pancreatic Surgery definition of post-pancreatectomy hemorrhage in a high-volume center. Surgery 2012;151:612–20.

81. Welsch T, Eisele H, Zschäbitz S, et al. Critical appraisal of the International Study Group of Pancreatic Surgery (ISGPS) consensus definition of postoperative hemorrhage after pancreatoduodenectomy. Langenbecks Arch Surg 2011;396: 783–91.

82. Correa-Gallego C, Brennan MF, D'Angelica MI, et al. Contemporary experience with postpancreatectomy hemorrhage: results of 1,122 patients resected between 2006 and 2011. J Am Coll Surg 2012;215:616–21.

83. Wellner UF, Kulemann B, Lapshyn H, et al. Postpancreatectomy hemorrhage-incidence, treatment, and risk factors in over 1,000 pancreatic resections. J Gastrointest Surg 2014;18:464–75.

84. Yekebas EF, Wolfram L, Cataldegirmen G, et al. Postpancreatectomy hemorrhage: diagnosis and treatment. Ann Surg 2007;246:269–80.

85. Eckardt AJ, Klein F, Adler A, et al. Management and outcomes of haemorrhage after pancreatogastrostomy versus pancreatojejunostomy. Br J Surg 2011;98: 1599–607.

86. Rajarathinam G, Kannan DG, Vimalraj V, et al. Post pancreaticoduodenectomy haemorrhage: outcome prediction based on new ISGPS clinical severity grading. HPB (Oxford) 2008;10:363–70.

87. Ansari D, Tingstedt B, Lindell G, et al. Hemorrhage after major pancreatic resection: incidence, risk factors, management, and outcome. Scand J Surg 2016. [Epub ahead of print].

88. Asai K, Zaydfudim V, Truty M, et al. Management of a delayed post-pancreatoduodenectomy haemorrhage using endovascular techniques. HPB (Oxford) 2015;17:902–8.

89. Roulin D, Cerantola Y, Demartines N, et al. Systematic review of delayed postoperative hemorrhage after pancreatic resection. J Gastrointest Surg 2011;15: 1055–62.

90. Beyer L, Bonmardion R, Marciano S, et al. Results of non-operative therapy for delayed hemorrhage after pancreaticoduodenectomy. J Gastrointest Surg 2009;13:922–8.

91. Tien YW, Wu YM, Liu KL, et al. Angiography is indicated for every sentinel bleed after pancreaticoduodenectomy. Ann Surg Oncol 2008;15:1855–61.

92. Limongelli P, Khorsandi SE, Pai M, et al. Management of delayed postoperative hemorrhage after pancreaticoduodenectomy: a meta-analysis. Arch Surg 2008; 143:1001–7.

93. Tol JA, Busch OR, Van Delden OM, et al. Shifting role of operative and nonoperative interventions in managing complications after pancreatoduodenectomy: what is the preferred intervention? Surgery 2014;156:622–31.

94. Brodsky JT, Turnbull AD. Arterial hemorrhage after pancreatoduodenectomy. The "sentinel bleed". Arch Surg 1991;126:1037–40.

Definition and Management of Borderline Resectable Pancreatic Cancer

 CrossMark

Jason W. Denbo, MD, Jason B. Fleming, MD*

KEYWORDS

- Borderline resectable pancreatic cancer • Definitions • Management
- Pancreatic ductal adenocarcinoma

KEY POINTS

- Pretreatment evaluation of patients can aid in accurate communication and treatment planning for patients with borderline resectable pancreatic cancer; many patients have technically resectable tumors but are not adequate candidates for surgery.
- Imaging using contrast-enhanced computed tomography is necessary to stage the patient and evaluate extrapancreatic extent of the primary tumor.
- Even though small variations in the definition of borderline resectable tumors exist, the surgeon remains responsible for the complete and safe resection of the primary tumor.
- Safe surgical resection requires detailed preoperative knowledge of pertinent vascular anatomy, careful retroperitoneal dissection, and vascular isolation before vascular resection if necessary.

INTRODUCTION

Recent genetic studies have shown that initial clinical evaluation of pancreatic ductal adenocarcinoma (PDAC) occurs very late in the natural history of the disease,[1] because only 10% to 20% of patients present with surgically resectable disease.[2–5]

Nevertheless, the possibility of a potentially curative surgical resection provides a powerful impetus toward surgical resection of all possible patients. The impetus must be governed by the discipline and insight necessary to perform a safe and oncologically effective pancreatic resection, which is just one part of a multidisciplinary effort engineered to achieve long-term patient survival.

Over the last several decades, particularly at high-volume centers, the postoperative mortality following pancreaticoduodenectomy (PD) has decreased from 30% to 1%.[6] However, despite these advances in surgical safety, patients with PDAC have

Disclosure: The authors have nothing to disclose.
Department of Surgical Oncology, The University of Texas MD Anderson Cancer Center, 1400 Pressler Street, Unit 1484, Houston, TX 77030, USA
* Corresponding author.
E-mail address: jbflemin@mdanderson.org

Surg Clin N Am 96 (2016) 1337–1350
http://dx.doi.org/10.1016/j.suc.2016.07.008
0039-6109/16/© 2016 Elsevier Inc. All rights reserved.

surgical.theclinics.com

not benefited from improved long-term survival when surgery is used as initial therapy.[3,6–8] Furthermore, despite multiple trials showing a survival benefit with adjuvant therapy,[7,9–11] up to 47% of patients treated with up-front surgical resection fail to receive any adjuvant therapy,[12] usually because of delayed postoperative recovery or early disease recurrence.[13,14] These pitfalls of surgery as primary therapy are amplified in borderline resectable (BR) patients for whom careful staging, meticulous patient evaluation, and preoperative therapy are necessary to identify the subset of patients most likely to benefit from the aggressive surgical procedures necessary for complete surgical resection.

IDENTIFICATION OF BORDERLINE RESECTABLE PATIENTS

Any patients with PDAC evaluated by a pancreatic surgeon may require a high-risk surgical procedure that offers the only chance of cure. A new diagnosis of PDAC is often made in patients with multiple underlying medical conditions of variable significance with respect to the risks of pancreatectomy. This high-stakes clinical scenario mandates that the surgeon uses an organized approach to ensure a thorough and efficient initial evaluation. The anatomic relationship of the tumor and critical vessels as determined by a pancreas protocol computed tomography (CT) scan is of crucial significance, but other nonanatomic factors must also be evaluated, such as suspicion for extrapancreatic disease, comorbidities, and functional status. Using this approach, the whole patient and not just tumors are classified as potentially resectable or borderline candidates for surgical resection of the primary tumor.

Our center has developed a systematic approach in which all patients with localized PDAC receive a physical examination, a review of laboratory studies, and radiographic imaging as part of a comprehensive evaluation in a surgical clinic. These data are then collated using a system denoted by the acronym ABC in which A refers to tumor anatomic considerations for surgery, B to cancer biology or stage; and C to patient condition or performance status and fitness for surgery (**Fig. 1**). In the course of treatment planning and communication across our multidisciplinary care team, patients are classified as clinically resectable (CR) or BR using the common nomenclature BR-A, BR-B, or BR-C.[15,16] BR-A patients have no major comorbidities, no clinical findings that are suspicious for extrapancreatic disease, and meet anatomic imaging criteria for a BR tumor, as outlined later. BR-B patients have no major comorbidities or anatomic imaging criteria for a borderline resectable tumor, and have clinical findings suspicious for extrapancreatic disease: (1) indeterminate liver lesions, (2) serum carbohydrate antigen 19-9 (CA19-9) level greater than or equal to 1000 U/mL in the setting of a normal bilirubin level, or (3) biopsy-proven involvement of regional lymph nodes. BR-C patients are advanced in age ($\geq$80 years old) or possess severe comorbidities requiring extensive evaluation or optimization, or depressed performance status (Eastern Cooperative Oncology Group [ECOG] $\geq$2). They may or may not have clinical findings suspicious for extrapancreatic disease.

In practice, the fitness of each patient for pancreatic surgery is evaluated first (see **Fig. 1**). Patients who are too frail for surgery secondary to uncorrectable comorbidities do not need to undergo extensive evaluation for surgical resection or consideration for preoperative therapy because surgical resection will not be the end result. These patients can therefore be efficiently triaged for palliative therapy or supportive care. If the patient is not currently fit for surgery, but has a potentially reversible condition, then medical optimization or prehabilitation during preoperative therapy is the goal. These patients are referred to as BR-C and are generally older (median age, 75 years) with a higher ECOG status (44% ECOG 2) usually secondary to

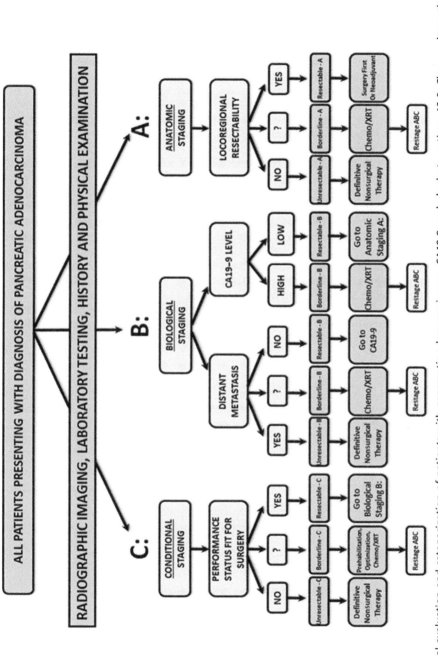

Fig. 1. Initial evaluation and categorization of patients with pancreatic adenocarcinoma. CA19-9, carbohydrate antigen 19-9; Chemo, chemotherapy; XRT, X-ray therapy.

cardiopulmonary disease (63%).[15] If the patient is fit for surgery, biological staging is next. Evidence of distant metastases on radiographic imaging is a contraindication to resection, but in many cases there are suspicious radiographic findings, but not diagnostic for distant metastatic disease. These patients are termed BR-B and receive chemotherapy followed by restaging. Similarly, patients with a high CA19-9 level (1,000 U/mL) even with negative imaging are considered BR-B and receive chemotherapy followed by restaging. In addition, local anatomic factors related to the primary tumor are considered in patients who are without metastases and are fit for surgery, which necessitates careful review of radiographic image using standard anatomic criteria designed to categorize tumors as resectable, borderline, or locally advanced. Patients who are fit for surgery with no evidence or suspicion of metastases and borderline tumors are considered BR-A, and usually receive chemotherapy plus or minus chemoradiation and restaging before proceeding with surgical resection.

Clinical application of this approach to the initial evaluation identifies that at least 50% of patients have borderline clinical features. When treated preoperatively, only 37% of BR-C patients can be expected to undergo resection, whereas the others fail to reach surgical resection because of poor performance status (31%) or interval identification of metastatic disease (26%). BR-C patients who undergo resection experienced a median survival of 38.6 months versus 13.3 months ($P = .02$) for those not receiving surgery. Roughly 46% of BR-B patients receive surgical resection after preoperative therapy and an equal portion (46%) have distant metastases precluding surgery. The loss of performance status is uncommon (4.9%) in BR-B patients. Resection conferred a 33-month median survival versus 11.8 months in those patients unable to proceed to resection ($P<.001$). Of note, local progression was rarely observed during preoperative therapy in either BR-B or BR-C patients (2.6%)[15,16] (**Fig. 2**). Management of patients with BR type A is considered later.

IMAGING

All patients with apparent localized disease are evaluated with a contrast-enhanced CT scan, which provides essential information about the presence of regional or distant metastases and the site and local extent of the primary tumor. This evaluation allows the surgeon to determine whether the patient has a resectable tumor and the likelihood of achieving a margin-negative resection. Multidetector row CT is the

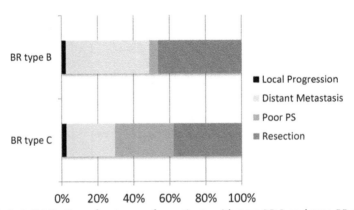

Fig. 2. Typical distribution of outcomes for patients with type BR-B and type BR-C treated with preoperative therapy. Identification of distant metastases or poor performance status (PS) is most common in patients with BR-B or BR-C, respectively.

most widely used staging modality for pancreas cancer and a workhorse for new patient evaluation. When performed and interpreted correctly, it provides valuable staging for both distant and regional metastases as well as local extrapancreatic extension of the primary tumor to adjacent critical vascular structures.[17] The National Comprehensive Cancer Network (NCCN) recommends that all patients with suspicion for PDAC have a dedicated pancreas protocol CT scan as part of the initial evaluation (Version 2.2015). At MD Anderson Cancer Center (MDACC), a pancreas protocol CT scan uses water as a negative oral contrast agent and starts with precontrast imaging from the dome of the liver extending caudally to include the entire liver reconstructed to 2.5-mm slice thickness. Next, 125 mL of iodinated contrast is administered intravenously at a rate of 3 to 5 mL/s. The pancreas phase/arterial phase uses bolus tracking and images are obtained 10 seconds after a Hounsfield unit value of 100 is reached in the aorta at the level at the celiac axis from the dome of the liver to the iliac crests. Images for the portal venous phase are obtained at a 20-second delay from the pancreas phase. Hepatic metastases are usually best visualized on the portal venous phase. Delayed images are obtained 15 seconds after the portal venous phase. The images are reconstructed to 2.5-mm slice thickness for imaging review and at 0.625-mm or 1.25-mm slice thickness to create coronal and sagittal reformatted images.[18]

The primary pancreatic tumor is best seen on the pancreas phase of the CT scan and is usually a hypodense mass, because the surrounding normal pancreatic parenchyma enhances. The pancreas phase/arterial phase illuminates the branches of the celiac axis and superior mesenteric artery (SMA), enabling clinicians to identify important arterial anatomy variants and discern whether the tumor has any arterial involvement. As many as 40% to 45% of patients have variants of normal hepatic arterial anatomy, which are of vital importance to appreciate on preoperative imaging because these variants can affect operative planning.[19] A replaced or accessory right hepatic artery is present in up to 15% of patients, and most commonly arises from the SMA and courses posterior to the pancreas and posterolateral to the bile duct. An additional 2.5% of patients have a replaced common hepatic artery (CHA) that arises from the SMA and follows a similar path to a replaced or accessory right hepatic artery. The superior mesenteric vein (SMV) and portal vein (PV) are best evaluated on the portal venous phase. The initial staging CT scan has 94% sensitivity and 84% specificity for determining vascular involvement, and the surgeon should carefully note the tumor-vein interface, vein contour, and/or deformity; there are multiple classification schemes that predict venous involvement based on imaging characteristics and these should be used for operative planning.[20–23] In addition, the surgeon should identify the location and relationship of the gastroepiploic vein, colic veins, inferior mesenteric vein (IMV), and jejunal/ileal branches of the SMV because these have variable courses and the drainage pattern directly affects the surgical options for reconstruction of the SMV-PV confluence, which can be expected in more than 40% of cases. Terminology that describes vascular involvement has become standardized and is reviewed in detail later. Vascular involvement of less than or equal to 180° of the circumference of the vessel is termed abutment. Vascular involvement greater than 180° of the circumference of the vessel is termed encasement. Properly staging patients and determining potential vascular involvement is a cornerstone of treatment planning and its importance cannot be overstated.[24]

DEFINITIONS OF RESECTABILITY

As patient assessment, imaging, and multidisciplinary treatment techniques for patients with localized PDAC were refined in the late 1990s, it became evident that this patient group included a spectrum of primary tumor types from removable to unresectable. To allow common classification, the multidisciplinary team at MDACC developed imaging criteria that are still in use that define CR tumors by (1) absence of extrapancreatic disease; (2) clear tissue plane between the tumor and the celiac axis, hepatic artery, and SMA; (3) a patent SMV-PV confluence, abutment, or encasement is allowed as long as the vessel is patent.[4,16,25] Locally advanced (LA) tumors are defined by (1) encasement of the celiac axis; (2) encasement of the hepatic artery with no options for vascular reconstruction; (3) encasement of the SMA greater than 180°; (4) occlusion of the SMV-PV confluence with no options for vascular reconstruction.[4,16,25] Patients who were classified as CR based on these imaging criteria were likely candidates for an R0 resection, whereas patients with LA tumors were unlikely to respond to chemotherapy and/or chemoradiation to a degree that would allow surgical resection; however, improved response to systemic therapy is occurring more frequently and has allowed patients with advanced tumors to undergo resection.

At present, NCCN defines resectable PDAC as a tumor with no contact of celiac axis, SMA, or CHA, and no contact with the SMV-PV or less than or equal to 180° contact without vein contour irregularity (Version 2.2015). LA PDAC of the head/uncinate process is a tumor that contacts the SMA greater than 180°, the celiac axis greater than 180°, the first jejunal SMA branch, the most proximal draining jejunal vein, or has unreconstructable SMV-PV involvement or occlusion. Tumors of the body/tail are LA when there is contact of greater than 180° with the SMA or celiac axis, contact with the aorta, or unreconstructable SMV-PV involvement or occlusion (Version 2.2015).

In 2001, Mehta and colleagues[26] described a group of marginally resectable patients who were treated with chemoradiation preoperatively in order to downstage the tumor and increase the likelihood of a margin-negative resection. Marginally resectable was defined as a tumor in which the perivascular fat plane was absent over 180° of the SMA, SMV, or PV and persisted for a length greater than 1 cm.[26] The NCCN adopted the term BR in 2006 to describe patients with localized tumors who blurred the distinction between CR and LA tumors. These patients were thought to be at higher risk of a margin-positive resection if up-front surgery was used; thus the NCCN suggested the use of preoperative therapy.

Over the last several years, several groups developed specific radiographic features to define BR PDAC. At MDACC, the imaging criteria used to define a BR tumor are (1) abutment of the celiac axis; (2) abutment of the hepatic artery or short-segment encasement; (3) abutment of the SMA less than or equal to 180°; (4) short-segment occlusion of the SMV-PV confluence amenable to resection and reconstruction.[4,16,25] The American Hepato-Pancreato-Biliary Association (AHPBA), the Society of Surgical Oncology (SSO), and the Society for Surgery of the Alimentary Tract (SSAT) define BR PDAC as tumors with no abutment or encasement of the celiac axis, short-segment abutment or encasement of the CHA amenable to reconstruction, abutment less than 180° of the SMA, or abutment with or without impingement or narrowing of the SMV-PV or encasement with or without occlusion with suitable vein proximal and distal to allow resection and reconstruction.[27,28] The difference between the MDACC and AHPBA/SSO/SSAT definitions depends on the extent of SMV-PV involvement that differentiates BR from resectable tumors. The NCCN definition for BR PDAC has changed multiple times over the years, but currently includes tumors of the head/uncinate process that contact the CHA without extension to the celiac axis or the hepatic artery bifurcation, contact less than or equal to 180° of the SMA, contact greater than 180° of the SMV or PV, contact less than or equal to 180° with a contour irregularity or thrombosis of the SMV-PV with suitable vessel proximal and distal that allows venous resection and reconstruction, or contact with inferior vena cava. Tumors of the body/tail are classified as BR when there is contact of less than or equal to 180° with the celiac axis or contact of greater than 180° with the celiac axis without involvement of the aorta and an intact and uninvolved gastroduodenal artery (Version 2.2015) (**Table 1**).

A current multi-institutional treatment trial investigating preoperative FOLFIRINOX (folinic acid, fluorouracil, irinotecan, oxaliplatin) and chemoradiation defines BR PDAC as radiographically localized tumors with 1 or more of the following: (1) an interface between the tumor and SMV-PV of greater than or equal to 180°, (2) short-segment occlusion of the SMV-PV with normal vein above and below that is amenable to resection and reconstruction, (3) short-segment interface between the tumor and hepatic artery with normal artery proximal and distal that is amenable to resection and reconstruction, (4) interface between the celiac axis or the SMA less than 180°.[29]

Although no consensus definition for BR has been reached, common themes can be appreciated. All BR criteria include statements regarding the ability or inability of the surgeon to reconstruct the SMV-PV or the hepatic artery involved with tumor. These statements imply that anatomic resectability depends heavily on the judgment and experience of the surgeon. The importance of this expertise cannot be overemphasized. In contrast, another common theme of borderline criteria is the exclusion of tumors involving greater than 180° of the SMA: a practice largely derived from the concept that tumor involvement of the nerves and periadventitial tissue reflects an aggressive tumor biology that likely cannot be overcome through surgical technique alone.

MANAGEMENT

Despite differences in definitions of BR PDAC, there is agreement that these patients are at a higher risk for margin-positive resection, and that preoperative therapy is prudent. Since initially described by Rich and Evans[30] in 1995, the potential benefits of preoperative therapy have been itemized and include (1) early treatment of

Table 1
Definitions of BR PDAC

	MDACC	AHPBA/SSO/SSAT	NCCN
CA	Abutment	No abutment or encasement	Contact ≤180°
CHA	Abutment of short-segment encasement	Short-segment abutment or encasement amenable to reconstruction	Contact without extension to celiac axis or hepatic artery bifurcation amenable to resection and reconstruction
SMA	Abutment <180°	Abutment <180°	Contact ≤180°
SMV/PV	Short-segment occlusion amenable to resection and reconstruction	Abutment >180° or occlusion amenable to resection and reconstruction	Contact of >180°, contact of ≤180° with irregularity of vein or thrombosis amenable to resection and reconstruction

Abbreviations: CA, celiac axis; CH, common hepatic artery; SMA, superior mesenteric artery; SMV/PV, superior mesenteric vein/portal vein.

micrometastatic disease; (2) higher proportion of patients receiving multimodal therapy; (3) select patients with localized disease and more favorable tumor biology, who are most likely to benefit from surgical resection; (4) increased likelihood of an R0 resection; and (5) smaller radiation fields with well-oxygenated tissue. At MDACC, all patients with BR PDAC receive chemotherapy, chemoradiation, or both before surgical resection. Chemotherapy regimens have continued to evolve over the years; currently, most patients receive either gemcitabine with nab-paclitaxel or FOLFIRINOX. External beam radiation therapy is used and consists of 50.5 Gy delivered in 28 fractions or 30 Gy in 10 fractions with a concomitant radiosensitizing dose of 5-fluorouracil, gemcitabine, or capecitabine. The most common treatment sequence for BR PDAC is 2 to 4 months of chemotherapy, followed by chemoradiation, and a 6-week treatment break before surgical resection. Patients are typically restaged every 2 months. Patients only undergo surgical resection if the operating surgeon and multidisciplinary treatment group reach consensus that pancreatectomy will safely achieve an R0 resection and provide a reasonable chance for cure.

Restaging should include a pancreas protocol CT scan and measurement of CA19-9. Katz and colleagues[31] evaluated the radiographic response, using response evaluation criteria in solid tumors (RECIST) criteria, of 129 patients with BR PDAC after completion of preoperative therapy (**Fig. 3**). The preoperative therapy consisted of gemcitabine-based chemotherapy followed by chemoradiation (30 Gy or 50.4 Gy) or chemoradiation alone. One-hundred and twenty-two patients completed therapy and were restaged, 84 (69%) had stable disease, 15 (12%) had a partial response, 23 (19%) had progressive disease (development of metastases, n = 21; primary tumor growth, n = 2), and no patient had a complete response. All patients were classified by the MDACC and AHPBA/SSO/SSAT definitions, and only 1 patient was downstaged, whereas approximately 80% remained at the same stage and 20% were upstaged.[31]

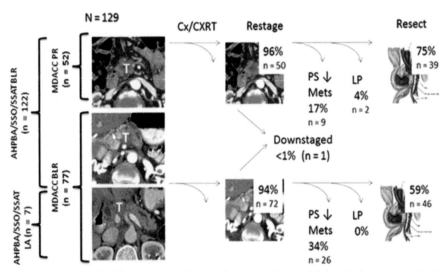

Fig. 3. Outcomes after preoperative therapy for 129 patients with borderline tumor criteria classified by AHPBA/SSO/SSAT and MDACC criteria. Regardless of criteria, local downstaging or progression is uncommon. After initial staging, 5 patients did not return for restaging for unclear reasons, possibly a decline in PS. BLR, borderline resectable; Cx, chemotherapy; CXRT, chemoradiation; LA, locally advanced; LP, local progression; PR, potentially resectable; PS, performance status.

The main purpose of a restaging CT scan is to rule out disease progression, not necessarily to look for downstaging. Donahue and colleagues[32] reported a series of patients with BR and LA pancreatobiliary malignancies who were treated with preoperative chemotherapy and were restaged with CT/MRI imaging, which only had a 71% sensitivity and 58% specificity for vascular involvement after completion of preoperative therapy.[32] Ferrone and colleagues[33] reported a series of patients with BR and LA PDAC treated with preoperative FOLFIRINOX with or without radiation therapy, and 30% were deemed resectable on posttreatment imaging. Most patients were still classified as LA (48%) and BR (22%), because there were no clear fat planes around the critical vascular structures. Nonetheless, an R0 resection was achieved in 92% of the patients.[33] Current cross-sectional imaging does not differentiate viable tumor from fibrosis.

Another important data point to consider during a restaging visit is the CA19-9 level. Tzeng and colleagues[34] compared pretreatment and posttreatment CA19-9 levels in patients with BR PDAC. All patients had a pretreatment CA19-9 level greater than or equal to 40 U/mL and a total bilirubin level less than or equal to 2 mg/dL. A decline in CA19-9 level was seen in 116 (82%) patients and 47 (33%) had normalization of CA19-9. Posttreatment CA19-9 level was a predictor of failure to undergo pancreatectomy. Normalization of CA19-9 level was associated with improved median overall survival in resected (38 vs 26 months, $P<.02$) and unresected patients (15 vs 11 months, $P = .02$).[34] After completion of preoperative chemotherapy/chemoradiation, patients without evidence of radiographic disease progression and a decrease in CA19-9 level should undergo attempted surgical resection, if medically fit for an operation.

The application of these management approaches is described in a recent report in which 160 patients with BR PDAC (BR-A 84, BR-B 44, BR-C 32) were followed prospectively. One-hundred and twenty-five (78%) patients completed induction therapy and a restaging evaluation. Forty-three patients were determined to not be surgical candidates: poor performance status (n = 10), distant disease progression (n = 16), and unresectable local-regional disease (n = 17). Seventy-nine patients were taken to the operating room, 9 were found to have radiographically occult distant metastases, 4 had LA disease, and the other 66 underwent a grossly complete resection of the primary tumor; 53% of the patients underwent restaging. Most underwent a PD (86%), 27% required an SMV-PV resection, and an additional 3% required a hepatic artery resection. An R0 resection was achieved in 94% of the patients, 4 patients had microscopically positive margins (2 SMA, 1 pancreatic duct, 1 bile duct). Twenty-six (39%) patients had nodal metastases. A partial or complete pathologic response (<50% remaining viable tumor cells) was seen in 56% of patients, and 4 patients (6%) had a complete pathologic response. Considering the cohort of 160 patients, 41% of patients underwent resection; the resection rates for BR-A, BR-B, and BR-C were 38%, 50%, and 38%, respectively. The median overall survival for the cohort was 18 months, with a 5-year survival of 18%. For the 66 patients who completed all therapy, the median survival was 40 months with a 5-year survival of 36%.[16] Together, these prospective data provide support for planned and ongoing single-institution and multi-institutional prospective studies evaluating this multidisciplinary approach for patients with BR PDAC.

SURGICAL TECHNIQUE

Once the decision to perform surgical resection is reached, the surgeon must adhere to certain principles necessary for safe and oncologically effective pancreatectomy, so that the patient has a chance for cure. There are several variables associated with improved patient survival after up-front surgical resection of localized PDAC. These variables include smaller tumor diameter, histologic grade (well differentiated or moderate differentiation), absence of lymph node metastases, negative surgical margins, and receipt of adjuvant therapy.[3,6,7] Although many of these variables are outside a surgeon's control, pathologically negative margins and a patient's ability to receive therapy after surgery are heavily influenced by surgical technique and postoperative morbidities. However, in large series, up to 42% of patients underwent a margin-positive PD.[2,6] A recent rapid autopsy series of patients with localized PDAC showed that 80% of patients treated with up-front surgical resection died with local recurrence, and 15% died of local recurrence alone.[35] Of note, 5 of 6 patients who underwent a positive-margin PD recurred locally.[35] A positive margin pancreatectomy should be viewed as a failure of patient selection, treatment strategy, and/or surgical technique. Routine use of planned segmental resection of the SMV-PV during PD was initially described in 1996 as a safe method of achieving negative margins when the primary tumor and SMV-PV interface were obliterated. Importantly, no difference in tumor biology or cancer-related outcome were observed suggesting that loss of the dissection plane between tumor and SMV-PV is an anatomic consequence more than an indicator of aggressive tumor biology.[36]

Performing a PD for a BR-A tumor requires a high level of technical expertise. The principles of oncologic and vascular surgery must simultaneously be applied in order to achieve the following surgical objectives:

1. Maintenance of hepatic artery blood flow
2. Exposure and meticulous dissection of the SMA
3. Preservation of portal venous flow from the stomach, spleen, and intestines, while minimizing the risk of sinistral portal hypertension[37]

Tumor encasement of the SMV-PV confluence is challenging, because it limits the exposure of the proximal SMA. During a procedure without vascular involvement, after the SMV-PV is freed from the pancreas and uncinate process, the venous confluence is retracted to the patient's left, so the proximal SMA can be exposed; this maneuver is not possible when there is encasement of the SMV-PV. When the SMV-PV is encased, division of the splenic vein allows retraction of the SMV-PV to the patient's right. Next, the periadvential plane on the SMA is accessed sharply caudal to the tumor and followed cephalad to the proximal portion of the SMA. After division of the remainder of the retroperitoneal tissues, the tumor and specimen are attached by only the SMV-PV confluence. After obtaining proximal and distal vascular control and heparinizing the patient, the vein is resected at a level to ensure negative margins but also being cognizant to preserve as much vein as possible. Portal venous flow can be restored with a primary venous anastomosis, vein patch, or internal jugular interposition, depending on the defect after venous resection. Resection of infiltrating tumors commonly requires ligation of the 3 main veins that drain the stomach: the coronary, right gastric, and right gastroepiploic veins. Venous outflow from the stomach can be comprised, especially after splenic vein ligation. If the IMV drains directly into the SMV, then we perform a splenorenal shunt to prevent sinistral hypertension. If the IMV drains into the splenic vein, then we do not perform a shunt, and rely on retrograde flow through the IMV.[38] Arterial resection can be necessary for tumors in the head of the pancreas that extend cephalad along the gastroduodenal artery to involve the common or proper hepatic arteries. In addition, an aberrant right hepatic artery or CHA arising from the SMA can easily be involved by a tumor in the head. The same principals discussed earlier for venous resection apply to arterial resection. After arterial resection, hepatic artery flow is restored with a saphenous vein interposition graft or polytetrafluoroethylene graft.[37,39]

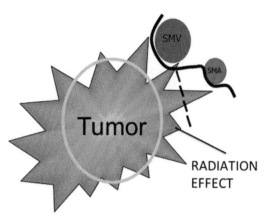

Fig. 4. The microscopic extent of pancreatic adenocarcinoma in the pancreatic head with respect to the SMV and SMA. The effect of radiation on tumor periphery is noted. The dark line represents the line of retroperitoneal surgical resection necessary to achieve a negative margin. (*Adapted from* a drawing courtesy of RA Wolff.)

The SMA margin is the margin that is most frequently positive after a PD.[40,41] As previously mentioned, the Johns Hopkins rapid autopsy series revealed that 80% of patients had evidence of local recurrence, and 15% had isolated local recurrence.[35] This finding highlights the importance of adherence to the surgical principals outlined earlier. Katz and colleagues[42] evaluated recurrence patterns in 194 patients with CR and BR PDAC with respect to the use of preoperative chemoradiation and SMA margin status. Fifteen (8%) patients had an R1 resection; the SMA margin was the most commonly involved margin. An additional 40 (22%) patients had a negative margin, but the margin distance was less than or equal to 1 mm. Patients who received preoperative chemoradiation had longer SMA margin distances ($P = .01$). Patients who underwent up-front surgical resection and had an SMA margin distance less than or equal to 1 mm had the highest overall (82%), locoregional (36%), and distant (50%) recurrence rates. CT scan overestimated the distance between the cancer and the SMA in 73% of cases. Liu and colleagues[43] found that the SMA margin distance is an independent predictor of both disease-free and overall survival in patients with PDAC treated with preoperative therapy. Adherence to meticulous surgical technique with periadvential SMA dissection and preoperative chemoradiation should be used to maximize the SMA margin (**Fig. 4**).

SUMMARY

Patients with BR PDAC represent a heterogeneous group of patients at high risk of regional and distant recurrence after therapy. The first step is to evaluate, accurately identify, and stage, so that a treatment plan can be derived accordingly for each patient. A multidisciplinary approach using preoperative chemotherapy and/or chemoradiation is necessary to select patients who are most likely to benefit from pancreatectomy. In the patients receiving surgery, a safe and oncologically sound resection of the primary tumor is achieved through meticulous retroperitoneal dissection and vascular resection if necessary. Postoperative recovery that allows additional systemic therapy provides patients with the greatest opportunity for long-term survival.

REFERENCES

1. Yachida S, Jones S, Bozic I, et al. Distant metastasis occurs late during the genetic evolution of pancreatic cancer. Nature 2010;467(7319):1114-7.
2. Cameron JL, Riall TS, Coleman J, et al. One thousand consecutive pancreaticoduodenectomies. Ann Surg 2006;244(1):10-5.
3. Lim JE, Chien MW, Earle CC. Prognostic factors following curative resection for pancreatic adenocarcinoma: a population-based, linked database analysis of 396 patients. Ann Surg 2003;237(1):74-85.
4. Varadhachary GR, Tamm EP, Crane C, et al. Borderline resectable pancreatic cancer. Curr Treat Options Gastroenterol 2005;8(5):377-84.
5. Katz MH, Wang H, Fleming JB, et al. Long-term survival after multidisciplinary management of resected pancreatic adenocarcinoma. Ann Surg Oncol 2009; 16(4):836-47.
6. Winter JM, Cameron JL, Campbell KA, et al. 1423 pancreaticoduodenectomies for pancreatic cancer: a single-institution experience. J Gastrointest Surg 2006; 10(9):1199-210 [discussion: 210-1].
7. Oettle H, Post S, Neuhaus P, et al. Adjuvant chemotherapy with gemcitabine vs observation in patients undergoing curative-intent resection of pancreatic cancer: a randomized controlled trial. JAMA 2007;297(3):267-77.
8. Klinkenbijl JH, Jeekel J, Sahmoud T, et al. Adjuvant radiotherapy and 5-fluorouracil after curative resection of cancer of the pancreas and periampullary region: phase III trial of the EORTC gastrointestinal tract cancer cooperative group. Ann Surg 1999;230(6):776-82 [discussion: 82-4].
9. Neoptolemos JP, Dunn JA, Stocken DD, et al. Adjuvant chemoradiotherapy and chemotherapy in resectable pancreatic cancer: a randomised controlled trial. Lancet 2001;358(9293):1576-85.
10. Oettle H, Neuhaus P, Hochhaus A, et al. Adjuvant chemotherapy with gemcitabine and long-term outcomes among patients with resected pancreatic cancer: the CONKO-001 randomized trial. JAMA 2013;310(14):1473-81.
11. Ueno H, Kosuge T, Matsuyama Y, et al. A randomised phase III trial comparing gemcitabine with surgery-only in patients with resected pancreatic cancer: Japanese Study Group of Adjuvant Therapy for Pancreatic Cancer. Br J Cancer 2009;101(6):908-15.
12. Hsu CC, Herman JM, Corsini MM, et al. Adjuvant chemoradiation for pancreatic adenocarcinoma: the Johns Hopkins Hospital-Mayo Clinic collaborative study. Ann Surg Oncol 2010;17(4):981-90.
13. Tzeng CW, Tran Cao HS, Lee JE, et al. Treatment sequencing for resectable pancreatic cancer: influence of early metastases and surgical complications on multimodality therapy completion and survival. J Gastrointest Surg 2014;18(1): 16-24 [discussion: 5].
14. Labori KJ, Katz MH, Tzeng CW, et al. Impact of early disease progression and surgical complications on adjuvant chemotherapy completion rates and survival in patients undergoing the surgery first approach for resectable pancreatic ductal adenocarcinoma - a population-based cohort study. Acta Oncol 2016; 55(3):265-77.
15. Tzeng CW, Fleming JB, Lee JE, et al. Defined clinical classifications are associated with outcome of patients with anatomically resectable pancreatic adenocarcinoma treated with neoadjuvant therapy. Ann Surg Oncol 2012;19(6):2045-53.

16. Katz MH, Pisters PW, Evans DB, et al. Borderline resectable pancreatic cancer: the importance of this emerging stage of disease. J Am Coll Surg 2008;206(5): 833–46 [discussion: 46–8].

17. Fuhrman GM, Charnsangavej C, Abbruzzese JL, et al. Thin-section contrast-enhanced computed tomography accurately predicts the resectability of malignant pancreatic neoplasms. Am J Surg 1994;167(1):104–11 [discussion: 11–3].

18. Balachandran A, Bhosale PR, Charnsangavej C, et al. Imaging of pancreatic neoplasms. Surg Oncol Clin North Am 2014;23(4):751–88.

19. Delbeke D, Pinson CW. Pancreatic tumors: role of imaging in the diagnosis, staging, and treatment. J Hepatobiliary Pancreat Surg 2004;11(1):4–10.

20. Karmazanovsky G, Fedorov V, Kubyshkin V, et al. Pancreatic head cancer: accuracy of CT in determination of resectability. Abdom Imaging 2005;30(4):488–500.

21. Ishikawa O, Ohigashi H, Imaoka S, et al. Preoperative indications for extended pancreatectomy for locally advanced pancreas cancer involving the portal vein. Ann Surg 1992;215(3):231–6.

22. Loyer EM, David CL, Dubrow RA, et al. Vascular involvement in pancreatic adenocarcinoma: reassessment by thin-section CT. Abdom Imaging 1996; 21(3):202–6.

23. Tran Cao HS, Balachandran A, Wang H, et al. Radiographic tumor-vein interface as a predictor of intraoperative, pathologic, and oncologic outcomes in resectable and borderline resectable pancreatic cancer. J Gastrointest Surg 2014; 18(2):269–78 [discussion: 78].

24. Al-Hawary MM, Francis IR, Chari ST, et al. Pancreatic ductal adenocarcinoma radiology reporting template: consensus statement of the Society of Abdominal Radiology and the American Pancreatic Association. Gastroenterology 2014; 146(1):291–304 e1.

25. Varadhachary GR, Tamm EP, Abbruzzese JL, et al. Borderline resectable pancreatic cancer: definitions, management, and role of preoperative therapy. Ann Surg Oncol 2006;13(8):1035–46.

26. Mehta VK, Fisher G, Ford JA, et al. Preoperative chemoradiation for marginally resectable adenocarcinoma of the pancreas. J Gastrointest Surg 2001;5(1): 27–35.

27. Callery MP, Chang KJ, Fishman EK, et al. Pretreatment assessment of resectable and borderline resectable pancreatic cancer: expert consensus statement. Ann Surg Oncol 2009;16(7):1727–33.

28. Landry J, Catalano PJ, Staley C, et al. Randomized phase II study of gemcitabine plus radiotherapy versus gemcitabine, 5-fluorouracil, and cisplatin followed by radiotherapy and 5-fluorouracil for patients with locally advanced, potentially resectable pancreatic adenocarcinoma. J Surg Oncol 2010;101(7):587–92.

29. Katz MH, Marsh R, Herman JM, et al. Borderline resectable pancreatic cancer: need for standardization and methods for optimal clinical trial design. Ann Surg Oncol 2013;20(8):2787–95.

30. Rich TA, Evans DB. Preoperative combined modality therapy for pancreatic cancer. World J Surg 1995;19(2):264–9.

31. Katz MH, Fleming JB, Bhosale P, et al. Response of borderline resectable pancreatic cancer to neoadjuvant therapy is not reflected by radiographic indicators. Cancer 2012;118(23):5749–56.

32. Donahue TR, Isacoff WH, Hines OJ, et al. Downstaging chemotherapy and alteration in the classic computed tomography/magnetic resonance imaging signs of vascular involvement in patients with pancreaticobiliary malignant tumors: influence on patient selection for surgery. Arch Surg 2011;146(7):836–43.

33. Ferrone CR, Marchegiani G, Hong TS, et al. Radiological and surgical implications of neoadjuvant treatment with FOLFIRINOX for locally advanced and borderline resectable pancreatic cancer. Ann Surg 2015;261(1):12–7.

34. Tzeng CW, Balachandran A, Ahmad M, et al. Serum carbohydrate antigen 19-9 represents a marker of response to neoadjuvant therapy in patients with borderline resectable pancreatic cancer. HPB (Oxford) 2014;16(5):430–8.

35. Iacobuzio-Donahue CA, Fu B, Yachida S, et al. DPC4 gene status of the primary carcinoma correlates with patterns of failure in patients with pancreatic cancer. J Clin Oncol 2009;27(11):1806–13.

36. Fuhrman GM, Leach SD, Staley CA, et al. Rationale for en bloc vein resection in the treatment of pancreatic adenocarcinoma adherent to the superior mesenteric-portal vein confluence. Pancreatic Tumor Study Group. Ann Surg 1996;223(2):154–62.

37. Katz MH, Lee JE, Pisters PW, et al. Retroperitoneal dissection in patients with borderline resectable pancreatic cancer: operative principles and techniques. J Am Coll Surg 2012;215(2):e11–8.

38. Katz MH, Fleming JB, Pisters PW, et al. Anatomy of the superior mesenteric vein with special reference to the surgical management of first-order branch involvement at pancreaticoduodenectomy. Ann Surg 2008;248(6):1098–102.

39. Tseng JF, Raut CP, Lee JE, et al. Pancreaticoduodenectomy with vascular resection: margin status and survival duration. J Gastrointest Surg 2004;8(8):935–49 [discussion: 49–50].

40. Raut CP, Tseng JF, Sun CC, et al. Impact of resection status on pattern of failure and survival after pancreaticoduodenectomy for pancreatic adenocarcinoma. Ann Surg 2007;246(1):52–60.

41. Katz MH, Merchant NB, Brower S, et al. Standardization of surgical and pathologic variables is needed in multicenter trials of adjuvant therapy for pancreatic cancer: results from the ACOSOG Z5031 trial. Ann Surg Oncol 2011;18(2): 337–44.

42. Katz MH, Wang H, Balachandran A, et al. Effect of neoadjuvant chemoradiation and surgical technique on recurrence of localized pancreatic cancer. J Gastrointest Surg 2012;16(1):68–78 [discussion: 78–9].

43. Liu L, Katz MH, Lee SM, et al. Superior mesenteric artery margin of posttherapy pancreaticoduodenectomy and prognosis in patients with pancreatic ductal adenocarcinoma. Am J Surg Pathol 2015;39(10):1395–403.

Techniques of Vascular Resection and Reconstruction in Pancreatic Cancer

George Younan, MD, Susan Tsai, MD, MHS, Douglas B. Evans, MD,
Kathleen K. Christians, MD*

KEYWORDS

- Pancreaticoduodenectomy • Vascular resection • Vascular reconstruction • Whipple

KEY POINTS

- Accurate staging and stage-specific therapy are used by a multidisciplinary team.
- Neoadjuvant treatment response (in contrast to disease progression) is associated with increased survival duration and predicts successful surgery.
- Vascular resections, whether venous or arterial, must be planned events (in contrast to an intraoperative surprise) for best possible outcomes.
- In situations of cavernous transformation of the portal vein, diversion of mesenteric flow before beginning the portal dissection is critically important to the performance of a safe operation.
- Revascularization of the common hepatic artery during an Appleby procedure lowers the risk of biliary/hepatic ischemia and gastric atony.

INTRODUCTION

Vascular resection during pancreatectomy was performed within two decades from Whipple and coworkers[1] first description of pancreaticoduodenectomy (PD) in 1935. The concept of "regional pancreatectomy" subsequently led by Fortner in the early 1970s failed to improve outcomes because wide tissue and lymphatic clearance around the tumor did not improve patient survival.[2–5] Vascular resections are currently performed to obtain an R0 margin during PD when the only area that prevents a gross complete resection of the tumor is vascular involvement otherwise amenable to

Conflict of Interest: None.
Pancreatic Cancer Program, Division of Surgical Oncology, Department of Surgery, Medical College of Wisconsin, 9200 W Wisconsin Ave, Milwaukee, WI 53226, USA
* Corresponding author. Department of Surgery, Medical College of Wisconsin, 9200 West Wisconsin Avenue, Milwaukee, WI 53226.
E-mail address: kchristi@mcw.edu

Surg Clin N Am 96 (2016) 1351–1370
http://dx.doi.org/10.1016/j.suc.2016.07.005
surgical.theclinics.com

reconstruction. Even in the pre–neoadjuvant treatment era, venous resections for isolated vein involvement conferred a 2-year survival benefit.[6–8] After the American Hepato-Pancreato-Biliary Association/Society of Surgical Oncology consensus statement in 2009, PD with venous resection and reconstruction became the standard of care in the treatment of pancreatic adenocarcinoma.[9] Arterial resection and reconstruction during PD was also part of the early regional pancreatectomy approach; however, enthusiasm for these procedures was lost because of technical difficulties of the operation, resulting in higher morbidity and mortality. With the improved surgical techniques available in specialized centers, arterial resections in appropriately selected patients have once again been adopted and proven to be safe.[10–12]

In addition to technical advances in surgery, advances in systemic chemotherapy have also resulted in improved response rates and prolonged survival.[13–18] Patients with borderline resectable pancreatic adenocarcinoma should be offered neoadjuvant systemic chemotherapy and/or chemoradiation based on all nationally recognized guidelines.[16,18,19] Multiple centers are now also starting to offer neoadjuvant therapy for resectable pancreatic cancer, representing a shift in the treatment paradigm in recognition of significantly improved survival rates recently reported with this approach.[17] The improved response rate to current chemotherapy regimens (FOLFIRINOX, gemcitabine-abraxane, GTX) has rendered patients, initially deemed unresectable, to be considered for resection.[13,14] There are increasing numbers of reports touting the positive effect of neoadjuvant therapy on margin status, lymph node positivity, and tumor response.[16] Neoadjuvant therapy allows for selection of patients with biologically responsive tumors to be considered for major vascular resection and reconstruction with curative intent.[17]

This article describes the technical aspects of these major operations, including accurate preoperative staging and planning, the technical aspects of venous and arterial resection and reconstruction during pancreatectomy, and key points of the perioperative care of these patients.

PREOPERATIVE PLANNING

Inherent in the planning for vascular resection during pancreatectomy is preoperative staging and the delineation of vascular involvement by the tumor. A computed tomography (CT)-based staging system for pancreatic cancer has been developed at the Medical College of Wisconsin and cited in national consensus guidelines (**Table 1**).[9,20,21] A multidisciplinary team approach to any new diagnosis of pancreas cancer is the foundation of success.[18] All team members follow the same principles to optimize and efficiently administer all intended parts of the treatment program. Key principles of this program are discussed next.

Clinical Staging

High-definition cross-sectional imaging is the mainstay for defining tumor-vessel relationships and aberrant vascular anatomy. Multidetector, dual-phase, contrast-enhanced CT provides accurate clinical staging based on reproducible anatomic relationships. The tumor is defined and classified as being resectable, borderline resectable, locally advanced A/B, or metastatic.[13] In a resectable tumor, there is no evidence of arterial involvement (abutment or encasement) and tumor-induced narrowing of the portal vein (PV), superior mesenteric vein (SMV), or PV-SMV confluence, if present, is less than 50% (**Fig. 1**). Borderline resectable tumors include tumors with abutment of the superior mesenteric artery (SMA) and celiac artery (CA) of 180° or less and/or short-segment encasement of the common hepatic artery (CHA) amenable for

Table 1
CT-based staging system for pancreatic cancer from the Medical College of Wisconsin

	RPC	BRPC	LAPC-A	LAPC-B
Tumor-artery relationship	No arterial abutment of CA, SMA, or HA	CA/SMA abutment <180°, HA abutment or short-segment encasement without CA involvement	SMA encasement >180° but <270°, CA encasement >180° without involvement of aorta, HA encasement involving the CA with target for reconstruction	SMA encasement >270°, CA encasement >180° with involvement of aorta, HA encasement involving the CA without target for reconstruction
Tumor-vein relationship	Vein (PV, SMV, PV-SMV) abutment and/or narrowing <50%	Vein (PV, SMV, PV-SMV) narrowing >50% with target for reconstruction	Vein (PV, SMV, PV-SMV) narrowing >50% without target for reconstruction	Vein (PV, SMV, PV-SMV) narrowing >50% without target for reconstruction
Extrapancreatic disease	No evidence of distant metastasis	Suspicious, nondiagnostic evidence of metastasis	No evidence of distant metastasis	No evidence of distant metastasis

Abbreviations: BRPC, borderline resectable pancreas cancer; CA, celiac artery; HA, hepatic artery; LAPC-A, locally advanced pancreas cancer type A; LAPC-B, locally advanced pancreas cancer type B; PV, portal vein; RPC, resectable pancreas cancer; SMA, superior mesenteric; SMV, superior mesenteric vein.
Data from Refs.[9,20,21]

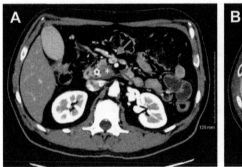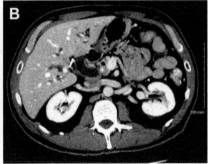

Fig. 1. Computed tomography axial images of resectable pancreas cancer. (*A*) Tumor in the uncinate process of the pancreas (*asterisk*); a fat plane is present between the tumor and the superior mesenteric artery (SMA, *red arrow*), and the SMV (*blue arrow*). (*B*) There is less than 50% lateral tumor abutment of the SMV and no extension to the SMA.

reconstruction. Tumors in this category also include those that narrow the SMV greater than 50% or those with short-segment occlusion of the PV, SMV, or SMV-PV confluence, with a proximal and distal venous target to allow for reconstruction. Patients who have indeterminate extrapancreatic lesions on CT scan that are worrisome, but not proven to be metastases, are also classified as borderline resectable tumors. Patients with a borderline performance status (surgical candidacy is a question at the time of diagnosis because of disease-related factors or patient comorbidities) are also considered borderline resectable because performance status alone has been correlated with disease progression and survival (**Fig. 2**).[19] In locally advanced tumors, there is greater than 180° (encasement) of the SMA or CA, nonreconstructable hepatic artery encasement, or encasement/occlusion of the PV, SMV, or SMV-PV confluence that is not amenable to reconstruction. We recently further divided locally advanced tumors into types A and B. Type A tumors can potentially be resected after a favorable response to neoadjuvant treatment. These tumors have greater than 180° but less than 270° encasement of the SMA (pancreatic head and uncinate tumors), or greater than 180° encasement of the CA without involvement of the aorta (usually pancreatic body tumors). Anything beyond these parameters is classified as locally advanced type B, and patients with these tumors are not typically considered for surgery regardless of the extent of treatment response following neoadjuvant therapy (**Figs. 3** and **4**).

Tissue Diagnosis and Biliary Drainage

Initiation of chemotherapy or radiotherapy is based on a tissue diagnosis of cancer and normalization of liver function tests, in particular, serum bilirubin. Therefore, an experienced gastroenterology team with on-site cytopathology is required for an endoscopic ultrasound-guided fine-needle aspiration biopsy of the tumor. Once the tissue diagnosis is confirmed, endoscopic retrograde cholangiopancreatography with placement of a durable self-expandable metallic biliary stent is completed.[22]

Restaging and Treatment Response

Patients are enrolled in stage-specific chemotherapy and/or chemoradiation protocols whenever possible. Patients with resectable pancreas cancer receive chemotherapy or chemoradiation before surgery. Patients with borderline resectable disease, by definition, have more advanced disease and require more complex operations. These

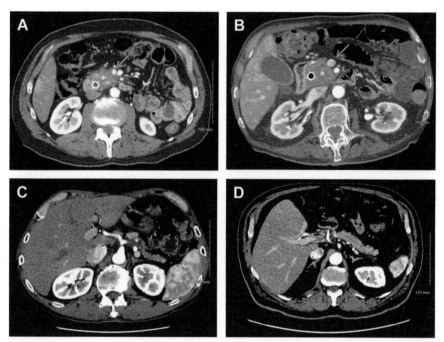

Fig. 2. Computed tomography axial images representing borderline resectable pancreas cancer. (*A*) Narrowing of greater than 50% of the SMV (*blue arrow*). (*B*) Abutment of the SMA (*red arrow*) of less than 180°. (*C*) CA (*red arrow*) abutment of less than 180°. (*D*) Short-segment encasement of the CHA (*red arrow*) amenable to reconstruction. Tumor is marked by *asterisk*.

patients are therefore treated with an extended period of induction therapy, usually including radiation. Most tumor-vessel relationships remain unchanged after neoadjuvant therapy despite a reduction in overall tumor size. Patients are evaluated and restaged with CT and tumor markers after completion of each phase of their neoadjuvant treatment program. Progression toward surgery depends on the favorable response of the disease (lack of distant disease progression) and the local tumor (absence of local progression and it is hoped a response as measured by a decrease in tumor diameter) to neoadjuvant therapy. We have defined treatment response based on three criteria: (1) clinical, (2) biochemical, and (3) radiographic response.

Patients are then classified into responders, nonresponders, and those with stable disease. Clinical assessment includes performance status and pain. We use serum levels of CA 19-9 for biochemical assessment of tumor response (additional serum markers are under active investigation). The CA 19-9 level is measured in all patients after diagnosis (and after normalization of their serum bilirubin) and is also rechecked at each restaging evaluation. A decrease in CA 19-9 levels has been associated with improved survival.[23,24] An increase of CA 19-9 at restaging is often an accurate marker of disease progression. Clinicians should have a low threshold to expand the restaging work-up before surgery in the event of a rising CA 19-9. Finally, radiographic restaging is completed after each phase of neoadjuvant therapy (usually every 2 months) and before surgery (within 4 weeks of surgery) to reassess tumor-vessel relationships as a guide to the possible need for vascular resection/reconstruction. A CT scan is also required after any endoscopic intervention to assess for possible inflammatory (pancreatitis) changes post–endoscopic retrograde cholangiopancreatography that

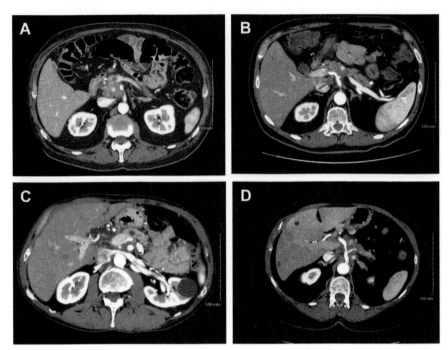

Fig. 3. Computed tomography axial images representing locally advanced pancreas cancer. (*A*) Locally advanced type A tumor with SMA (*arrow*) encasement greater than 180° but less than 270°. (*B*) Locally advanced type A tumor with celiac axis (*red arrow*) encasement greater than 180° without involvement of the aorta. (*C*) Locally advanced type B tumor with SMA (*arrow*) encasement greater than 270°. (*D*) Locally advanced type B tumor with celiac axis (*arrow*) encasement extending to the aorta. Tumor is marked by *asterisk*.

may delay surgery; we would never operate on a patient after an interventional procedure in the absence of a repeat CT scan.

Patients are seen in clinic for their final restaging just before surgery. Medical clearance with explicit definition and optimization of comorbidities is obtained with special

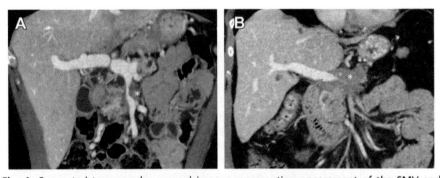

Fig. 4. Computed tomography coronal images representing encasement of the SMV and SMV-PV confluence. (*A*) Greater than 50% narrowing of the SMV-PV confluence (*arrow*) with a distal vein suitable for reconstruction. (*B*) Greater than 50% narrowing of the SMV-PV confluence, however without a distal vein that is suitable for reconstruction. Tumor is marked by *asterisk*.

reference to cardiac function. Attention is also paid to routine health maintenance and we prefer that patients have had a colonoscopy within the last 5 to 10 years based on personal/family history. Additional individualized imaging pertaining to specific clinical scenarios is obtained (ie, MRI or PET scans to rule out metastatic disease). Patients are consented for pancreatectomy and feeding jejunostomy tube insertion. Consent is also obtained for the harvest of the internal jugular vein and/or saphenous vein for vascular reconstruction. Venous mapping studies may be obtained preoperatively if needed. All patients undergo light bowel preparation the day before surgery.

SURGICAL APPROACH

Prophylactic antibiotics are given within an hour of the incision time. Central venous access is avoided in the left neck to preserve the internal jugular conduit for venous reconstruction. If the patients have power ports used for chemotherapy, these are accessed in the preoperative holding area for use during the operation. The left neck and groin are prepared along with the abdomen if vascular resection is anticipated. We perform a detailed "time out" procedure during which we review important tumor-vessel considerations and rereview the CT images. A detailed preoperative note completed by the attending surgeon reviews indications for surgery and the planned operative approach. A diagnostic laparoscopy is always performed before an open exploration to rule out extrapancreatic disease that is radiologically occult and thereby avoid an open laparotomy that provides no oncologic benefit to the patient.[25] Pancreatectomies are performed as we have described previously.[26] Nuances pertaining to anatomy and surgical techniques for vascular resection and reconstruction are described next.

Venous Resection and Reconstruction

Venous anatomy
Understanding the mesenteric venous anatomy during pancreatectomy is critical. The SMV joins the splenic vein posterior to the pancreas neck to form the PV. The SMV drains the midgut through two first-order branches; the proximal small bowel is drained by the jejunal branch and the distal small bowel and proximal colon are drained by the ileal branch. The jejunal branch normally arises from the posteromedial aspect of the SMV and courses posterior to the SMA, whereas the ileal branch travels in a cranial-caudal direction in the anterior root of the small bowel mesentery. The inferior mesenteric vein (IMV) drains the distal colon and travels in a cranial-caudal direction, just lateral to the ligament of Treitz, frequently joining the distal splenic vein. The IMV may, however, enter the SMV directly, just below the SMV-PV confluence. The common trunk of the SMV has two early anterior branches at the level of the transverse mesocolon: the middle colic vein and the gastroepiploic vein, which may arise separately, or together, as the gastrocolic trunk of Henle (**Fig. 5**).[27]

Reconstruction guidelines: portal vein and superior mesenteric vein
When pancreatic tumors involve the PV, SMV, or PV-SMV confluence, venous resection and reconstruction are required.[9] High-quality axial imaging with three-dimensional vascular reconstructions helps to accurately predict vascular involvement and allows the surgeon to plan the operation with the goal of avoiding intraoperative technical misadventures. The types of venous resection and reconstruction have been published[8,28] and are classified as follows: lateral venorrhaphy and primary repair (VR0), tangential resection with saphenous vein patch (VR1), segmental resection with splenic vein ligation and either primary anastomosis (VR2) or an interposition

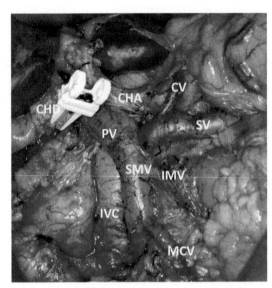

Fig. 5. Intraoperative photograph of mesenteric venous anatomy. In this particular patient, the IMV drains directly into the SMV. CHD, common hepatic duct; CV, coronary vein; IVC, inferior vena cava; MCV, middle colic vein; SV, splenic vein.

graft (VR3), or segmental resection with splenic vein preservation and either primary anastomosis (VR4) or an interposition graft (VR5) (**Fig. 6**).

At the time of operation, surgical judgment is used to decide if venous resection is needed or if the tumor in the pancreatic head can be separated from the PV, SMV, or

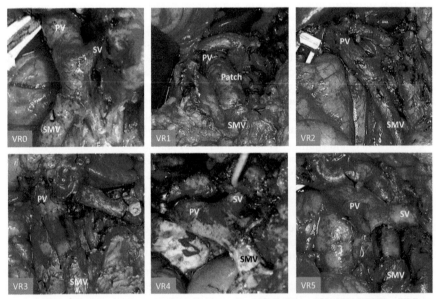

Fig. 6. Types of venous reconstructions: lateral venorrhaphy and primary repair (VR0), tangential resection with saphenous vein patch (VR1), segmental resection with splenic vein ligation and either primary anastomosis (VR2) or an interposition graft (VR3), or segmental resection with splenic vein preservation and either primary anastomosis (VR4) or an interposition graft (VR5).

the PV-SMV confluence without leaving residual disease on or within the vein. Sometimes this requires obtaining proximal and distal control followed by a trial dissection. If the tumor does not separate from the vein, then venous resection is needed. We frequently use an artery (SMA)-first approach, which requires cutting through tissue medial to the SMV down to the level of the SMA and removing all of the soft tissue to the right of the SMA (**Fig. 7**).[29] This leaves the PD specimen attached to the patient only at the site of tumor-vein adherence. Historically, this approach involved ligation of the splenic vein to not only gain improved access to the SMA but also to allow primary repair of the PV or SMV. If the splenic vein is preserved, an interposition graft is needed if the resected vein segment is more than 2 to 3 cm; otherwise, the reconstruction is often placed on undo tension (which can predispose to thrombosis and occlusion). Autologous vein harvesting adds time to the procedure. The left internal jugular vein harvest is technically straight forward, associated with minimal morbidity, and probably the quickest and easiest option (compared with the left renal vein or the saphenous vein). We do not use the left renal vein even though a second incision is not necessary, because the conduit frequently does not provide enough length for interposition grafting.[30] Proximal and distal control of the PV or SMV is obtained with vascular clamps positioned 2 to 3 cm above and below the level of intended resection. We routinely use inflow occlusion on the SMA and systemic heparinization during the repair to prevent small bowel edema, which would make the biliary and pancreatic reconstructions unnecessarily difficult.[8,30] Vein reconstruction is completed with interrupted 6-0 prolene. The final result should consist of a near perfect size match of the interposition graft between the proximal and distal venous targets and tension-free anastomoses. When a patch is used, it must match the contour and size of the initial resected vein.[30] We want to emphasize the need for perfection in venous reconstruction; this is a low-flow system that results in thrombosis if not done well (**Fig. 8**).

Splenorenal shunting

The splenic vein may require ligation when (1) the SMV-PV confluence is encased by tumor, (2) the splenic vein is ligated for improved exposure of the proximal SMA, or (3) when increased length is needed for primary anastomosis of the SMV to the PV.[31]

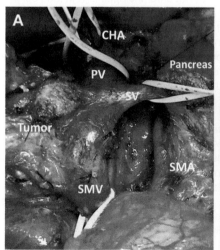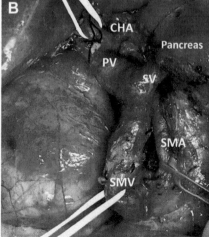

Fig. 7. An artery first approach was used to safely resect a tumor adherent to the portal vein (PV). (*A*) Tumor attached to the SMV. (*B*) View of the same anatomy after the tumor has been removed.

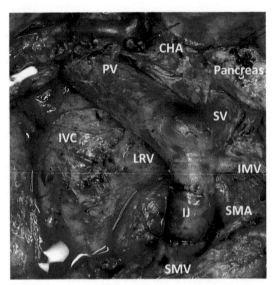

Fig. 8. Perfection in venous reconstruction is emphasized in this picture delineating a near perfect size match of the interposition graft between the proximal and distal venous targets and a tension-free anastomosis. IJ, internal jugular vein graft.

The IMV usually drains into the splenic vein but can empty into the SMV at or just below the SMV-PV confluence, in up to 30% of patients. When the splenic vein is ligated, blood flow returning from the spleen is usually diverted through the IMV (retrograde) away from the spleen to decompress the splenic vein. However, when the IMV does not empty into the splenic vein, splenic vein ligation can result in gastric and esophageal varicosities and sinistral portal hypertension; a risk factor for upper gastrointestinal hemorrhage. We usually avoid reanastomosis of the splenic vein to the reconstructed SMV-PV confluence because this may add tension and/or cause distortion of the repair. Thus, when the IMV does not enter the splenic vein (and splenic vein ligation is necessary), we have created a distal splenic vein to left renal vein anastomosis referred to as the splenorenal shunt of Warren.[32] The end of the splenic vein is anastomosed to the side of the left renal vein allowing for decompression of the splenic circulation and thereby avoiding sisnistral portal hypertension.[8,31] However, we ligate the splenic vein only when necessary; we prefer to preserve the PV-splenic vein confluence when it is not involved by tumor because we believe that this leads to augmentation of portal flow and increased long-term graft patency rates (**Fig. 9**).[30]

Portal venous cavernous transformation and mesocaval shunting

Chronic (in contrast to acute/immediate) PV occlusion causes cavernous transformation of the PV and creation of large venous collaterals around the pancreatic head, which pose a significant bleeding risk. Venous resection in this setting adds technical complexity to PD for an otherwise operable pancreatic tumor.[33] In this scenario, we have used mesocaval shunting to safely divert all mesenteric blood flow before attempting the portal dissection. Early in the procedure, but after the SMV is identified below the pancreatic neck (an area usually free of varices), the left internal jugular vein is harvested. A temporary mesocaval shunt is then created between the infrapancreatic SMV and the adjacent inferior vena cava, using an IJ interposition graft (**Fig. 10**).[33,34]

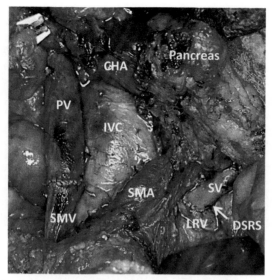

Fig. 9. A distal splenorenal shunt (DSRS, *white arrow*) is created by ligating the SV at the PV-SMV confluence and sewing the SV into the left renal vein (LRV).

Additional procedures may be necessary to control mesenteric blood flow, including early splenic artery ligation when performing a total pancreatectomy, or preoperative splenic artery embolization if direct access to the splenic vein is thought to be too difficult at the time of operation; the goal is total diversion of portal flow until the specimen is removed. The bile duct, PV, and other associated structures may also be stapled to decrease blood loss during the tumor resection. It is important to mention that each step of this complicated operation is carefully planned preoperatively to avoid any surgical misadventure and result in the best possible outcome.

Management of jejunal and ileal branches of the superior mesenteric vein

Variations of the venous anatomy are common and add complexity to the procedure. In 20% of the population, the jejunal branch crosses anterior, as opposed to posterior, to the SMA. An anterior jejunal vein provides easier access to the vein in cases of tumor involvement, but is usually associated with other venous anomalies. These variations may include the lack of a main SMV trunk, drainage of the IMV directly into the jejunal branch, or variable inferior pancreaticoduodenal venous branches arising from the ileal branch of the SMV. As a general rule, one of the two first-order SMV branches, whether the jejunal branch or the ileal branch, may be sacrificed without the need for reconstruction if it is encased by tumor and if the other branch is of appropriate caliber for reconstruction. For example, we usually prefer that the ileal branch be larger in transverse diameter than the SMA (as seen on preoperative axial imaging) to improve patency of the SMV-PV reconstruction (the distal venous target should be 1.5 times the diameter of the SMA if possible). When ligation of one of the first-order SMV branches is required during PD, it adds significantly to the complexity of the operation. If interposition grafting is needed, we use the internal jugular vein for the conduit and the ileal branch is always preferred for the distal target (as opposed to the jejunal branch). The ileal branch has a thicker wall relative to the jejunal branch and its anatomic location facilitates a safe distal anastomosis. In contrast, the jejunal branch in its usual anatomic location courses posterior to the SMA.[27] Ligation of both of these

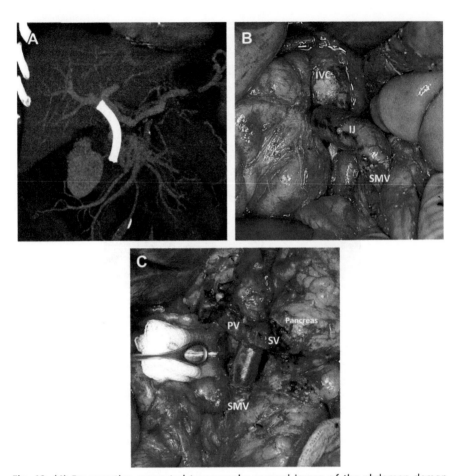

Fig. 10. (A) Preoperative computed tomography coronal image of the abdomen demonstrating the mesenteric venous anatomy and cavernous transformation of the PV. (B) An IJ vein is used as a temporary mesocaval shunt during pancreaticoduodenectomy. (C) IJ vein being used as an interposition graft between the SMV and the PV after removal of the specimen.

branches is not tolerated when the pancreatic head and accompanying venous collaterals are removed and results in acute bowel ischemia and necrosis (**Fig. 11**).[26]

Arterial Resection and Reconstruction

Arterial anatomy

Although venous resection and reconstruction is now routinely done for pancreatic cancer, arterial resection continues to be an area of significant controversy. Patients with arterial involvement, who were previously considered unresectable, are now selectively being considered for resection if they show adequate response to induction therapy.[10] Arterial abutment of the SMA or the CA, or even short-segment encasement of the CHA, are considered in the category of borderline resectable tumors.[13] Planned arterial resection is performed with acceptable outcomes when done in appropriately selected patients and may improve long-term survival.[10]

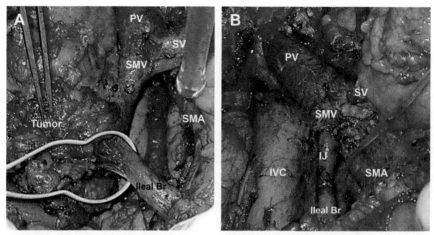

Fig. 11. Intraoperative photograph of a pancreatic tumor involving the inferior part of the SMV. (*A*) Tumor still attached after ligation of the first jejunal branch. The tumor was resected en bloc with a part of the inferior SMV. (*B*) IJ graft used to reconstruct the ileal branch into the SMV.

Visceral arteries are circumferentially covered by a perineural sheath, which is not present around visceral mesenteric veins. Tumors that involve this sheath tend to spread longitudinally through this neural layer. There is a natural plane between the arterial adventitia and this nerve sheath, which allows resection of the tumor without arterial resection in many patients. Additionally, preoperative chemoradiation has been shown to sterilize the periphery of these tumors, resulting in R0 margins even in the presence of arterial abutment.[13,16,35] One caveat to this finding is when a tumor encases the whole circumference of an artery; dissection then requires cutting through tumor to reach this per-adventitial plane, which is considered oncologically unacceptable (at least at the time that this article is being written, understanding the rapidly changing environment of pancreatic cancer treatment).[13]

Superior mesenteric artery

The SMA margin is undoubtedly the most technically challenging and the most commonly positive margin following PD and, therefore, the most common site of local disease recurrence. High-quality preoperative axial imaging is accurate in defining the tumor-artery relationship. Steps of the dissection of the SMA margin have been previously published by our group.[26] We classify SMA abutment of 180° or less as being borderline resectable, and encasement of greater than 180° to be locally advanced, with a recent subclassification of the locally advanced tumors into type A and type B. Type A tumors have encasement of the SMA greater than 180° but less than or equal to 270°. These tumors are potentially operable if they respond to neoadjuvant therapy. The one caveat is the morbidity of skeletonization of the SMA at the time of operation. This may result in rapid gastrointestinal transit caused by denervation of the mid-gut as the autonomic nerves that regulate small bowel motility are divided. Total parenteral nutrition may be required along with agents to slow gastrointestinal motility. SMA resection and reconstruction is not yet considered acceptable in pancreas cancer surgery because of risk of intestinal ischemia and death and the profound nutritional depletion that would occur in most patients (because of complete denervation of the entire mid-gut (**Fig. 12**).[13]

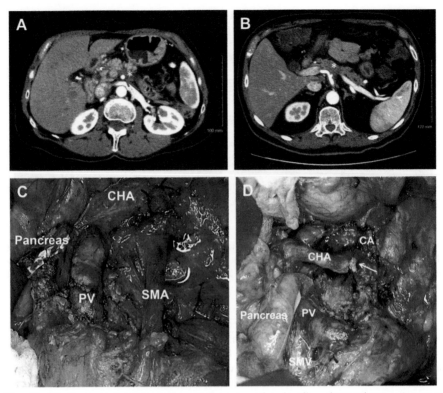

Fig. 12. (*A*) Computed tomography axial image of a locally advanced type A tumor involving greater than 180° of the SMA, (*blue arrow*) SMV, (*red arrow*) SMA, (*asterisk*) tumor. (*B*) Locally advanced type A tumor involving greater than 180° of the CA. Both tumors were microdissected off the SMA and the CA, respectively, (*red arrow*) celiac axis, (*asterisk*) tumor. (*C, D*) Intraoperative photographs of the respective tumors after being resected; *arrow* points to the splenic artery stump.

Celiac artery

The Appleby procedure evolved as an answer to the question of resection of the CA because of tumor encasement.[12,36] Patients with cancers of the pancreatic body being considered for celiac axis resection must manifest disease stability or improvement following neoadjuvant therapy.[10] Resection of pancreatic body tumors with concurrent celiac axis resection relies on retrograde blood flow though the gastroduodenal artery (GDA) and the pancreatic arcade, providing hepatic arterial blood flow through the proper hepatic artery and gastric perfusion through the right gastric and right gastroepiploic arteries. Preoperative CT imaging is of major importance in surgical planning for these procedures. We prefer a "supercharged" Appleby procedure when the celiac axis is resected.[10] A reversed saphenous vein graft is used as an interposition graft between the CA stump and the distal CHA before it divides into the GDA and the proper hepatic artery. Interposition grafting augments hepatic and gastric blood flow and may enhance gastric emptying. Supercharging theoretically prevents delayed gastric emptying resulting from relative gastric ischemia when the left gastric artery needs to be resected with the CA.[10] The presence of a replaced right hepatic artery during an Appleby procedure would preclude the need for supercharging the hepatic arterial flow but would obviously not affect gastric perfusion; if the left gastric artery is resected, some degree of gastric atony may occur in the absence of a larger head of pressure in the right gastric and right gastroepiploic arteries (**Fig. 13**).[10]

In cases of CA stenosis, it is critically important when performing PD to test the hepatic arterial flow with compression of the GDA before ligation of this artery. If the flow in the CHA is diminished or absent with a test clamp of the GDA, the celiac axis is dissected and freed from a compressing median arcuate ligament (which is usually the cause). If this does not improve blood flow, then a reversed saphenous vein interposition graft is used to augment hepatic arterial flow.[26]

Common hepatic artery and anatomic variations

Encasement of a short segment of the CHA is classified as borderline resectable disease if arterial reconstruction is possible. This is usually encountered with tumors of the head or neck of the pancreas that require PD. We use a reversed saphenous vein graft to reconstruct the CHA.[10] This interposition graft is anastomosed to the CHA stump arising from the celiac axis (**Fig. 14**). We have also used the right renal artery as an inflow source to revascularize the CHA if the CHA stump is friable and not useable; the aorta can also be used as an inflow source (**Fig. 15**).

Variations in mesenteric arteries are a common occurrence and plans should be made preoperatively to address anomalies should the need arise. Preoperative imaging is critical to allow for accurate assessment of the hepatic arterial anatomy including replaced or accessory right hepatic arteries arising from the SMA. Such vessels travel posterior to the PV and common bile duct and they may abut the tumor, although they most commonly course cephalad to the pancreas and associated neoplasm. An accessory right hepatic artery can be ligated without any consequence; however, a replaced right hepatic artery should be revascularized (**Fig. 16**). The same principle also applies to a replaced CHA where all of the blood flow to the liver is derived from the SMA. Proximal bile duct perfusion comes from the hepatic arterial system (usually the right hepatic artery) and therefore to prevent ischemia to a newly formed biliary-enteric anastomosis, revascularization of the CHA (or right hepatic artery) is required.

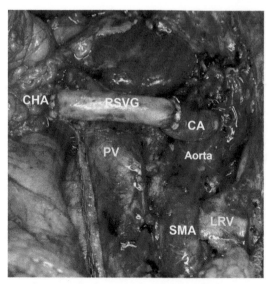

Fig. 13. Intraoperative photograph of a supercharged Appleby procedure where a reversed saphenous vein graft (RSVG) is used between the CA stump and the CHA.

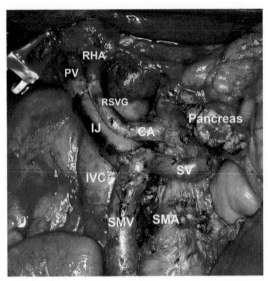

Fig. 14. Intraoperative photograph of a revascularization of the right hepatic artery (RHA) from the CA stump using an RSVG.

For reconstruction, we have most commonly used a reversed saphenous vein graft as an interposition graft between the proximal and distal parts of the resected vessel.[10,26]

POSTOPERATIVE CARE

Postpancreatectomy patients are most commonly admitted to the surgical ward the day of surgery with the exception of patients who undergo total pancreatectomy, whom we prefer to watch one night in the surgical intensive care unit for blood sugar

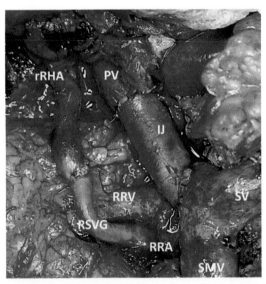

Fig. 15. Intraoperative photograph of a revascularization of a replaced right hepatic artery (rRHA) from the right renal artery (RRA) using an RSVG.

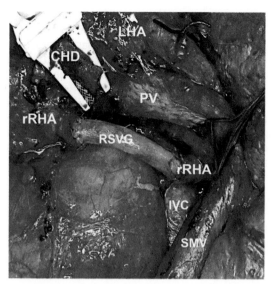

Fig. 16. Intraoperative photograph of a revascularization of a replaced rRHA using an RSVG.

monitoring. The average hospital stay on the surgical floor is 7 to 8 days. A postpancreatectomy pathway for PD patients has been used for many years and provides clear expectations for recovery on a daily basis. Patients are placed on a pain protocol regimen consisting of a patient-controlled anesthesia pump, scheduled oral gabapentin, and intravenous acetaminophen. Scheduled ketorolac is also given starting on postoperative Day 1 after proof of adequate renal function and stable blood counts. The intravenous pain regimen is switched to an enteral route, whether given orally or as a solution through the feeding jejunostomy tube following return of bowel function. All patients receive a soft nasogastric tube during surgery that is usually removed on postoperative Day 2 or 3. In patients showing early signs of delayed gastric emptying, promotility agents may be used as needed. The diet is then advanced daily from clear liquids to full liquids to a low-residue diet. Most of our patients have feeding jejunostomy tubes placed at the time of PD or total pancreatectomy and enteral feeds are started as early as the second postoperative day at a very slow rate.

Thrombosis of the vascular reconstruction rarely occurs in the acute postoperative setting if the surgery is done correctly. However, thrombosis may occur over time, with or without the appearance of disease recurrence. Most published series report 80% to 90% long-term patency rates of autologous conduits.[6,30,37] We reported a 90% 1-year patency rate in 43 patients who had venous resection and reconstruction.[30] There are no guidelines, however, on the optimal pharmacologic management of patients after vascular resection and reconstruction. Our patients receive 300 mg of aspirin rectally, and prophylactic heparin (5000 units two or three times a day), beginning on postoperative day zero. Enteric coated oral aspirin is initiated once the patients are started on a diet and they are discharged home on 325 mg/day; the heparin is discontinued at the time of hospital discharge.

SUMMARY

Vascular resection and reconstruction during pancreatectomy add to the level of complexity of a procedure known to require mastery of surgical technique. With the increase in the number of venous resections during PD and the acceptance and safety of arterial resections, the pancreas surgeon is required to select the appropriate patient and medically optimize them, understand and plan the procedure preoperatively, prepare the site of a vascular conduit to be harvested, and have sufficient skills in vascular surgery to perform complex vascular work as it pertains to pancreatectomy. The incorporation of newer systemic chemotherapy protocols in the treatment of pancreas cancer has led to an improvement in survival of affected patients; when such therapies are given before surgery, more patients with complex tumor-vessel anatomy are being considered for surgery. Importantly, complex pancreatic surgery for cancer, especially operations that involve vascular resection and reconstruction, should be considered only as part of a clearly defined multidisciplinary approach to this disease.

REFERENCES

1. Whipple AO, Parsons WB, Mullins CR. Treatment of carcinoma of the ampulla of Vater. Ann Surg 1935;102(4):763–79.
2. Yeo CJ, Cameron JL, Lillemoe KD, et al. Pancreaticoduodenectomy with or without distal gastrectomy and extended retroperitoneal lymphadenectomy for periampullary adenocarcinoma. Part 2: randomized controlled trial evaluating survival, morbidity, and mortality. Ann Surg 2002;236(3):355–66 [discussion: 366–8].
3. Farnell MB, Pearson RK, Sarr MG, et al. A prospective randomized trial comparing standard pancreatoduodenectomy with pancreatoduodenectomy with extended lymphadenectomy in resectable pancreatic head adenocarcinoma. Surgery 2005;138(4):618–28 [discussion: 628–30].
4. Nguyen TC, Sohn TA, Cameron JL, et al. Standard vs. radical pancreaticoduodenectomy for periampullary adenocarcinoma: a prospective, randomized trial evaluating quality of life in pancreaticoduodenectomy survivors. J Gastrointest Surg 2003;7(1):1–9 [discussion: 9–11].
5. Pedrazzoli S, DiCarlo V, Dionigi R, et al. Standard versus extended lymphadenectomy associated with pancreatoduodenectomy in the surgical treatment of adenocarcinoma of the head of the pancreas: a multicenter, prospective, randomized study. Lymphadenectomy Study Group. Ann Surg 1998;228(4):508–17.
6. Tseng JF, Raut CP, Lee JE, et al. Pancreaticoduodenectomy with vascular resection: margin status and survival duration. J Gastrointest Surg 2004;8(8):935–49 [discussion: 949–50].
7. Raut CP, Tseng JF, Sun CC, et al. Impact of resection status on pattern of failure and survival after pancreaticoduodenectomy for pancreatic adenocarcinoma. Ann Surg 2007;246(1):52–60.
8. Christians KK, Lal A, Pappas S, et al. Portal vein resection. Surg Clin North Am 2010;90(2):309–22.
9. Evans DB, Farnell MB, Lillemoe KD, et al. Surgical treatment of resectable and borderline resectable pancreas cancer: expert consensus statement. Ann Surg Oncol 2009;16(7):1736–44.
10. Christians KK, Pilgrim CH, Tsai S, et al. Arterial resection at the time of pancreatectomy for cancer. Surgery 2014;155(5):919–26.
11. Aosasa S, Nishikawa M, Noro T, et al. Total pancreatectomy with celiac axis resection and hepatic artery restoration using splenic artery autograft interposition. J Gastrointest Surg 2016;20(3):644–7.

12. Yamamoto Y, Sakamoto Y, Ban D, et al. Is celiac axis resection justified for T4 pancreatic body cancer? Surgery 2012;151(1):61–9.

13. Evans DB, George B, Tsai S. Non-metastatic pancreatic cancer: resectable, borderline resectable, and locally advanced-definitions of increasing importance for the optimal delivery of multimodality therapy. Ann Surg Oncol 2015;22(11): 3409–13.

14. Evans DB, Ritch PS, Erickson BA. Neoadjuvant therapy for localized pancreatic cancer: support is growing? Ann Surg 2015;261(1):18–20.

15. Christians KK, Evans DB. Additional support for neoadjuvant therapy in the management of pancreatic cancer. Ann Surg Oncol 2015;22(6):1755–8.

16. Christians KK, Tsai S, Mahmoud A, et al. Neoadjuvant FOLFIRINOX for borderline resectable pancreas cancer: a new treatment paradigm? Oncologist 2014;19(3): 266–74.

17. Christians KK, Heimler JW, George B, et al. Survival of patients with resectable pancreatic cancer who received neoadjuvant therapy. Surgery 2016;159(3): 893–900.

18. Evans DB, Crane CH, Charnsangavej C, et al. The added value of multidisciplinary care for patients with pancreatic cancer. Ann Surg Oncol 2008;15(8): 2078–80.

19. Katz MH, Pisters PW, Evans DB, et al. Borderline resectable pancreatic cancer: the importance of this emerging stage of disease. J Am Coll Surg 2008;206(5): 833–46 [discussion: 846–8].

20. Appel BL, Tolat P, Evans DB, et al. Current staging systems for pancreatic cancer. Cancer J 2012;18(6):539–49.

21. Tempero MA, Malafa MP, Behrman SW, et al. Pancreatic adenocarcinoma, version 2.2014: featured updates to the NCCN guidelines. J Natl Compr Canc Netw 2014;12(8):1083–93.

22. Aadam AA, Evans DB, Khan A, et al. Efficacy and safety of self-expandable metal stents for biliary decompression in patients receiving neoadjuvant therapy for pancreatic cancer: a prospective study. Gastrointest Endosc 2012;76(1): 67–75.

23. Katz MH, Varadhachary GR, Fleming JB, et al. Serum CA 19-9 as a marker of resectability and survival in patients with potentially resectable pancreatic cancer treated with neoadjuvant chemoradiation. Ann Surg Oncol 2010;17(7): 1794–801.

24. Aldakkak M, Christians KK, Krepline AN, et al. Pre-treatment carbohydrate antigen 19-9 does not predict the response to neoadjuvant therapy in patients with localized pancreatic cancer. HPB (Oxford) 2015;17(10):942–52.

25. Jayakrishnan TT, Nadeem H, Groeschl RT, et al. Diagnostic laparoscopy should be performed before definitive resection for pancreatic cancer: a financial argument. HPB (Oxford) 2015;17(2):131–9.

26. Christians KK, Tsai S, Tolat PP, et al. Critical steps for pancreaticoduodenectomy in the setting of pancreatic adenocarcinoma. J Surg Oncol 2013;107(1):33–8.

27. Katz MH, Fleming JB, Pisters PW, et al. Anatomy of the superior mesenteric vein with special reference to the surgical management of first-order branch involvement at pancreaticoduodenectomy. Ann Surg 2008;248(6):1098–102.

28. Tseng JF, Tamm EP, Lee JE, et al. Venous resection in pancreatic cancer surgery. Best Pract Res Clin Gastroenterol 2006;20(2):349–64.

29. Leach SD, Davidson BS, Ames FC, et al. Alternative method for exposure of the retropancreatic mesenteric vasculature during total pancreatectomy. J Surg Oncol 1996;61(2):163–5.

30. Krepline AN, Christians KK, Duelge K, et al. Patency rates of portal vein/superior mesenteric vein reconstruction after pancreatectomy for pancreatic cancer. J Gastrointest Surg 2014;18(11):2016–25.

31. Pilgrim CH, Tsai S, Tolat P, et al. Optimal management of the splenic vein at the time of venous resection for pancreatic cancer: importance of the inferior mesenteric vein. J Gastrointest Surg 2014;18(5):917–21.

32. Warren WD. Cirrhosis and portal hypertension: selection of patients for shunt and shunt for the patient. Am J Dig Dis 1964;9:906–17.

33. Christians KK, Riggle K, Keim R, et al. Distal splenorenal and temporary mesocaval shunting at the time of pancreatectomy for cancer: initial experience from the Medical College of Wisconsin. Surgery 2013;154(1):123–31.

34. Pilgrim CH, Tsai S, Evans DB, et al. Mesocaval shunting: a novel technique to facilitate venous resection and reconstruction and enhance exposure of the superior mesenteric and celiac arteries during pancreaticoduodenectomy. J Am Coll Surg 2013;217(3):e17–20.

35. Kang CM, Chung YE, Park JY, et al. Potential contribution of preoperative neoadjuvant concurrent chemoradiation therapy on margin-negative resection in borderline resectable pancreatic cancer. J Gastrointest Surg 2012;16(3):509–17.

36. Appleby LH. The coeliac axis in the expansion of the operation for gastric carcinoma. Cancer 1953;6(4):704–7.

37. Chu CK, Farnell MB, Nguyen JH, et al. Prosthetic graft reconstruction after portal vein resection in pancreaticoduodenectomy: a multicenter analysis. J Am Coll Surg 2010;211(3):316–24.

Management of Locally Advanced Pancreatic Cancer

Robert C.G. Martin II, MD, PhD

KEYWORDS

- Stage 3 pancreatic cancer • Locally advanced pancreatic cancer • Treatment
- Algorithm

KEY POINTS

- The optimal management of these patients is evolving quickly with the advent of newer chemotherapeutics, radiation, and nonthermal ablation modalities.
- For patients with locally advanced pancreatic cancer (stage III), the addition of irreversible electroporation to conventional chemotherapy and radiation therapy results in substantially prolonged survival compared with historical controls.
- The CORRECT and ACCURATE diagnosis for locally advanced pancreatic cancer must be based on high-quality, thin cut (<2mm) cross-sectional imaging, which demonstrates tumor abutment into the celiac/superior mesenteric arteries (>180 degrees) and/or encasement of the superior mesenteric/portal venous system that is not reconstructable.

INTRODUCTION

Pancreatic ductal adenocarcinoma is one of the most aggressive cancers and is the fourth most frequent tumor-related cause of death in the Western world.[1] Locally advanced disease is difficult to control, and limited improvement in outcomes has been achieved in the last 30 years despite the advances in diagnostic modalities and therapeutic options. For all stages combined, the 1-year survival rate is 20%, and the overall 5-year survival rate has remained dismally poor at 5%.[2] Complete surgical resection remains the only potentially curative treatment of pancreatic cancer. Advanced T stage of pancreatic adenocarcinoma is defined according to the involvement of the superior mesenteric artery (SMA), the celiac axis, long-segment portal vein occlusion, or their combination on cross-sectional imaging.[3,4]

Surgical resection offers the only chance of long-term disease control for nonmetastatic exocrine pancreatic cancer. However, only 15% to 20% of patients have potentially resectable disease at diagnosis; approximately 40% have distant metastases, and another 30% to 40% have locally advanced unresectable tumors. Typically,

Disclosures: The author is a paid consultant for Angiodynamics.

Division of Surgical Oncology, University of Louisville, School of Medicine, 315 East Broadway, M10, Room #312, Louisville, KY 40202, USA

E-mail address: Robert.Martin@louisville.edu

Surg Clin N Am 96 (2016) 1371–1389
http://dx.doi.org/10.1016/j.suc.2016.07.010
0039-6109/16/© 2016 Elsevier Inc. All rights reserved.

patients with locally advanced unresectable pancreatic cancer have tumor invasion into adjacent critical structures, particularly the celiac artery and SMA. Pancreatic tumors become symptomatic at a very advanced stage; therefore, a small percentage (15%–20%) of patients may undergo therapeutic resection. In the remaining patients, there might be either advanced locoregional disease without distant metastases (expected survival of 6–12 months) or locoregional disease with distant metastases (expected survival of 3–6 months).[5]

Chemoradiation therapy (CRT) provides short-term disease control. Most chemotherapeutic regimens do not prolong survival greatly, and only recently did gemcitabine-associated CRT seem to offer a modest survival benefit of 3 months.[6,7] FOLFIRINOX (5-fluorouracil [5FU], leucovorin, irinotecan, and oxaliplatin) recently showed better response and survival rates in stage 3 and 4 patients; however, long-term results from ongoing trials for stage 3 alone are not yet available.[8] The usefulness of radiation therapy (RT) was also assessed; however, the results were not significant.[7,9]

Considering the limited duration of effect of CRT, there is a clear need for an adjunctive or consolidative local treatment to provide greater durable local control to provide pain relief and possibly improve overall survival in patients with locally advanced pancreatic cancer (LAPC). Image-guided ablation techniques, such as radiofrequency ablation, microwave ablation, high-intensity focused ultrasonography, and irreversible electroporation (IRE), have been proposed as new treatment options in such cases.

CRITERIA FOR UNRESECTABILITY

An assessment of resectability should be made based on a thin cut (0.5–1 mm), triple-phase contrast-enhanced computed tomography (CT) scan and/or dynamic MRI. These minimal quality standards must be met to accurately and definitively stage patients at initial diagnosis. A detailed discussion of CT and magnetic resonance assessment of resectability is found elsewhere in this issue.

The accuracy of a single-phase diagnostic CT scan at thicker cuts (ie, 5 or 7 mm) is only 40% to 50% for assessing the presence of metastatic disease to the liver or peritoneum and even less accurate for assessing abutment and/or encasement of the portal venous and arterial structures.[10,11] Regardless of when a suboptimal referral CT scan was performed, it should be repeated for accurate initial staging. A diagnostic laparoscopy is also commonly performed to evaluate for subradiologic occult peritoneal or liver metastases. This procedure should be performed before any local nonsystemic therapy is being considered or if there are equivocal findings on CT or MRI. This procedure is critical because even these subtle changes seen on CT can have significant overall survival effects (**Table 1**).

Proper determination of the disease extent on imaging studies at the time of staging is one of the most important steps in optimal patient management. Given the variability in expertise and definition of disease extent among different practitioners, as well as a frequent lack of reporting of pertinent imaging findings, adoption of a standardized template for radiology reporting, using universally accepted and agreed-on terminology for solid pancreatic neoplasms, is needed. A recent consensus statement describing the standardization reporting template was developed under the joint sponsorship of the Society of Abdominal Radiologists and the American Pancreatic Association.[12] This standardized template is discussed in detail elsewhere in this issue. Adoption of this standardized reporting template can improve the decision-making process for the management of patients with pancreatic ductal adenocarcinoma by providing a complete and accurate assessment of disease staging to optimize treatment recommendations. A standardized imaging template can also

Table 1
Radiologic criteria for defining resectability

Stage Classification	% at Diagnosis	5-y Survival (%)	Median Overall Survival (mo)
Localized	10	26	15–19
Locally advanced/unresectable	40	10	7–12
Metastatic	50	2	3–6

improve the decision-making process for the management of patients with LAPC as well as facilitate research and clinical trial design by providing consistent staging and assessment of resectability.

TREATMENT ALGORITHM

The overall treatment algorithm (**Fig. 1**) for LAPC should only be initiated after accurate staging has been obtained. Following the confirmation of stage 3 LAPC, systemic chemotherapy that is known to be active in LAPC should be considered. Two active regimens are available and should be initiated to confirm 3 major factors: first and foremost, the biology of the disease. Second the overall and potentially surgical fitness of the patient. Third, the responsiveness of the tumor to chemotherapy and the ability of the tumor to be downsized to potentially resectable disease. Following this induction therapy for 3 to 4 months, repeat staging is completed to evaluate the stage of disease and then to decide on local consolidative therapy. The options for local treatment can include surgical resection if downsized to borderline resectable, RT, or IRE. These therapies are discussed at length later.

Systemic Chemotherapy

The development of combination chemotherapy regimens such as FOLFIRINOX[8,13] and gemcitabine with nab-paclitaxel[14,15] in the setting of metastatic disease produced

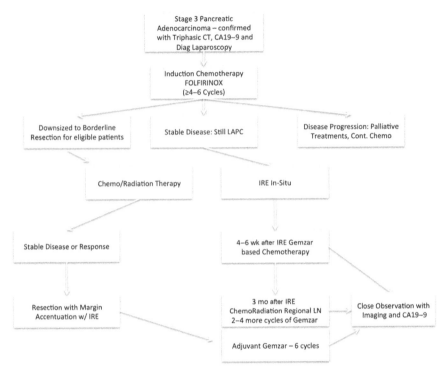

Fig. 1. Proposed treatment algorithm for LAPC that uses trimodality therapy. CA19-9, carbohydrate antigen 19-9; Chemo, chemotherapy; Cont, continue; Diag, Diagnostic; LN, lymph node; w/, with.

significantly higher objective response rates than are seen with gemcitabine alone (23% with nab-paclitaxel plus gemcitabine and 39% with FOLFIRINOX vs approximately 10% with gemcitabine alone) and has led to their use as the chemotherapy of choice in the initial treatment of patients with LAPC.

All patients with LAPC who have been appropriately staged as described earlier should undergo an initial period of chemotherapy (3–4 months) rather than immediate RT or chemoradiotherapy. This bias/recommendation is consistent with consensus-based guidelines from the National Comprehensive Cancer Network (NCCN) and the European Society of Medical Oncology (ESMO). The optimal regimen should include either FOLFIRINOX or gemcitabine with nab-paclitaxel. If a patient is not an appropriate candidate for this therapy at initial presentation (secondary to malnutrition, physical limitation, social support) then an attempt (<4 weeks) should be made to try to improve on these limitations. If this short-term improvement is not achieved, then initiating gemcitabine monotherapy is an acceptable but less than optimal (based on response rates) alternative. For patients with acceptable functional status (eg, Groningen Frailty Indicator or The Vulnerable Elders Survey [VES-13]),[16,17] a total bilirubin level that is less than or equal to 1.5 times the upper limit of normal, and who are able to tolerate it, induction treatment with FOLFIRINOX is the optimal option.

For patients who undergo appropriate induction chemotherapy, do not develop metastatic disease, and do not have local progression, then a local consolidative therapy can be considered (see **Fig. 1**).

However, an alternative acceptable approach is to continue chemotherapy until optimal response and/or lack of tolerance. Exceptional care needs to be continued if this pathway is chosen. Allowing for significant loss of functional status while maintaining chemotherapy could impede the patient from moving to the next step in therapy and require a long period (>10 weeks) off all therapy, thus putting the initial response obtained in jeopardy. Therefore, the author recommends restaging at 8-week intervals with repeat functional status evaluation so that stopping induction chemotherapy can be achieved with minimal delay to the next step in a patient's therapy.

Gemcitabine alone

The data to support the use of gemcitabine alone in LAPC is limited and comes from 2 recent trials conducted in mixed populations of patients with both locally advanced and metastatic disease. In a global phase III trial comparing gemcitabine with and without tipifarnib in 688 patients with locally advanced (n = 164) or metastatic pancreatic cancer, the median survival of patients with locally advanced disease in both groups was 10.5 months.[18] A randomized comparison between gemcitabine with or without irinotecan in 360 patients (51 with locally advanced disease) reported a median survival duration of 11.7 and 9.8 months in the patients with locally advanced disease in the gemcitabine alone and gemcitabine/irinotecan arms, respectively.[19] A longer median survival duration (15 months) was reported in a Japanese phase II trial of single-agent gemcitabine that was limited to 50 patients with locally advanced, nonmetastatic pancreatic cancer.[20] When these median survival rates are evaluated it is apparent that the overall survival is similar to or better than those reported in series of patients treated with chemoradiotherapy (discussed later).

Combination regimens

Recent data have shown improved overall survival as well as enhanced downsizing of LAPC with combination regimens compared with monotherapy.[21–23] These enhanced response rates have led to higher resection rates in certain patients with LAPC based on type of vascular involvement as well as to greater consolidative therapy with surgery and nonthermal ablation.[13,24]

The challenge remains that these more active regimens lead to enhanced toxicity, and thus appropriate patient selection is critically important. Because of the enhanced toxicity, the author prefers induction with FOLFIRINOX at an attenuated dose to start and then dose escalate after the third to fourth cycles based on tolerance. In addition, it is common to decrease the bolus 5FU in marginally functional patients in order to reduce the toxicity. Gemcitabine plus nab-paclitaxel can also be used, but the author has not seen as robust a downsizing and thus prefers FOLFIINOX as induction therapy with the goal to leave gemcitabine plus nab-paclitaxel for later therapy when needed.

The optimal number of courses of induction chemotherapy is described earlier and is critical to maintaining a patient's functional status and optimal response.

Many institutions have used induction FOLFIRINOX for patients with locally advanced pancreatic cancer, and the available data on the safety and efficacy of this approach for LAPC continue to grow.[13,25,26] The overall response rates of the primary tumor are encouraging, leading to greater use of surgical resection and local ablation with acceptable perioperative morbidity and mortality, similar to patients undergoing resection first.[27]

Key to the use of induction chemotherapy is the finding that postchemotherapy imaging may unreliable at predicting resectability in patients treated with up-front FOLFIRINOX. This finding has been shown in recent studies in which radiologic local advancement was shown but surgical resection was achieved in a large percentage of patients.[24,26] Surgical resectability was most commonly achieved in patients with

SMA alone or celiac axis alone involvement, compared with patients with unreconstructable venous involvement. Ferrone and colleagues[24] showed that 19 patients who received induction FOLFIRINOX as initial treatment of LAPC underwent resection with a 92% R0 resection. High-quality posttreatment CT as described earlier should still be performed after 2 to 3 months of induction chemotherapy to assess for M1 disease. CT or MRI has not been found to definitively confirm T4 (locally advanced) disease in all cases, and an assessment of resectability should be made intraoperatively with both ultrasonography and precise surgical dissection.[28]

Based on the lack of robust response rates for the primary tumor, the use of gemcitabine alone for induction therapy in LAPC is not endorsed. The use of gemcitabine plus nab-paclitaxel has not been reported in LAPC that has undergone resection. A recent phase II trial evaluating neoadjuvant gemcitabine plus oxaliplatin in patients with initially unresectable (n = 18) or borderline resectable (n = 15) nonmetastatic pancreatic cancer showed that 40% (far more in the borderline group than the LAPC group) had sufficient tumor regression to undergo operative resection, which was complete (R0) in 69%.[29]

Radiation Therapy

For patients who do not progress following initial chemotherapy some form of local consolidative therapy (RT or ablative therapy) can be considered. The type of chemotherapy with RT has not been universally agreed on and remains one of the limitations with RT. A common CRT is external beam RT (EBRT) plus concomitant low-dose infusional 5FU or gemcitabine as a radiation sensitizer. This approach is also consistent with published guidelines from the NCCN and ESMO, but lacks true long-term durable local disease control. Stereotactic body radiotherapy (SBRT) is another option based on its ease of dosing, but there remain no trials establishing the comparable efficacy (depending on how this is defined) of SBRT versus standard fractionation EBRT in LAPC.

Stereotactic body radiotherapy

SBRT is capable of precisely delivering high doses of radiation to small tumor volumes. SBRT uses real-time tracking of implanted fiducials to integrate organ motion into real-time therapy.

SBRT has been evaluated in an increasing number of clinical studies as an alternative approach to conventionally fractionated EBRT with concurrent chemotherapy for the management of locally advanced disease. However, the benefit of SBRT compared with EBRT remains unproved, because it is not clear that median survival is better than would be expected with other forms of therapy, and toxicity has been worse in some studies.[30,31]

As an example, a recent single-institution trial included 22 patients with locally advanced, unresectable pancreatic cancer who were treated with SBRT (45 Gy divided into 3 doses of 15 Gy over 5–10 days).[32] Acute toxicity was pronounced, with deterioration of performance status, nausea, and increased pain seen at 14 days. Four patients developed severe gastric mucositis or ulceration, and 1 patient had a nonfatal stomach perforation. Six patients developed local tumor progression, and median survival was only 6 months.

Chang and colleagues[33] presented 62 patients with LPAC treated with SBRT (single fraction of 25 Gy). The overall survival rates at 6 months (56%) and 12 months (21%) were limited. The 12-month rate of late toxicity (mostly ulceration of the gastrointestinal tract) was 25%. The late mucosal toxicity was even higher (44%) in a second prospective trial from the same institution of 16 patients who were treated with single-fraction SBRT (25 Gy) using SBRT between cycles 1 and 2 of gemcitabine.[34]

The risk of these local toxicities did not outweigh the benefits by an improvement in overall survival. The median survival durations reported in these 3 studies (6–7 months) does not compare favorably with the median overall survivals seen in modern phase II studies of chemotherapy alone or conventionally fractionated chemoradiation in patients with locally advanced disease ($\geq$10 months) or compared with trimodality therapy with chemotherapy, conventional RT, and IRE.[26]

Despite it being clearly preferable for patients to receive 3 to 5 treatments over a 1-week to 2-week period rather than 28 to 30 treatments over 6 weeks, the overall outcomes of improvement are far from definitive, and the potential for long-term toxicity with SBRT remains a concern. In experienced centers, SBRT could be considered an alternative to conventional fractionation chemoradiotherapy if the true goals of the SBRT are described: local tumor control only versus local regional (ie, tumor and regional lymph nodes) control. However, until randomized trials comparing SBRT with conventional chemoradiotherapy are completed, the place of SBRT in the therapeutic armamentarium for LAPC will remain uncertain.

CHEMORADIATION THERAPY

Infusional 5FU was used in an Eastern Cooperative Oncology Group (ECOG) trial, which randomly assigned 114 patients to RT (59.4 Gy) alone or with concurrent infusional 5FU (1000 mg/m^2 daily on days 2 through 5 and 28–31) plus mitomycin (10 mg/m^2 on day 2).[35] The addition of chemotherapy to RT provided no benefit in terms of response rate (9% vs 6%), median disease-free survival (DFS; 5 vs 5.1 months), or overall survival (7.1 vs 8.4 months, respectively). However, a recent pooled analysis of trials found that the length of survival with chemoradiotherapy was significantly increased relative to radiotherapy alone (hazard ratio for death, 0.69; 95% confidence interval, 0.51–0.94).[36] A recent meta-analysis of 21 studies also confirmed that 5FU-based chemoradiotherapy improved overall survival compared with RT alone.[37] These studies evaluating chemoradiotherapy (with or without subsequent chemotherapy) versus chemotherapy alone concluded that there was no survival benefit (and greater toxicity) for chemoradiotherapy compared with chemotherapy alone.[36,37] The limitations of both of these reviews was driven by the vast differences in chemotherapy regimen and RT dose, as well as small sample size.

The most compelling reason for initial chemotherapy is based on the estimate that close to 30% of patients with LAPC are actually stage 4 with metastatic disease that was not visualized at initial diagnosis and becomes quickly apparent at the 2-month to 4-month follow-up imaging.[9] Thus, the rationale of initial chemotherapy allows better patient selection for those who may benefit from consolidative local therapy.[38,39]

As an example, this strategy was evaluated in a retrospective series of 181 patients with LAPC who had been treated with gemcitabine-based chemotherapy alone as part of phase II and III trials conducted by the European Groupe Cooperateur Multidisciplinaire en Oncologie (GERCOR).[9] In each protocol, chemotherapy was initially given for 3 months, and the decision to continue it or administer chemoradiotherapy (55 Gy EBRT with concurrent infusional 5FU) was left to the discretion of the investigator. Among the 128 patients who did not progress after 3 months of chemotherapy and who retained an adequate performance status, 72 received chemoradiotherapy, whereas 56 continued with chemotherapy. When the two groups were compared, chemoradiotherapy was associated with significant improvement in median progression-free survival (10.8 vs 7.4 months with chemotherapy) and overall survival (15 vs 11.7 months).

However, the efficacy of this approach could not be confirmed in the international locally advanced pancreatic (LAP) 07 trial, a randomized 2 × 2 factorial design study in which 442 patients with LAPC and an ECOG performance status of 0 to 2 were randomly assigned to gemcitabine with or without erlotinib. At the end of 4 months, patients with controlled disease were randomly assigned to 2 additional months of chemotherapy or chemoradiotherapy (54 Gy EBRT plus concurrent capecitabine 1600 mg/m^2/ d). In a preliminary report presented at the 2013 American Society of Clinical Oncology annual meeting, at a median follow-up of 36 months, chemoradiotherapy was not superior to continuing chemotherapy (median overall survival 15.3 vs 16.5 months).

RT as a single modality could be considered to palliate pain for patients who are not considered candidates for combined chemoradiotherapy because of medical comorbidities and whose pain is not adequately controlled with narcotic analgesics. Another option is celiac plexus nerve block.

ROLE OF SURGERY: RESECTION AND ELECTROPORATION

It is essential to restage and reevaluate the potential for resection after chemotherapy with or without chemoradiotherapy. The ability to perform an R0 resection is variable (15%–50%) based on the size and location of the LAPC.[24–26] Given that the current median survival of patients with LAPC remains at 10 to 12 months with chemotherapy and/or CRT, a surgery first for LAPC is not indicated. The principles of neoadjuvant/induction therapy for patients with LAPC must be followed to ensure that the longer term improvement in overall survival can be achieved. The challenge remains that patients treated with initial chemotherapy with or without RT are difficult to define with regard to response to this therapy.[40] All patients with LAPC who are responding to chemotherapy should be evaluated for potential resectability after induction treatment. The frequency with which patients respond or remain with stable disease that can lead to resection is encouraging, but needs to be enhanced.[41,42]

LOCAL ABLATIVE THERAPIES

When local ablative therapies are applied, chemical, thermal, or electrical energy is transferred to a specific area of soft tissue with the intent of complete tissue destruction or ablation.

Chemical ablation includes the use of ethanol or acetic acid, which induces coagulation necrosis of the tumor mass after direct injection/contact with these agents. With chemical ablation, there is always the risk of migration/injection into the arterial system with potentially fatal consequences, and its application in the treatment of pancreatic cancer is limited.[43]

Thermal ablation is based on the increase or decrease of tumor temperature. When heat is applied, a target temperature of more than 50°C is the goal, with temperatures ranging from 60°C to 100°C, and sometimes more. These temperatures result in a coagulative necrosis of the tissue via a thermal-based method of action. Cell death results from apoptosis and eventually coagulative necrosis, which occurs at temperatures greater than 50°C after 2 minutes. When cold is applied (cryoablation), temperatures lower than the tissue freezing edge are achieved. The target temperature is lower than −40°C, which in most tissues is necessary to cause necrosis of target cells.[44,45] There are several thermal ablation studies on the treatment of pancreatic cancer, mainly with the use of heat, and very limited studies on cryoablation in the literature.[46–48]

Electrical current ablation (IRE) is a technology that is based on the irreversible increase of permeability of the cellular membrane with the use of high-voltage (3000 V), short-pulse (70–90 microseconds) electric currents. IRE is one of the latest technological advances, and recent studies have been performed on its application in the local treatment of pancreatic cancer. Improvements in intraoperative imaging, electrodes, and ultrasonography technology have enabled the technology to accurately treat tumors.[49–51] IRE has been applied to patients who are not considered suitable for surgical resection and have received CRT with persistent disease. Thus it is designed to offer consolidative disease control, with symptom relief, control of pain, and definitive eradication of the lesion.

The inherent limitation for local ablative therapy for the pancreas is the heterogeneity of the tissue and the surrounding structures. This heterogeneity limits certain therapies because of the damage to healthy tissue, which can lead to complications such as pancreatitis, vascular thrombosis, or enteric damage. These concerns limit the use of certain techniques and augment others.

IRREVERSIBLE ELECTROPORATION

IRE represents a new nonthermal injury[52] ablative technique with advantages through the ability to definitively treat a soft tissue tumor with a decreased risk of thermal damage to vital structures adjacent to pancreatic tissue.[49,51] The technique uses a series of short (70–90 microseconds), high-voltage (2250–3000 V) pulses that are applied between 2 electrodes that are spaced 1.5 to 2.2 cm apart. These pulses increase the permeability of the cell membrane, which induces electrolyte disturbances across the cell, leading to cell death via apoptosis.[53,54] Reversible electroporation has been used in basic science laboratories as a technique that allows the transfer of genetic material or intracellular delivery of drugs.[55–57] The technique of reversible electroporation has a certain threshold to which the electrical energy induces permanent cell membrane porosity, leading to irreversible permeabilization.[58] The IRE technique influences only the intracellular environment and not the extracellular matrix, thus allowing for cell repopulation and avoidance of luminal strictures of vital structures.[53,59–61]

Bower and colleagues[49] reported the first initial use of IRE in a chronic non–tumor-bearing porcine pancreatic model. Six 70-kg to 80-kg pigs underwent a general anesthesia procedure and through a midline incision either two or three 19-gauge monopolar or one 16-gauge bipolar electrode were placed under ultrasonography guidance to avoid mechanical damage and to ensure bracketing of the vital structures. The electrodes were placed within the pancreatic tissue at a distance of 1 mm from the portal vein or the mesenteric artery. Monopolar electrodes were spaced at 1.5 and 2 cm. The electroporation generator was the NanoKnife system (AngioDynamics, Queensbury, NY), which used an energy output of a maximum of 3000 V and maximum current of 50 A. The system is used with cardiac synchronization in order to deliver electrical pulses during the refractory phase of the cardiac rhythm and not during the vulnerable phase in order to prevent cardiac arrhythmias. The goal of treatment is to deliver enough pulses (range 110–220) in groups of 10 in order to see a change in resistance of the target tissue.[62] All animals tolerated the IRE procedure of the pancreas, and the animals had a transient (peak at 48 hours) increase in pancreatic enzyme levels (normalized at 72 hours in most animals). The animals were survived to 72 hours, 7 days, and 14 days after the procedure. Pathology showed complete electroporation with nonthermal injury–induced necrosis of pancreatic cells adjacent to vascular structures. There was no evidence of thermal injury to the vessels or bile ducts. The investigators were able to conclude from this preliminary study that IRE might be used in the ablation of pancreatic tissue without significant risk of pancreatitis or vascular thrombosis. Attention to the safe and efficacious use is essential, because misuse or lack of attention can lead to high current energy delivery, which could result in thermal injury.

The initial clinical use of IRE was reported by Martin and colleagues[63] in which 27 patients, with a median age of 61 years, underwent IRE. Eight patients underwent margin accentuation with IRE combined with left-sided resection (N = 4) or pancreatic head resection (n = 4). Nineteen patients had in situ IRE, in which the primary tumor is completely treated without removal of the tumor. All patients underwent successful IRE, with intraoperative imaging confirming effective delivery of therapy. All 27 patients showed non–clinically relevant increase of their amylase and lipase levels, which peaked at 48 hours and returned to normal at 72 hours postprocedure. There was one 90-day mortality. No patient showed evidence of clinical pancreatitis or fistula formation. After all patients completed 90-day follow-up, there was 100% ablation success. The investigators concluded that IRE ablation of LAP tumors is a safe and feasible primary local treatment in unresectable, locally advanced disease.

Martin and colleagues[64] reported on a larger study of 54 patients who underwent combination of chemotherapy, CRT with consolidative IRE, compared with a control group of chemotherapy/CRT for LAPC. All patients were confirmed stage 3 LAPC based on staging CT and/or MRI because of encasement of the SMA, celiac axis, or long-segment occlusion of the superior mesenteric vein (SMV)/portal vein. IRE was performed through an open midline incision or in a laparoscopic fashion. After a median follow-up time of 15 months, 15 of the 54 patients appeared to have local disease recurrence. The adverse events that were IRE related were 2 cases of bile leakage and 2 cases of duodenal leakage. However, the duodenal leaks occurred after the removal of a duodenal stent and placement of the IRE needle. The 90-day mortality in the IRE patients was 1 (2%). In comparing IRE patients with standard therapy, there was an improvement in local progression-free survival (14 vs 6 months, $P = .01$), distant progression-free survival (15 vs 9 months, $P = .02$), and overall survival (20 vs 13 months, $P = .03$). The investigators concluded that IRE as a consolidative therapy for locally advanced pancreatic tumors remains safe. In appropriate patients who have undergone standard induction therapy for a minimum of 4 months, IRE can achieve greater local palliation and potential improved overall survival compared with standard chemoradiation-chemotherapy treatments.

Dunki-Jacobs and colleagues[52] also recently published on the temperature effects and the ability to treat around metal structures such as metal biliary stents, clips, and fiducials. In vivo continuous temperature assessments of 86 different IRE procedures were performed on porcine liver, pancreas, kidney, and retroperitoneal tissue. Tissue temperature was measured continuously throughout IRE by means of 2 thermocouples placed at set distances ($\leq$0.5 cm and 1 cm) from the IRE probes within the treatment field. Thermal injury was defined as a tissue temperature of 54°C lasting at least 10 seconds. Tissue type, pulse length, probe exposure length, number of probes, and retreatment were evaluated for associations with thermal injury. In addition, IRE ablation was performed with metal clips or metal stents within the ablation field to determine their effect on thermal injury. An increase in tissue temperature beyond the animals' baseline temperature (median 36.0°C) was generated during IRE in all tissues studied, with the greatest increase found at the thermocouple placed within 0.5 cm in all instances. On univariate and multivariate analysis, ablation in kidney tissue (maximum temperature, 62.8°C), ablation with a pulse length setting of 100 microseconds (maximum, 54.7°C), probe exposure of at least 3.0 cm (maximum 52.0°C), and ablation with metal within the ablation field (maximum, 65.3°C) were all associated with a significant risk of thermal injury. Care should be taken because animal data have confirmed that inappropriate use of IRE can lead to thermal energy (>52°C for 10 seconds) and thermal injury.[52] This thermal injury can occur based on tissue type (pancreas vs liver vs kidney), probe exposure lengths, pulse lengths, and proximity to metal. Awareness of probe placement regarding proximity to critical structures as well as probe exposure length and pulse length are necessary to ensure safety and prevent thermal injury. A probe exposure of 2.5 cm or less for liver IRE, and 1.5 cm or less for pancreas, with maximum pulse length of 90 microseconds results in safe and nonthermal energy delivery with spacing of 1.5 to 2.6 cm between probe pairs.

Similar work has also been performed to adequately define a clinical end point for IRE.[62] Because intraoperative ultrasonography evaluation of successful pancreatic tumor ablation using irreversible IRE is difficult secondary to edematous changes that occur, a more specific end point for electroporation was needed. The IRE generator provides feedback by reporting current (amperage), which can be used to calculate changes in tumor tissue resistance. The investigators used a change in resistance to predict successful tumor ablation during IRE for pancreatic cancers.

All patients undergoing pancreatic IRE from March 2010 to December 2012 were evaluated using a prospective database. Intraoperative information, including change in tumor resistance during ablation and slope of the resistance curve, were used to evaluate effectiveness of tumor ablation in terms of local failure or recurrence (LFR) and DFS. A total of 65 patients underwent IRE for LAPC. Median follow-up was 23 months. LFR was seen in 17 patients at 3, 6, or 9 months post-IRE. Change in tumor tissue resistance and the slope of the resistance curve were both significant in predicting LFR ($P = .02$ and $P = .01$, respectively). The median local DFS was 5.5 months in patients who had recurrence compared with 12.6 months in patients who did not recur ($P = .03$). Neither mean change in tumor tissue resistance nor the slope of the resistance curve significantly predicted overall DFS. Mean change in tumor tissue resistance and the slope of the resistance curve could be used intraoperatively to assess successful tumor ablation during IRE. Larger sample size and longer follow-up are needed to determine whether these parameters can be used to predict DFS.

All of these factors lead to the most recent data for the use of IRE in LAPC by Martin and colleagues[65]. From July 2010 to October 2014, patients with radiographic stage III LAPC were treated with IRE and monitored under a multicenter, prospective, independent review board–approved registry. Perioperative 90-day outcomes, local failure, and overall survival were recorded. A total of 200 patients with LAPC underwent IRE alone (n = 150) or pancreatic resection plus IRE for margin enhancement (n = 50). All patients underwent induction chemotherapy, and 52% received CRT as well, for a median of 6 months (range, 5–13 months) before IRE. IRE was successfully performed in all patients. Thirty-seven percent sustained complications, with a median grade of 2 (range, 1–5). Median length of stay was 6 days (range, 4–36 days). With a median follow-up of 29 months, 6 patients (3%) experienced local recurrence. Median overall survival was 24.9 months (range, 4.9–85 months). The investigators concluded that, in patients with LAPC, the addition of IRE to conventional chemotherapy and RT results in substantially prolonged survival compared with historical controls. These results suggest that ablative control of the primary tumor may prolong survival.

Because most reports of IRE use have been through an open midline laparotomy, another option is the use of a percutaneous access approach. Narayanan and colleagues[66] performed a study of 14 patients who received CT-guided percutaneous treatment with IRE for LAPC. The indications for treatment were downstaging of the locally advanced cancer, control of local recurrence after previous Whipple procedure, and/or intolerance to systemic chemotherapy. All patients had received previous cycles of chemotherapy and 10 of 14 also received previous RT. The median tumor size treated was 3.3 cm (range, 2.5–7). In 6 cases, the tumor was located in the pancreatic head; in 7 cases it was located in the body, and in 1 case it was located in the uncinate process. In 3 cases, small-volume metastatic disease was present, whereas patients with extensive metastatic disease were not included in the study. No severe complications occurred after the procedure. Complications included pneumothorax, a small subcutaneous hematoma, and self-limiting pancreatitis. There were 4 deaths during the course of the follow-up; however, no deaths were attributed to the procedure. Three other patients with intolerance to chemotherapy showed stable disease and did not require any further treatment. The median overall survival was reported as 6 months. With these results, the investigators concluded that patients with metastatic disease do not seem to benefit from IRE and that patients with extensive varices need to be excluded from a percutaneous approach, thus indicating that a safe CT window is not enough for percutaneous IRE of LAPC.

The importance of avoiding incomplete electroporation as well as avoiding IRE in patients with metastatic disease cannot be overstated. A recent report from Philips and colleagues[67] created the first ever heterotopic murine pancreatic cancer model by inoculating BALB/c nude mice in the hind limb with a subcutaneous injection of Panc-1 cells, an immortalized human pancreatic adenocarcinoma cell line. Tumors were allowed to grow from 0.75 to 1.5 cm and then treated with the goal of complete ablation or partial ablation using standard IRE settings. Animals were recovered and survived for 2 (n = 6), 7 (n = 6), 14 (n = 6), 21 (n = 6), 30 (n = 8), and 60 (n = 8) days. All 40 animals/tumors underwent successful IRE under general anesthesia with muscle paralysis. The mean tumor volume of the animals undergoing ablation was 1447.6 ± 884 mm^3. On histology, in the 14-day, 21-day, 30-day, and 60-day survival groups, the entire tumor was nonviable, with a persistent tumor nodule completely replaced by fibrosis. In the group treated with partial ablation, incomplete electroporation /recurrences (N = 10 animals) were seen, of which 66% had confluent tumors and this was a significant predictor of recurrence ($P<.001$). Recurrent tumors were also significantly larger (mean, 4578 mm^3 $\pm$ standard deviation 877 mm^3 vs completed electroporated tumors 925.8 ± 277 mm^3, $P<.001$). Recurrent tumors had a steeper growth curve (slope = 0.73) compared with primary tumors (0.60, $P = .02$). Recurrent tumors also had a significantly higher percentage of epithelial cell adhesion molecule expression, suggestive of stem cell activation. The investigators concluded that tumors that recur after incomplete electroporation show a biologically aggressive behavior that could be more resistant to standard-of-care chemotherapy. Clinical correlation of these data is limited, but should be considered when IRE of pancreatic cancer is being considered.

The established technique for IRE of LAPC has been published. Martin[28,68] reported on the optimal technique for both the LAPC of the pancreatic head (**Fig. 2**) and LAPC of the pancreatic neck/body (**Fig. 3**). A representative case would involve a patient who presents with LAPC of the pancreatic head who has been treated with induction chemotherapy, who now has a mass of less than 3.5 cm, with clear vascular involvement (see **Fig. 2**). Given the size of the tumor, at least 4 needles would be placed in a bracketing fashion, covering the entire tumor and the vital structures, which in this case would include the SMA, SMV, and the bile duct.

Similar presentation can occur with LAPC of the neck, which should be treated with induction chemotherapy. After appropriate selection, the needle placement again is in a bracketed fashion to cover the entire tumor and the vital structures that the tumor invades (see **Fig. 3**). After optimal needle placement, with precise spacing,[69] the energy is delivered between the probes in a sequential fashion until a change in resistance is seen.[62]

However, there is a learning curve with IRE that cannot be underestimated. A recent analysis by Philips and colleagues[70] evaluated 150 consecutive patients over

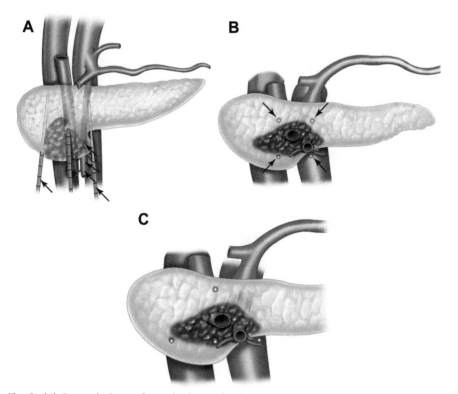

Fig. 2. (*A*) Coronal plane of standard 4-probe (*arrows*) technique with SMA encasement. Care should be taken so that the needles are not placed past the extent of tumor involvement, thus preventing injury to the aorta. (B) Axial plane of classic 4 probe box (*arrows*) technique for a locally advanced pancreatic head tumor with SMA and SMV encasement with 4 probes bracketing the tumor and the SMA with maximum probe exposure of 1 cm. (*C*) Axial image of LAPC of the pancreatic head with a triangle IRE probe configuration, which is sometimes required because the posterior/retroperitoneal extension is wider than the anterior apex of the tumor. (*From* Martin RCG, O'Connor R. The role of irreversible electroporation and other ablative techniques in patients with borderline resectable pancreatic cancer. New York: Springer; 2015; with permission.)

7 institutions from September 2010 to July 2012, divided these into 3 groups (A [first 50 patients treated], B [second 50], and C [third 50 patients treated]), and analyzed for outcomes. Over time, complex treatments of larger lesions and lesions with greater vascular involvement were performed without a significant increase in adverse effects or impact on local relapse-free survival. This evolution showed the safety profile of IRE and speed of graduation to more complex lesions, which was greater than 5 cases per institution.

In addition, the CT imaging post-IRE also continues to evolve. Because IRE is fairly new to locoregional therapy, post-IRE imaging findings are limited.[71] In a recent review by our institution for less than 30-day imaging, 3 distinct abnormalities are seen (**Fig. 4**).

The most common finding overall was of direct vascular change; specifically, that of a significant postprocedural narrowing in caliber (estimated to be at least 50%) or even occlusion of a major peripancreatic vessel. The portal vein and confluence, SMA, and

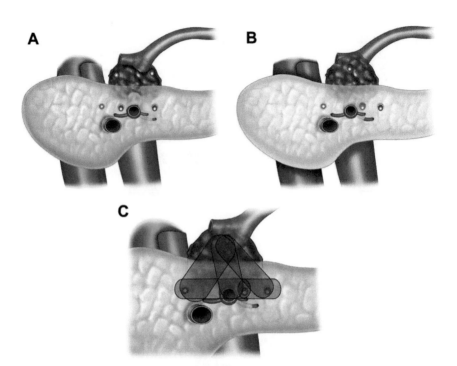

Fig. 3. (*A*) Axial plane of classic 5 probe technique for a locally advanced pancreatic midbody tumor with just celiac encasement and SMA involvement with probes bracketing the tumor and the celiac axis with maximum probe exposure of 1 cm. (*B*) Axial plane of this same 4 probe technique. (*C*) Example of energy delivery that occurs between probes for a total of 6 probes with IRE energy delivered. (*From* Martin RCG, O'Connor R. The role of irreversible electroporation and other ablative techniques in patients with borderline resectable pancreatic cancer. New York: Springer; 2015; with permission.)

SMV were the most commonly affected. A few occurrences involving the celiac artery and hepatic artery were also noted. In 8 instances there was development of significant intravascular thrombus, and 6 pseudoaneurysms were identified. Indirect vascular findings manifested as end-organ infarcts were seen in 4 cases, all involving the spleen. The clinical correlations with these findings were minor or were asymptomatic in all patients and did not require further medical or surgical therapy.

The next most common category of findings was related to the gastrointestinal tract, most frequently with a nonspecific edematous appearance to the bowel wall, most commonly the stomach, as well as adjacent bowel loops in several cases. However, potentially more ominous findings related to the gastrointestinal tract, in descending order of frequency, include bowel perforation, portal venous gas, gastrointestinal hemorrhage, and pneumatosis intestinalis.

The remaining findings were associated with postoperative fluid collections within the abdominopelvic cavity, including 9 rim-enhancing fluid collections suspicious for abscess formation and 8 bland-appearing fluid collections. Biliary findings were infrequent, with 2 cases of common bile duct dilatation and 1 case of bile duct obstruction.

For longer term imaging post-IRE, the postablation bed is larger than the original ablated tumor. This ablation zone may get smaller (because of decreased edema and hyperemia) in the following months and, more importantly, remains stable provided there is no recurrence.[71] The evaluation of response rates for IRE using response evaluation

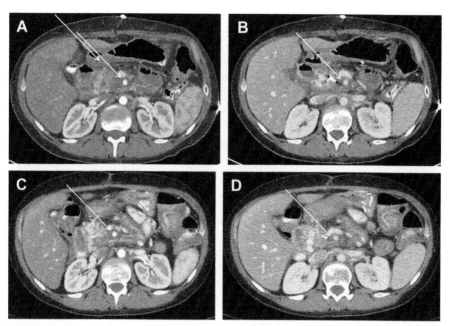

Fig. 4. Immediate postoperative scans in arterial (*A*) and venous phases (*B*) showing an increase in hazy soft tissue in the postablation bed (*white arrows*) and continued encirclement of SMA. Two-month postoperative scans in arterial (*C*) and venous (*D*) phases showing similar irregular, hazy, amorphous soft tissue stranding but with decreased size of the postablation zone (*white arrow*) consistent with no recurrence.

criteria in solid tumors (RECIST) criteria is limited given the lack of true decrease in size based on the pancreatic tumor stroma, fibrosis, and vasculature. Thus a complete response of IRE has been defined with no residual solid enhancing tumor and free of metastasis. Partial response is a decrease of 30% or more of the solid enhancing mass, and stable disease is less than 30% decrease or less than 20% increase compared with the first follow-up scan, which is performed at 3 months post-IRE. In cases of recurrent disease there is increased size of the ablation bed, mass effect, and new or worsening vascular encasement or occlusion.

CT imaging remains the best current imaging modality to assess post-IRE ablation changes. Serial imaging over at least 2 to 6 months must be used to detect recurrence by comparing with prior studies in conjunction with clinical and serum studies. Larger imaging studies are underway to evaluate for a more ideal imaging modality for this unique patient population.

SUMMARY

LAPC is a distinct disease with a clearly different biology from stage 4 pancreatic cancer. Separating these two entities allows the appropriate treatment of both patient subsets. Surgical evaluation at the time of diagnosis in conjunction with high-quality imaging is required, along with repeated evaluation at intervals of 2 to 3 months while on induction chemotherapy. Only after the biology of the disease is determined (lack of progression within the first 4–6 months) should any type of local therapy (RT or IRE) be considered. IRE can have a clear role in the local control of stage 3 and borderline resectable pancreatic adenocarcinoma only if used responsibly with the highest technical quality with extensive knowledge of IRE clinical end points and management of LAPC. The use of IRE in such a manner compares favorably with historical treatment of LAPC with chemotherapy and/or CRT and argues for its continued investigation as part of a multidisciplinary treatment plan. However, challenges related to intraprocedural targeting and posttreatment surveillance remain in 2016 and present limitations to the wider expansion of this technology.

REFERENCES

1. Spinelli GP, Zullo A, Romiti A, et al. Long-term survival in metastatic pancreatic cancer. A case report and review of the literature. JOP 2006;7(5):486–91.
2. Jemal A, Thomas A, Murray T, et al. Cancer statistics, 2002. CA Cancer J Clin 2002;52(1):23–47.
3. Callery MP, Chang KJ, Fishman EK, et al. Pretreatment assessment of resectable and borderline resectable pancreatic cancer: expert consensus statement. Ann Surg Oncol 2009;16(7):1727–33.
4. Varadhachary GR, Tamm EP, Abbruzzese JL, et al. Borderline resectable pancreatic cancer: definitions, management, and role of preoperative therapy. Ann Surg Oncol 2006;13(8):1035–46.
5. Ghaneh P, Kawesha A, Howes N, et al. Adjuvant therapy for pancreatic cancer. World J Surg 1999;23(9):937–45.
6. Hu J, Zhao G, Wang HX, et al. A meta-analysis of gemcitabine containing chemotherapy for locally advanced and metastatic pancreatic adenocarcinoma. J Hematol Oncol 2011;4:11.
7. Loehrer PJ Sr, Feng Y, Cardenes H, et al. Gemcitabine alone versus gemcitabine plus radiotherapy in patients with locally advanced pancreatic cancer: an Eastern Cooperative Oncology Group trial. J Clin Oncol 2011;29(31):4105–12.
8. Conroy T, Desseigne F, Ychou M, et al. FOLFIRINOX versus gemcitabine for metastatic pancreatic cancer. N Engl J Med 2011;364(19):1817–25.
9. Huguet F, Andre T, Hammel P, et al. Impact of chemoradiotherapy after disease control with chemotherapy in locally advanced pancreatic adenocarcinoma in GERCOR phase II and III studies. J Clin Oncol 2007;25(3):326–31.
10. Shoup M, Winston C, Brennan MF, et al. Is there a role for staging laparoscopy in patients with locally advanced, unresectable pancreatic adenocarcinoma? J Gastrointest Surg 2004;8(8):1068–71.
11. Liu RC, Traverso LW. Diagnostic laparoscopy improves staging of pancreatic cancer deemed locally unresectable by computed tomography. Surg Endosc 2005;19(5):638–42.
12. Al-Hawary MM, Francis IR, Chari ST, et al. Pancreatic ductal adenocarcinoma radiology reporting template: consensus statement of the Society of Abdominal Radiology and the American Pancreatic Association. Radiology 2014;270(1): 248–60.
13. Blazer M, Wu C, Goldberg RM, et al. Neoadjuvant modified (m) FOLFIRINOX for locally advanced unresectable (LAPC) and borderline resectable (BRPC) adenocarcinoma of the pancreas. Ann Surg Oncol 2015;22(4):1153–9.
14. Von Hoff DD, Ervin T, Arena FP, et al. Increased survival in pancreatic cancer with nab-paclitaxel plus gemcitabine. N Engl J Med 2013;369(18):1691–703.
15. Seufferlein T, Bachet JB, Van Cutsem E, et al. Pancreatic adenocarcinoma: ESMO-ESDO Clinical Practice Guidelines for diagnosis, treatment and follow-up. Ann Oncol 2012;23(Suppl 7):vii33–40.

16. Saliba D, Elliott M, Rubenstein LZ, et al. The Vulnerable Elders Survey: a tool for identifying vulnerable older people in the community. J Am Geriatr Soc 2001; 49(12):1691–9.

17. Tegels JJ, de Maat MF, Hulsewe KW, et al. Value of geriatric frailty and nutritional status assessment in predicting postoperative mortality in gastric cancer surgery. J Gastrointest Surg 2014;18(3):439–45 [discussion: 445–36].

18. Van Cutsem E, van de Velde H, Karasek P, et al. Phase III trial of gemcitabine plus tipifarnib compared with gemcitabine plus placebo in advanced pancreatic cancer. J Clin Oncol 2004;22(8):1430–8.

19. Rocha Lima CM, Green MR, Rotche R, et al. Irinotecan plus gemcitabine results in no survival advantage compared with gemcitabine monotherapy in patients with locally advanced or metastatic pancreatic cancer despite increased tumor response rate. J Clin Oncol 2004;22(18):3776–83.

20. Ishii H, Furuse J, Boku N, et al. Phase II study of gemcitabine chemotherapy alone for locally advanced pancreatic carcinoma: JCOG0506. Jpn J Clin Oncol 2010;40(6):573–9.

21. Andriulli A, Festa V, Botteri E, et al. Neoadjuvant/preoperative gemcitabine for patients with localized pancreatic cancer: a meta-analysis of prospective studies. Ann Surg Oncol 2012;19(5):1644–62.

22. Rose JB, Rocha FG, Alseidi A, et al. Extended neoadjuvant chemotherapy for borderline resectable pancreatic cancer demonstrates promising postoperative outcomes and survival. Ann Surg Oncol 2014;21(5):1530–7.

23. Kadera BE, Sunjaya DB, Isacoff WH, et al. Locally advanced pancreatic cancer: association between prolonged preoperative treatment and lymph-node negativity and overall survival. JAMA Surg 2014;149(2):145–53.

24. Ferrone CR, Marchegiani G, Hong TS, et al. Radiological and surgical implications of neoadjuvant treatment with FOLFIRINOX for locally advanced and borderline resectable pancreatic cancer. Ann Surg 2015;261(1):12–7.

25. Kwon D, McFarland K, Velanovich V, et al. Borderline and locally advanced pancreatic adenocarcinoma margin accentuation with intraoperative irreversible electroporation. Surgery 2014;156(4):910–20.

26. Martin RC 2nd, Kwon D, Chalikonda S, et al. Treatment of 200 locally advanced (stage III) pancreatic adenocarcinoma patients with irreversible electroporation: safety and efficacy. Ann Surg 2015;262(3):486–94.

27. Boone BA, Steve J, Krasinskas AM, et al. Outcomes with FOLFIRINOX for borderline resectable and locally unresectable pancreatic cancer. J Surg Oncol 2013; 108(4):236–41.

28. Martin RC. Irreversible electroporation of locally advanced pancreatic head adenocarcinoma. J Gastrointest Surg 2013;17(10):1850–6.

29. Sahora K, Kuehrer I, Eisenhut A, et al. NeoGemOx: Gemcitabine and oxaliplatin as neoadjuvant treatment for locally advanced, nonmetastasized pancreatic cancer. Surgery 2011;149(3):311–20.

30. Koong AC, Christofferson E, Le QT, et al. Phase II study to assess the efficacy of conventionally fractionated radiotherapy followed by a stereotactic radiosurgery boost in patients with locally advanced pancreatic cancer. Int J Radiat Oncol Biol Phys 2005;63(2):320–3.

31. Didolkar MS, Coleman CW, Brenner MJ, et al. Image-guided stereotactic radiosurgery for locally advanced pancreatic adenocarcinoma results of first 85 patients. J Gastrointest Surg 2010;14(10):1547–59.

32. Hoyer M, Roed H, Sengelov L, et al. Phase-II study on stereotactic radiotherapy of locally advanced pancreatic carcinoma. Radiother Oncol 2005;76(1):48–53.

33. Chang DT, Schellenberg D, Shen J, et al. Stereotactic radiotherapy for unresectable adenocarcinoma of the pancreas. Cancer 2009;115(3):665–72.

34. Schellenberg D, Goodman KA, Lee F, et al. Gemcitabine chemotherapy and single-fraction stereotactic body radiotherapy for locally advanced pancreatic cancer. Int J Radiat Oncol Biol Phys 2008;72(3):678–86.

35. Cohen SJ, Dobelbower R, Lipsitz S, et al. A randomized phase III study of radiotherapy alone or with 5-fluorouracil and mitomycin-C in patients with locally advanced adenocarcinoma of the pancreas: Eastern Cooperative Oncology Group study E8282. Int J Radiat Oncol Biol Phys 2005;62(5):1345–50.

36. Sultana A, Tudur Smith C, Cunningham D, et al. Systematic review, including meta-analyses, on the management of locally advanced pancreatic cancer using radiation/combined modality therapy. Br J Cancer 2007;96(8):1183–90.

37. Huguet F, Girard N, Guerche CS, et al. Chemoradiotherapy in the management of locally advanced pancreatic carcinoma: a qualitative systematic review. J Clin Oncol 2009;27(13):2269–77.

38. Krishnan S, Rana V, Janjan NA, et al. Induction chemotherapy selects patients with locally advanced, unresectable pancreatic cancer for optimal benefit from consolidative chemoradiation therapy. Cancer 2007;110(1):47–55.

39. Arvold ND, Ryan DP, Niemierko A, et al. Long-term outcomes of neoadjuvant chemotherapy before chemoradiation for locally advanced pancreatic cancer. Cancer 2012;118(12):3026–35.

40. Donahue TR, Isacoff WH, Hines OJ, et al. Downstaging chemotherapy and alteration in the classic computed tomography/magnetic resonance imaging signs of vascular involvement in patients with pancreaticobiliary malignant tumors: influence on patient selection for surgery. Arch Surg 2011;146(7):836–43.

41. Massucco P, Capussotti L, Magnino A, et al. Pancreatic resections after chemoradiotherapy for locally advanced ductal adenocarcinoma: analysis of perioperative outcome and survival. Ann Surg Oncol 2006;13(9):1201–8.

42. Turrini O, Viret F, Moureau-Zabotto L, et al. Neoadjuvant chemoradiation and pancreaticoduodenectomy for initially locally advanced head pancreatic adenocarcinoma. Eur J Surg Oncol 2009;35(12):1306–11.

43. Jurgensen C, Schuppan D, Neser F, et al. EUS-guided alcohol ablation of an insulinoma. Gastrointest Endosc 2006;63(7):1059–62.

44. Goel R, Anderson K, Slaton J, et al. Adjuvant approaches to enhance cryosurgery. J Biomech Eng 2009;131(7):074003.

45. Robinson D, Halperin N, Nevo Z. Two freezing cycles ensure interface sterilization by cryosurgery during bone tumor resection. Cryobiology 2001;43(1):4–10.

46. Spiliotis JD, Datsis AC, Michalopoulos NV, et al. Radiofrequency ablation combined with palliative surgery may prolong survival of patients with advanced cancer of the pancreas. Langenbecks Arch Surg 2007;392(1):55–60.

47. Date RS, Siriwardena AK. Radiofrequency ablation of the pancreas. II: Intraoperative ablation of non-resectable pancreatic cancer. A description of technique and initial outcome. JOP 2005;6(6):588–92.

48. Siriwardena AK. Radiofrequency ablation for locally advanced cancer of the pancreas. JOP 2006;7(1):1–4.

49. Bower M, Sherwood L, Li Y, et al. Irreversible electroporation of the pancreas: definitive local therapy without systemic effects. J Surg Oncol 2011;104(1):22–8.

50. Habash RW, Bansal R, Krewski D, et al. Thermal therapy, part III: ablation techniques. Crit Rev Biomed Eng 2007;35(1-2):37–121.

51. Charpentier KP, Wolf F, Noble L, et al. Irreversible electroporation of the pancreas in swine: a pilot study. HPB (Oxford) 2010;12(5):348–51.

52. Dunki-Jacobs EM, Philips P, Martin Ii RC. Evaluation of thermal injury to liver, pancreas and kidney during irreversible electroporation in an in vivo experimental model. Br J Surg 2014;101(9):1113–21.
53. Davalos RV, Mir IL, Rubinsky B. Tissue ablation with irreversible electroporation. Ann Biomed Eng 2005;33(2):223–31.
54. Al-Sakere B, Andre F, Bernat C, et al. Tumor ablation with irreversible electroporation. PLoS One 2007;2(11):e1135.
55. Granot Y, Rubinsky B. Mass transfer model for drug delivery in tissue cells with reversible electroporation. Int J Heat Mass Transf 2008;51(23-24):5610–6.
56. Escobar-Chavez JJ, Bonilla-Martinez D, Villegas-Gonzalez MA, et al. Electroporation as an efficient physical enhancer for skin drug delivery. J Clin Pharmacol 2009;49(11):1262–83.
57. Prud'homme GJ, Glinka Y, Khan AS, et al. Electroporation-enhanced nonviral gene transfer for the prevention or treatment of immunological, endocrine and neoplastic diseases. Curr Gene Ther 2006;6(2):243–73.
58. Lee RC. Cell injury by electric forces. Ann N Y Acad Sci 2005;1066:85–91.
59. Rubinsky B, Onik G, Mikus P. Irreversible electroporation: a new ablation modality–clinical implications. Technol Cancer Res Treat 2007;6(1):37–48.
60. Edd JF, Horowitz L, Davalos RV, et al. In vivo results of a new focal tissue ablation technique: irreversible electroporation. IEEE Trans Biomed Eng 2006;53(7): 1409–15.
61. Maor E, Ivorra A, Leor J, et al. The effect of irreversible electroporation on blood vessels. Technol Cancer Res Treat 2007;6(4):307–12.
62. Dunki-Jacobs EM, Philips P, Martin RC 2nd. Evaluation of resistance as a measure of successful tumor ablation during irreversible electroporation of the pancreas. J Am Coll Surg 2014;218(2):179–87.
63. Martin RC 2nd, McFarland K, Ellis S, et al. Irreversible electroporation therapy in the management of locally advanced pancreatic adenocarcinoma. J Am Coll Surg 2012;215(3):361–9.
64. Martin RC 2nd, McFarland K, Ellis S, et al. Irreversible electroporation in locally advanced pancreatic cancer: potential improved overall survival. Ann Surg Oncol 2013;20(Suppl 3):S443–9.
65. Martin RCG, Kwon D, Chalikonda S, et al. Treatment of 200 locally advanced (Stage III) pancreatic adenocarcinoma patients with irreversible electroporation safety and efficacy. Ann Surg 2015;262:486–94.
66. Narayanan G, Hosein PJ, Arora G, et al. Percutaneous irreversible electroporation for downstaging and control of unresectable pancreatic adenocarcinoma. J Vasc Interv Radiol 2012;23(12):1613–21.
67. Philips P, Li Y, Li S, et al. Efficacy of irreversible electroporation in human pancreatic adenocarcinoma: advanced murine model. Mol Ther Methods Clin Dev 2015; 2:15001.
68. Martin RCG. Irreversible electroporation in locally advanced pancreatic adenocarcinoma of body/neck. J Gastrointest Oncol 2015;6(3):329–35.
69. Martin RCG. Use of irreversible electroporation in unresectable pancreatic cancer. Hepatobiliary Surg Nutr 2015;4(3):211–5.
70. Philips P, Hays D, Martin RC. Irreversible electroporation ablation (IRE) of unresectable soft tissue tumors: learning curve evaluation in the first 150 patients treated. PLoS One 2013;8(11):e76260.
71. Akinwande O, Ahmad SS, Van Meter T, et al. CT findings of patients treated with irreversible electroporation for locally advanced pancreatic cancer. J Oncol 2015; 2015:680319.

Management of Metastatic Pancreatic Adenocarcinoma

Ahmad R. Cheema, MD[a,b], Eileen M. O'Reilly, MD[c,d],*

KEYWORDS

- Pancreatic cancer • Metastatic disease • Gemcitabine • Nab-paclitaxel
- FOLFIRINOX • Targeted agents • Immune therapy

KEY POINTS

- Progress in the treatment of pancreatic ductal adenocarcinoma (PDAC) has been incremental, mainly ensuing from cytotoxic systemic therapy, which continues to be a standard of care for metastatic disease.
- Folinic acid, 5-fluorouracil (5-FU), irinotecan, and oxaliplatin (FOLFIRINOX) and gemcitabine plus nab-paclitaxel have emerged as new standard therapies, improving survival in patients with good performance status.
- Novel therapeutics targeting the peritumoral stroma and tumor-driven immune suppression are currently a major focus of research in metastatic disease.
- Identification of reliable and validated predictive biomarkers to optimize therapeutics continues to be a challenge.
- Continued efforts toward better understanding of tumor biology and developing new drugs are warranted because a majority of patients succumb within a year of diagnosis, despite an increasing number of therapeutic options available today.

INTRODUCTION

In the year 2016, there will be approximately 53,000 estimated new individuals diagnosed with PDAC in the United States, representing approximately 3% of all cancer

Financial Disclosures: None (A.R. Cheema). Research support: Sanofi Pharmaceuticals, Celgene, Astra-Zenica, MedImmune, Bristol-Myers Squibb, Incyte, Polaris, Myriad Genetics, Momenta Pharmaceuticals, OncoMed. Consulting: Celgene, MedImmune, Sanofi Pharmaceutical, Threshold Pharmaceuticals, Gilead, Merrimack (E.M. O'Reilly).
Funding support: Cancer Center Support Grant (P30 CA008748).
[a] Department of Medicine, Icahn School of Medicine at Mount Sinai, 1 Gustave Levy Pl, New York, NY 10029, USA; [b] Department of Medicine, Mount Sinai St. Luke's-West Hospital Center, 1111 Amsterdam Avenue, New York, NY 10025, USA; [c] Rubenstein Center for Pancreatic Cancer Research, Memorial Sloan Kettering Cancer Center, 300 East 66th Street, Office 1021, New York, NY 10065, USA; [d] Weill Cornell Medical College, 1300 York Avenue, New York, NY 10065, USA
* Corresponding author. Rubenstein Center for Pancreatic Cancer Research, Memorial Sloan Kettering Cancer Center, 300 East 66th Street, Office 1021, New York, NY 10065.
E-mail address: oreillye@mskcc.org

cases.[1] Despite the low incidence, pancreatic cancer is the fourth leading cause of cancer-related death among both men and women in the United States, with a high mortality-to-incidence ratio, and is expected to become the second leading cause of cancer-related mortality by 2030.[2,3] PDAC is the most common histologic subtype, found in more than 85% of cases. Surgical resection is curative in a minority of patients; however, 70% to 80% of patients have unresectable disease, with more than 50% having distant metastases at the time of initial diagnosis, where the treatment goals are to control disease, palliate symptoms, and prolong survival.[2] For PDAC, the expected 5-year survival for all patients is approximately 6% to 7% and less for patients who are diagnosed with metastatic disease de novo.[2,4] Putative explanations for poor outcomes are generally attributed to the asymptomatic early stages of the disease, lack of effective screening tools, early metastatic dissemination, relative resistance of the tumor to cytotoxic and targeted therapies, dense stroma, hypoxic microenvironment, and immune suppression.

Over the past several years, tangible improvements in outcomes have been observed in patients with metastatic PDAC with the increasing use of new chemotherapeutic regimens. Gemcitabine plus albumin-bound paclitaxel and FOLFIRINOX have generated median overall survivals (OSs) ranging from 8.5 to 11.1 months for patients with good performance status.[5,6] For patients with poor performance status, however, median OS is typically in the 3-month to 6-month range.

Through extensive research over the past decade, remarkable advances have been made in understanding the molecular pathogenesis and underpinnings of PDAC. Major advances include elucidation of genetic alterations present in PDAC as well as defining the role of signaling pathways, peritumoral stroma, and immune system in tumor initiation, spread, and resistance to systemic therapies. Therefore, various targeted and immune therapies have been designed and are currently being investigated. Despite encouraging results in phase I/II studies, substantial impact in outcomes has not yet been observed. Therefore, PDAC remains a serious challenge for patients, families, and the scientific community.

This review discusses the current management options for patients with metastatic PDAC, with particular emphasis on the current state of the art along with current clinical trials and a focus on novel agents and immune therapeutics.

FIRST-LINE SYSTEMIC THERAPY

Systemic therapy is the mainstay of treatment of patients with metastatic PDAC, with proved efficacy in terms of prolonging survival. Historically, 5-FU as a single agent or 5-FU–based regimens were the standard treatments for patients with advanced disease, until the advent of gemcitabine.[7,8]

Single-agent Gemcitabine

Gemcitabine is an S-phase–specific pyrimidine antimetabolite that is converted by cellular kinases into difluorodeoxycytidine triphosphate. This active metabolite then competes with deoxycytidine to inhibit DNA synthesis.[9] In 1997, gemcitabine was approved by the US Food and Drug Administration (FDA) as monotherapy for metastatic PDAC after Burris and colleagues[10] demonstrated that gemcitabine was superior to 5-FU in patients with baseline Karnofsky performance scale score (KPS) greater than or equal to 50%; 126 patients with advanced PDAC were randomized to receive either gemcitabine (1000 mg/m^2 over 30 minutes weekly for 7 weeks, followed by a week of rest, and then weekly for 3 of 4 weeks) or weekly bolus of 5-FU (600 mg/m^2). Clinical benefit response, the principal endpoint of this trial, defined by composite assessment of pain (pain intensity/analgesia consumption), KPS, and dry weight gain, was observed in 23.8% of patients receiving gemcitabine compared with 4.8% in those receiving 5-FU (P = .022). Furthermore, median OS was also better for gemcitabine arm (5.65 vs 4.41 months, P = .0015). Based on the results of this trial, gemcitabine was established as a standard of care for first-line chemotherapy in patients with metastatic PDAC.

To enhance the efficacy of gemcitabine, conventional dosing over 30 minutes versus fixed dose rate (FDR), 10 mg/m^2/min, administration has been evaluated. Based on a phase I and pharmacokinetics study, which demonstrated saturation of deoxycytidine kinase enzyme, which catalyzes conversion of gemcitabine to its active metabolite, it was hypothesized that slower/prolonged infusion (FDR) could maximize the intracellular accumulation of active metabolite and enhance the antitumor activity.[11] A phase III randomized trial did not, however, demonstrate improvements in symptoms, median OS, progression-free survival (PFS), or 1-year or 2-year survival rates in patients who received FDR gemcitabine compared with standard-dose gemcitabine.[12]

Gemcitabine Combination Therapies

Given the positive outcomes with single-agent gemcitabine, numerous clinical trials investigated gemcitabine-based combination therapies in an attempt to improve the efficacy over single-agent therapy. Until recently, however, the results have been largely disappointing. Although gemcitabine combination therapies were observed to be safe and associated with better response rates, no statistically significant improvement in OS, the principal endpoint of most studies, was shown (**Table 1**). In meta-analyses, however, a survival benefit with some gemcitabine-based combinations, mainly fluoropyrimidine and platinum agents, over gemcitabine monotherapy was identified,[13–15] providing some support for the use of gemcitabine combinations in patients with a good functional status.

Several studies have also investigated gemcitabine-based polychemotherapy regimens comprising multiple cytotoxic drugs. One such study (randomized phase III, n = 99) was conducted by Reni and colleagues,[16] who demonstrated superior outcomes in terms of 4-month PFS (primary endpoint) with cisplatin, epirubicin, 5-FU, and gemcitabine (PEFG) combination therapy over single-agent gemcitabine. Even though outcome was favorable in the PEFG group, hematological toxicity was concerning with significant number of patients developing greater than or equal to grade 3 neutropenia and thrombocytopenia. Although this study favored the use of intensified chemotherapy, it did not receive much endorsement due to the limitations, including small sample size and principal endpoint of 4-month PFS (instead of OS), which made results difficult to generalize.

Gemcitabine Plus Erlotinib

Erlotinib, a tyrosine kinase (TYK) inhibitor of the epidermal growth factor receptor (EGFR), was the first drug to show survival benefit when administered in combination with gemcitabine. Moore and colleagues,[17] in 2007, conducted a phase III trial, including 569 patients, randomized to receive gemcitabine plus erlotinib (100 mg/d or 150 mg/d) or gemcitabine alone in patients with locally advanced and metastatic PDAC. The principal endpoint of the study was OS. An experimental group was observed to have improved outcomes in terms of OS and PFS compared with a gemcitabine-alone group. Even though the median survival time reached statistical significance, the advantage was marginal (6.24 months vs 5.9 months), and the clinical significance has been heavily debated over ensuing years. Patients who developed greater than or equal to grade 2 skin rash had a better median OS and 1-year survival rate compared with patients

Table 1
Selected phase 3 trials of gemcitabine-based therapies

Author, Year	No. of Patients	Treatment Arms	Median Progression-Free Survival (mo)	Median Overall Survival (mo)
Berlin et al,[119] 2002	327	Gemcitabine	2.2	5.4
		Gemcitabine + 5-FU	3.4	6.7
			$P = .02$	$P = .09$
Rocha Lima et al,[120] 2004	360	Gemcitabine	3.0	6.6
		Gemcitabine + irinotecan	3.5	6.3
			$P = .35$	$P = .79$
Louvet et al,[121] 2005	313	Gemcitabine	3.7	7.1
		Gemcitabine + oxaliplatin	5.8	9.0
			HR 1.29, $P = .04$	HR 1.20, $P = .13$
Oettle et al,[122] 2005	565	Gemcitabine	3.3	6.3
		Gemcitabine + pemetrexed	3.9	6.2
			$P = .11$	HR 0.98, $P = .85$
Abou-Alfa et al,[123] 2006	349	Gemcitabine	3.8	6.2
		Gemcitabine + exatecan	3.7	6.7
			$P = .22$	$P = .52$
Heinemann et al,[124] 2006	195	Gemcitabine	3.1	6.0
		Gemcitabine + cisplatin	5.3	7.5
			HR 0.75, $P = .05$	HR 0.80, $P = .15$
Herrmann et al,[125] 2007	319	Gemcitabine	3.9	7.2
		Gemcitabine + capecitabine	4.3	8.4
			$P = .10$	HR 0.87, $P = .23$
Moore et al,[17] 2007	569	Gemcitabine	3.7	5.9
		Gemcitabine + erlotinib	3.5	6.2
			HR 0.77, $P = .004$	HR 0.82, $P = .038$
Cunningham et al,[126] 2009	533	Gemcitabine	3.8	6.2
		Gemcitabine + capecitabine	5.3	7.1
			HR 0.78, $P = .004$	HR 0.86, $P = .08$
Poplin et al,[12] 2009	547	Gemcitabine	2.6	4.9
		Gemcitabine + oxaliplatin	2.7	5.7
			$P = .10$	HR 0.88, $P = .22$
Colucci et al,[127] 2010	400	Gemcitabine	3.9	8.3
		Gemcitabine + cisplatin	3.8	7.2
			HR 0.97, $P = .80$	HR 1.10, $P = .38$
Ueno et al,[128] 2013	554	Gemcitabine	4.1	8.8
		Gemcitabine + S1	5.7	10.1
			HR 0.66, $P<.001$	HR 0.88, $P = 0.15$

Data from Refs.[12,17,119–128]

with no skin rash (OS 10.5 vs 5.3 months, 1-year survival rate 43% vs 16%), and analysis of tumor specimens showed a nonstatistical trend for the benefit of gemcitabine and erlotinib in KRAS wild-type patients (hazard ratio [HR] = 0.66).[18] This trial led to FDA approval of erlotinib combined with gemcitabine as first-line therapy in metastatic PDAC; however, the modest activity, increased toxicity, and ambivalence about the clinical utility collectively limited its widespread use.

Given the superior survival in patients developing skin rash secondary to EGFR inhibition, a phase II study, Dose Escalation to Rash for Erlotinib Plus Gemcitabine (RACHEL), was conducted, where the erlotinib dose was escalated by 50 mg every

2 weeks to a maximum of 250 mg daily. Even though erlotinib dose escalation induced greater than or equal to grade 2 skin rash in 41.4% patients, no improvement in OS was noted over standard dose.[19]

Folinic Acid, 5-Fluorouracil, Irinotecan, and Oxaliplatin

In 2011, after the report of PRODIGE-4/ACCORD 11 (Partenarait de Recherche en Oncologie Digestive-4/Actions Concertées dans les Cancers Colo-Rectaux et Digestifs-11) trial, FOLFIRINOX emerged as a promising new regimen in the first-line setting. Encouraged by the efficacy and safety profile of these agents demonstrated in phase I/II studies, Conroy and colleagues[6] randomized 342 patients with good performance status (Eastern Cooperative Oncology Group [ECOG] 0–1) to FOLFIRINOX (folinic acid, 400 mg/m^2; irinotecan, 180 mg/m^2; oxaliplatin, 85 mg/m^2; and 5-FU, 400 mg/m^2) as bolus followed by 2400 mg/m^2 as 46-h continuous infusion, every 2 weeks or gemcitabine. The principal endpoint was OS, and response rate (RR), PFS, quality of life (QOL), and toxicity were secondary endpoints. The OS was significantly improved in patients who received FOLFIRINOX compared with gemcitabine (11.1 vs 6.8 months; HR 0.57; 95% CI, 0.45–0.73; $P<.001$). Equally encouraging improvements with FOLFIRINOX were noted in terms of 1-year survival rate (48.4% vs 20.6%), median PFS (6.4 vs 3.3 months; HR 0.47; 95% CI, 0.37–0.59; $P<.001$), and RR (31.6% vs 9.4%, $P<.001$). Even though the safety profile of FOLFIRINOX was less favorable (higher incidence of neutropenia, febrile neutropenia, thrombocytopenia, fatigue, diarrhea, sensory neuropathy, and alopecia), significantly improved global health status and delay in time to deterioration of (QOL) (assessed using European Organisation for Research and Treatment of Cancer QLQ-C30 questionnaire) were observed in FOLFIRINOX arm, which may reflect that disease-related symptoms likely influence the QOL more than treatment-related side effects. The QOL assessments were presented 2 years after the primary study, which also showed that age greater than 65, low albumin, and hepatic metastasis were associated with a poorer prognosis.[20]

After the results of this study, many single-institution and multi-institution studies confirmed the positive outcomes with FOLFIRINOX and the associated toxicity profile comparable to that reported in the parent trial.[21–23]

In an attempt to enhance the tolerability of this regimen, modified forms of FOLFIRINOX (ie, elimination of bolus 5-FU, modification of irinotecan and oxaliplatin doses, and administration of growth factors) have been evaluated and have shown to improve safety while preserving efficacy; however, data are limited and nonrandomized.[24–26]

Gemcitabine Plus Nab-Paclitaxel

Secreted protein acid rich in cysteine (SPARC), an albumin-binding protein, is present in the stromal fibroblasts within the pancreatic tumor microenvironment and its overexpression is recognized to promote cancer cell invasion and metastasis, hence is associated with poor prognosis.[27,28] To target the tumor stroma, nab-paclitaxel (albumin-bound paclitaxel) was developed and investigated in PDAC based on a rationale that it depletes the desmoplastic stroma by binding with SPAR and thus promotes intratumoral gemcitabine levels.[29] After the promising results of phase I/II studies showing improved OS (median OS 12.2 months) in patients treated with gemcitabine plus nab-paclitaxel, Von Hoff and colleagues[5] conducted a phase III trial (MPACT [Metastatic Pancreatic Adenocarcinoma Clinical Trial]), assigning 861 patients with KPS greater than or equal to 70% to gemcitabine plus nab-paclitaxel or gemcitabine alone.[30] Statistically significant improvement in survival was demonstrated in the combination treatment arm, with median OS of 8.5 months versus 6.7 months in gemcitabine arm. Improvements were also noted in the combination treatment group in terms of median PFS (5.5 vs 3.7 months), RR (23% vs7%), 1-year survival (35% vs 22%), and

2-year survival (9% vs 4%). Not surprisingly, the experimental arm had a greater incidence of greater than or equal to grade 3 adverse effects, including neutropenia, fatigue, peripheral neuropathy, and diarrhea. QOL data were not collected on this trial. Later, these results were validated by Goldstein and colleagues,[31] who demonstrated that 4% of patients survived greater than 3 years in the combination group versus none in the control arm.

Early phase I/II studies demonstrated a significant increase in OS in patients with high stromal SPARC expression.[30] Recent analysis of prospectively collected biospecimens from the MPACT trial did not, however, demonstrate any correlation of SPARC expression levels in tumor stroma, tumor epithelial cells, or plasma with OS in either treatment arm, arguing against the role of SPARC as a predictive or prognostic biomarker.[32] Gemcitabine/nab-paclitaxel has emerged as a regimen for adding novel therapeutics and multiple ongoing randomized trials are under way (see **Table 5**).

Folinic Acid, 5-Fluorouracil, Irinotecan, and Oxaliplatin Versus Gemcitabine/Nab-Paclitaxel

The recent development of 2 combination regimens has altered the therapeutic landscape for patients with metastatic PDAC. Both FOLFIRINOX and gemcitabine/nab-paclitaxel have shown improvement in OS over single-agent gemcitabine.[5,6] The optimal first-line choice of treatment remains a question, however, given no head-to-head comparison is available and cross-trial comparisons have significant limitations. The PRODIGE trial was conducted in a single country, included patients with ECOG less than or equal to 1 only and age less than or equal to 75 years, enrolled fewer patients than in MPACT trial, and had a greater percentage of patients with peritoneal metastasis. Despite the differences, patients who received gemcitabine alone in both trials had identical median OS (6.8 months in PRODIGE and 6.7 months in MPACT), suggesting that the patient populations were overall similar (**Table 2**). Even though FOLFIRINOX seems superior in terms of OS (11.1 vs 8.5 months), it is associated with potentially greater toxicity. Therefore, the first-line choice of treatment should be based on careful evaluation of patient's preference, comorbid conditions, age, ability to tolerate toxicity, willingness to have central venous access, and treatment cost. A neoadjuvant trial, S1505, by the Southwest Oncology Group (SWOG) is under way evaluating FOLFIRINOX versus gemcitabine/nab-paclitaxel in patients with resectable PDAC and will provide comparative information of the regimens in a nonmetastatic setting (NCT02562716).

National Comprehensive Cancer Network 2015 guidelines for first-line treatment of metastatic PDAC recommend either FOLFIRINOX or gemcitabine/nab-paclitaxel for patients with good performance status (ECOG ≤ 1, good pain management, patent biliary stent, and good nutritional status). Acceptable lower consensus options include gemcitabine plus erlotinib and gemcitabine plus capecitabine for patients with poorer performance status. Although less effective, single-agent gemcitabine remains an appropriate option for patients with poor performance status or when combination treatment is contraindicated for any reason.

Finally, given the possibly better safety profile of gemcitabine and nab-paclitaxel, it may serve as an appropriate chemotherapeutic backbone on which to add novel agents.

SECOND-LINE SYSTEMIC THERAPIES

Several agents have been investigated over the past decade, including taxanes, fluoropyrimidine, oxaliplatin, and pemetrexed, either as single agents or in combination regimens (eg, FOLFIRI3, FOLFOX4, FOLFIRINOX, CAPOX, and GEMOX).[33–44] Even

Table 2
Characteristics, outcomes, and greater than or equal to grade 3 adverse events in the PRODIGE-4 and MPACT trials

	PRODIGE-4 Trial		MPACT Trial	
	FOLFIRINOX	**Gemcitabine**	**Gemcitabine + Nab-Paclitaxel**	**Gemcitabine**
Number of patients	171	171	431	430
Median age, years (range)	61 (25–76)	61 (34–75)	62 (27–86)	63 (32–88)
Males, %	62	61.4	57	60
ECOG or KPS, (%)				
0 or 100	37.4	38.6	16	16
1 or 80/90	61.9	61.4	77	76
2 or 60/70	0.6	0	7	8
Primary head tumor, %	39.2	36.8	44	42
Liver involvement, %	87.6	87.7	85	84
Lung involvement, %	19.4	28.7	35	43
Peritoneal involvement, %	19.4	18.7	4	2
Response rate, %	31.6	9.4	23	7
Median PFS, months	6.4	3.3	5.5	3.7
Median OS, months	11.1	6.8	8.5	6.7
Neutropenia, %	45.7	21	38	27
Febrile neutropenia, %	5.4	1.2	3	1
Thrombocytopenia, %	9.1	3.6	13	9
Diarrhea, %	12.7	1.8	6	1
Peripheral neuropathy, %	9.0	0	17	1
Fatigue, %	23.6	17.8	17	7

Data from Von Hoff DD, Ervin T, Arena FP, et al. Increased survival in pancreatic cancer with nab-paclitaxel plus gemcitabine. N Engl J Med 2013;369(18):1691–703; and Conroy T, Desseigne F, Ychou M, et al. FOLFIRINOX versus gemcitabine for metastatic pancreatic cancer. N Engl J Med 2011;364(19):1817–25.

though trials have demonstrated potential efficacy of these regimens as second-line combinations, the results were mostly not generalizable due to the limitations of either study designs (mainly phase II, single arm) or small sample sizes. Fewer phase III trials have been conducted in the second-line setting.

Charite onkologie (CONKO)-01, one of few phase III trials in a second-line setting, has provided evidence for survival benefit with the oxaliplatin, folinic acid, and 5-FU (OFF) regimen over best supportive care alone in patients with gemcitabine-resistant PDAC.[45] After CONKO-01, the CONKO-003 trial evaluated the efficacy of oxaliplatin in the second-line setting by comparing OFF with folinic acid/leucovorin (5-FU/LV).[46] This study observed superior median OS with OFF (5.9 vs 3.3 months) and supported oxaliplatin-based regimens as standard second-line therapy. The PANCREOX trial failed, however, to demonstrate the superior efficacy of oxaliplatin-based regimens over FF in gemcitabine pretreated patients (**Table 3**).[47] Therefore, the role of oxaliplatin in a second-line setting remains a debated one.

Recently, MM-398, a nanoliposomal irinotecan, has emerged as a promising option after the results of the NAPOLI (Nanoliposomal Irinotecan with Fluorouracil and Folinic Acid in Metastatic Pancreatic Cancer After Previous Gemcitabine-Based

Table 3
Selected phase III clinical trials in the second-line and beyond setting

Author, Year	No. of Patients	Treatment Arms	Median Progression-Free Survival (mo)	Median Overall Survival (mo)
Pelzer et al,[45] 2011	46	BSC	NA	2.3
		OFF + BSC		4.8
				HR 0.45, P = .008
Oettle et al,[46] 2014	168	5-FU/LV	2.0	3.3
		OFF	2.9	5.9
			HR 0.68, P = .019	HR 0.66, P = .010
Gill et al,[47] 2014	108	5-FU/LV	2.9	9.9
		mFOLFOX6	3.1	6.1
			HR 1.00, P = .99	HR 1.78, P = .02
Wang-Gilliam et al,[50] 2016	417	5-FU/LV	1.5	4.2
		MM-398	2.7	4.9
		MM-398 + 5-FU/LV	3.1	6.1
			HR 0.56, P = .0001	HR 0.67, P = .012

Abbreviations: BSC, best supportive care; mFOLFOX6, modified FOLFOX6.
 Data from Refs.[45–47,50]

Therapy)-1 trial. This drug was designed based on the rationale that the nanoliposomal encapsulation allows prolonged blood circulation time and increased intratumoral levels of irinotecan and its active metabolite SN-38, potentially leading to better efficacy and reduced toxicity to normal tissues.[48,49] Wang-Gilliam and colleagues[50] conducted a global phase III randomized trial, including 417 patients who had progressed on gemcitabine-based therapy, administered in either an adjuvant, neoadjuvant, or metastatic disease setting. Patients were randomly assigned to receive liposomal irinotecan with or without 5-FU/LV or 5-FU/LV alone.[50] OS was the principal endpoint of the study. The combination of nanoliposomal irinotecan and 5-FU/LV demonstrated improved median OS compared with 5-FU/LV alone (6.1 vs 4.2 months; HR 0.67; 95% CI, 0.49–0.92; P = .012). Combination treatment also showed better efficacy in terms of median PFS (3.1 vs 1.5 months, P = .0001), PFS at 12 weeks (57% vs 26%), and objective RR (ORR) (16% vs 1%, P<.0001). In contrast, no difference in OS was observed between liposomal irinotecan alone and 5-FU/LV alone arms; thus, single-agent liposomal irinotecan is not a recommended option. Common greater than or equal to grade 3 toxicities in the combination arm included neutropenia, diarrhea, fatigue, and vomiting. The promising results from the NAPOLI-1 trial earned FDA approval for the combination of liposomal irinotecan and 5-FU/LV in patients with metastatic PDAC who have had prior progression on gemcitabine-based therapy in late 2015.

Because FOLFIRINOX and gemcitabine/nab-paclitaxel are increasingly used as first-line therapies, there is growing interest about the possibility of using them sequentially, after disease progression on the other. The feasibility of this approach has been suggested by recently published single-center and multicenter studies, with 1 study conducted in fit patients demonstrating remarkable improvement in OS to 18 months (from the time of diagnosis) in patients treated with gemcitabine/nab-paclitaxel after FOLFIRINOX failure.[51,52] Larger trials are needed, however, to validate these results. Overall, the past several years have seen several new treatment options approved for PDAC, indicating real, albeit incremental, improvements in outcome for this disease. Combination cytotoxic regimens are also being integrated into other disease settings, such as in adjuvant and locally advanced disease settings (NCT01964430, NCT01526135, NCT01921751).

NOVEL THERAPEUTICS

With the expanding knowledge of molecular and cellular pathways underlying PDAC growth and spread, a variety of novel agents have been designed and investigated. PDAC is characterized by mutations in key oncogenes and tumor suppressor genes, initially predominantly in the RAS proliferative pathway (primarily KRAS and rarely BRAF) and later in CDKN2A/RB/INK4A, TP53 and transforming growth factor (TGF)-β/SMAD4.[53–57] These mutations are thought to accumulate in a stepwise manner and mark the progression of precursors lesion into invasive adenocarcinoma. In addition, several cellular signaling pathways that are altered or dysregulated in PDAC have been defined, including DNA repair, cell cycle regulation, apoptosis, Wnt and Notch signaling.[58,59]

The KRAS oncogene is mutated in greater than 90% of PDAC cases and is one of the major drivers in the initiation and maintenance of PDAC. Mutation in KRAS results in constitutive activation of downstream signaling pathways, such as PI3K/AKT/mTOR and Mitogen activated protein kinase/Extracellular signal-related kinase (MAPK/ERK), which play crucial roles in carcinogenesis and metastasis.[60] Given that the direct therapeutic targeting of KRAS to date has been ineffective, research focus has moved to targeting downstream signal mediators of KRAS. The results have not been promising, however, thus far (**Table 4**). The failure of single targeted agents has led to the idea of dual targeting in hopes of overcoming tumor resistance, proposed as secondary to activation of other compensatory downstream pathways. The feasibility of this approach was recently supported by a phase II trial of combined erlotinib and MAPK/ERK kinase (MEK) inhibitor selumetinib in 46 patients with previously treated advanced PDAC, where combination treatment showed modest antitumor activity with median OS of 7.3 months.[61] Multiple other combination strategies are under investigation (NCT01449058).

Everolimus, a mammalian target of rapamycin inhibitor (mTOR), has shown promise in gastric cancer; however, results have been inconsistent in metastatic PDAC. Recently, Kordes and colleagues,[62] in a phase II study, demonstrated improved efficacy of everolimus in combination with capecitabine in the first-line setting (RR 6%, median OS 8.9 months). Previously, however, 2 small prospective studies assessing temsirolimus and a combination regimen of everolimus plus erlotinib did not produce encouraging results.[63] For the most part, combining targeted agents has led to limited efficacy.

Notch Signaling

Growing molecular evidence suggests implication of Notch signaling in pancreatic cancer initiation and maintenance because Notch overexpression leads to accumulation of undifferentiated precursor cells.[64,65] Two Notch ligands, JAGGED 2 and DLL4, have been shown to be overexpressed in PDAC, contributing to Notch activation.[66,67] Thus, inhibition of Notch pathway has been looked on as a viable therapeutic target, and encouraging results have already been observed in preclinical and early clinical studies assessing this strategy.[68–70] Despite the promising early results, a recent announcement has indicated that a randomized phase II trial evaluating the addition of OMP-59R5/placebo to gemcitabine/nab-paclitaxel is likely to meet futility.[71] Other ongoing trials are targeting other components of the Notch pathway.

Janus Kinase/Signal Transducer and Activator of Transcription Pathway

The role of the Janus kinase (JAK)/signal transducer and activator of transcription (STAT) pathway is well established in many human malignancies, including

Table 4
Selected phase III clinical trials of targeted agents

Author, Year	Study Design	N	Treatment Arms	Target	Median Progression-Free Survival (mo)	Median Overall Survival (mo)
Bramhall et al,[129] 2002	R, phase 3	239	Gemcitabine Gemcitabine + marimastat	MMP	3.2 3.0 HR 0.95, P = .68	5.4 5.4 HR 0.99, P = .95
Van Cutsem et al,[130] 2004	R, phase 3	688	Gemcitabine Gemcitabine + tipifarnib	MAPK	3.6 3.7 HR 1.03, P = .72	6.0 6.3 HR 1.03, P = .75
Philip et al,[131] 2010	R, phase 3	743	Gemcitabine Gemcitabine + cetuximab	MAPK	3.0 3.4 HR 1.07, P = .18	5.9 6.3 HR 1.06, P = .19
Ko et al,[61] 2016	S, phase 2	46	Selumetinib + erlotinib	MAPK	1.9	7.3
Infante et al,[132] 2014	R, phase 2	160	Gemcitabine Gemcitabine + trametinib	MAPK	3.5 3.7 HR 0.93, P = .35	6.7 8.4 HR 0.98, P = .45
Van Cutsem et al,[133] 2009	R, phase 3	607	Gemcitabine + erlotinib Gemcitabine + erlotinib + bevacizumab	VEGF	3.6 4.6 HR 0.73, P = .0002	6.0 7.1 HR 0.89, P = .54
Kindler et al,[134] 2010	R, phase 3	602	Gemcitabine Gemcitabine + bevacizumab	VEGF	2.9 3.8 P = .08	5.9 5.8 P = .95

Study	Design	N	Treatment	Target						
Kindler et al,[135] 2011	R, phase 3	632	Gemcitabine Gemcitabine + axitinib	VEGF	4.4 4.4 HR 1.01, P = .52			8.3 8.5 HR 1.01, P = .54		
Javle et al,[63] 2010	S, phase 2	16	Everolimus + erlotinib	mTOR	1.6			2.9		
Gonçalves et al,[136] 2012	R, Phase 3	104	Gemcitabine Gemcitabine + sorefenib	VEGFR PDGFR B-Raf	5.7 3.8 HR 1.04, P = .90			9.2 8.0 HR 1.27, P = .23		
Rougier et al,[137] 2013	R, phase 3	546	Gemcitabine Gemcitabine + ziv-aflibercept	VEGF	3.7 3.7 HR 1.02, P = .86			7.8 6.5 HR 1.17, P = .20		
Hurwitz et al,[76] 2015	R, phase 2	127	Capecitabine Capecitabine + ruxolitinb	JAK	1.5 1.7 HR 0.75, P = .14			4.2 4.5 HR 0.79, P = .25		

Abbreviations: MMP, matrix metalloproteinase; PDGFR, platelet-derived growth factor receptor; R, randomized; S, single arm; VEGF, vascular endothelial growth factor; VEGFR, vascular endothelial growth factor receptor.
  Data from Refs.[61,63,76,129–137]

PDAC.[72–74] JAKs (JAK1, JAK2, JAK3, and TYK2) are cytoplasmic TYKs, which, on activation, phosphorylate STAT transcription factors. This constitutive STAT activation leads to up-regulation of several cellular processes promoting cell proliferation, angiogenesis, and inflammation. Thus, activation of JAK/STAT has been associated with poor outcomes, providing a rationale for potential therapeutic targeting.[75] Recently, Hurwitz and colleagues[76] conducted a randomized phase II trial (RECAP) testing addition of ruxolitinib (JAK1/2 inhibitor) to capecitabine versus capecitabine alone in patients with gemcitabine refractory PDAC. Even though the primary endpoint of OS was not met in the overall group, a prespecified subgroup analysis showed that patients with evidence of systemic inflammation (defined by high serum C-reactive protein), had better OS than those without elevated C-reactive protein in the combination treatment arm. Moreover, combination treatment was well tolerated. These promising results prompted 2 phase III trials, JANUS1 and JANUS2, evaluating capecitabine with or without ruxolitinib as second-line therapy in metastatic disease (NCT02117479 and NCT02119663). Again, however, a recent press release has indicated that futility for the combination over capecitabine has been met and further development of ruxolitinib in solid tumors has ceased.[77]

ANTISTROMAL AGENTS

PDAC is characterized by an extremely dense microenvironment or desmoplastic stroma, which is a complex network of cellular elements within a protein-rich extracellular matrix.[78–81] This dense stroma has been postulated as creating a hypoxic environment not penetrable by current cytotoxic agents, thus protecting the tumor cells and promoting proliferation and metastasis.[82] Due to its potential oncogenic role, peritumoral stroma has been a focus of extensive research.

Pegylated Recombinant Human Hyaluronidase

The extracellular matrix PDAC is rich in hyaluronan, or hyaluronic acid (HA), which interacts with several cell surface receptors, most importantly CD44, and regulates TYK receptor–induced signaling pathways, thus promoting angiogenesis and tumor progression.[83] Also, the abundance of HA increases interstitial fluid pressure and leads to relative hypovascularity of the tumor, postulated as one of the major mechanisms of resistance to chemotherapies.[82] Enzymatic degradation by pegylated recombinant human hyaluronidase (PEGPH20) was found to decrease interstitial fluid pressure, re-expand the collapsed vasculature and enhance drug delivery, and thus improve survival in mouse models of PDAC.[82,84] The efficacy of PEGPH20 demonstrated in mouse model has prompted 2 randomized trials (SWOG S1313 and HALO 109–202) exploring PEGPH20 on the backbone of standard chemotherapeutic agents in the first-line setting. Promising interim results of the ongoing randomized phase 2 trial evaluating the addition of PEGPH20 to gemcitabine/nab-paclitaxel in patients with untreated metastatic PDAC were recently presented. The trial included 135 patients and demonstrated an improved median PFS, the principal endpoint, in patients with high-HA tumor treated with PEGPH20 combination compared with gemcitabine/nab-paclitaxel (9.2 vs 4.3 months, HR 0.39, $P = .05$). Patients in the combination arm also showed significant improvement in ORR (52% vs 24%, $P = .038$) and a trend toward improved OS (12 vs 9 months).[85] An excess of thromboembolic events was also seen in the trial on the experimental arm; however, the addition of low-molecular-weight heparin in the combination arm of PEGPH20 and gemcitabine/nab-paclitaxel seems to have mitigated this finding. A phase 3 trial of gemcitabine/nab-paclitaxel with/without PEGPH20 is ongoing in patients with metastatic PDAC without thromboses and with high HA using a similar low-molecular-weight heparin prophylactic strategy (NCT01839487, NCT02715804).

TH-302

Hypoxia in tumor microenvironment, a common feature of PDAC, confers resistance to chemotherapy. TH-302 is a hypoxia-activated prodrug that releases the DNA cross-linker bromo-isophosphoramide (Br-IPM) under hypoxic conditions. On activation, Br-IPM can exert cytotoxic effects by diffusing into the adjacent oxygenated tissues, the rationale for TH-302 development.[86,87] Based on the encouraging results of preclinical and phase II studies, a phase III trial (MAESTRO) was conducted to test TH-302 in combination with gemcitabine in previously untreated patients; however, results were disappointing[88] and further development of TH-302 in PDAC has ceased.

Targeting DNA Repair Pathways

BRCA1 and BRCA2 are the most common germline mutations in PDAC, and, more recently, mutations in PALB2 have also been identified. Numerous cellular roles have been attributed to BRCA1 and BRCA2, including repair of DNA double-stranded breaks (DSBs) by homologous recombination.[89,90] In the absence of functional BRCA1/2 or PALB2, however, these DSBs are repaired by error-prone nonhomologous end joining and single-strand annealing, leading to genomic instability.[91] Poly (ADP-ribose) polymerase (PARP) is an important enzyme that mediates repair of DNA single-stranded breaks (SSBs) and gaps, rescuing tumor cells from DNA damage. Considering PARP as a potential therapeutic target, especially in BRCA or PALB2 mutated tumors, PARP inhibitors (PARPi) have been designed and investigated. These inhibitors block the SSBs repair and induce DSBs, which in the absence of functional BRCA or PALB2, are not accurately repaired, resulting in cancer cell death.[92,93] BRCA-mutated tumor cells demonstrate susceptibility to platinum compounds as platinum compounds induce interstrand cross-links, which require repair by homologous recombination.[94] Encouraging results have been demonstrated in a phase II study evaluating olaparib, a PARPi, in patients with advanced pancreatic cancer.[95] Several other clinical trials in the advanced disease setting are under way (NCT01296763, NCT01585805, and NCT01296763) (**Table 5**).

IMMUNE THERAPIES

Immune therapy has been a subject of rapidly expanding interest in cancer research.[96] PDAC is generally considered immune resistant and several mechanisms have been hypothesized as playing a role. Because the genetic mutations/alterations accumulate, cancer cells secrete factors, such as interleukin (IL)-8, IL-10, TGF-β, and galectin 1, that recruit and activate immune suppressor cells (ie, regulatory T cells and myeloid-derived suppressor cells) and inhibit effector T cells.[97–99] Additionally, the cancer-associated fibroblasts in the tumor stroma recruit macrophages with suppressive phenotype and secrete fibroblast activation protein, which suppresses effector T cell function.[100] An extensive series of trials are under way evaluating a variety of immune-based approaches in PDAC.

VACCINES

Vaccine therapies have been a focus of attention and several strategies have been investigated, such as dendritic cell vaccines, whole cancer cell vaccines, DNA

Table 5
Selected ongoing clinical trials in advanced pancreatic ductal adenocarcinoma

Clinical Trial	Phase	Estimated Enrollment (n)	Treatments	Target
NCT01959139	Ib/II	138	mFOLFIRINOX ± PEGPH20	HA
NCT01839487	II	237	Gemcitabine + nab-paclitaxel ± PEGPH20	HA
NCT01621243	II	148	Gemcitabine + nab-paclitaxel ± M402	Antistromal
NCT01373164	I/II	168	Gemcitabine ± LY2157299	TGF-β
NCT01088815	II	80	Gemcitabine + nab-paclitaxel ± vismodegib	Hedgehog
NCT01485744	I	40	FOLFIRINOX + LDE225	Hedgehog
NCT01728818	II	117	Gemcitabine + afatinib	EGFR1, HER2, HER4
NCT01509911	II	80	Gemcitabine ± RX-0201	Angiogenesis
NCT01585805	II	70	Gemcitabine + cisplatin ± veliparib	PARP (BRCA+)
NCT01296763	I/II	18	ICM ± AZD2281 (olaparib)	DNA repair
NCT02395016	III	276	Gemcitabine ± nimotuzumab in KRAS wild-type	EGFR
NCT02101021	III	430	Gemcitabine + nab-paclitaxel ± momelotinib	JAK1/2
NCT02436668	II/III	326	Gemcitabine + nab-paclitaxel ± ibrutinib	TYK
NCT01222689	II	46	Erlotinib + AZD6244	MEK, TYK
NCT0200426	II	240	CRS-207 ± GVAX/CY vs chemotherapy	Mesothelin (vaccine)
NCT02243371	II	94	GVAX/CY + CRS-207 ± nivolumab	Vaccine
NCT01928394	I/II	410	Nivolumab ± ipilimumab	PD-1, CTLA-4
NCT01473940	Ib	28	Gemcitabine + ipilimumab	CTLA-4

Abbreviations: CY, cyclophosphamide; ICM, Irinotecan, Cisplatin, Mitomycin C; mFOLFIRINOX, modified FOLFIRINOX.

vaccines, and peptide vaccines, with limited activity overall.[101,102] Although early phase 1/II studies provided evidence for antitumor immune response with vaccine-based therapies, the results of subsequent phase III trials were not promising.[102,103]

An encouraging signal has been identified for a combination of GVAX, an irradiated granulocyte macrophage–colony-stimulating factor–secreting allogeneic pancreatic cancer vaccine, in combination with CRS-207, a recombinant, live-attenuated *Listeria* vaccine designed to secrete mesothelin. After a phase 1 study showing synergistic effect of GVAX and CRS-207, a phase II clinical trial randomized 90 previously treated metastatic PDAC patients to GVAX plus CRS-207 versus GVAX alone. Improved OS was observed in combination treatment arm compared with GVAX monotherapy (6.1 vs 3.9 months, $P = .002$). Furthermore, enhanced mesothelin-specific CD8 T-cell responses were associated with longer OS, regardless of treatment arms.[104,105] Several ongoing studies are evaluating GVAX and CRS-207 compared with chemotherapy and combined with or without a checkpoint inhibitor (NCT02004262 and NCT02243371).

CHECKPOINT BLOCKADE

Recently, targetable peptides, such as cytotoxic T-lymphocyte–associated antigen 4 (CTLA4), programmed death 1 (PD-1) immune checkpoint receptor, and PD ligand 1 have been identified, which inactivate the immune response. Ipilimumab, a fully humanized monoclonal antibody, inhibits CTLA4 and thus prevents the development of self-tolerance, maintaining antitumor T-cell response. Unfortunately, early clinical studies testing anti-CTLA4 and anti–PD-1 antibodies have not generated meaningful results.[106] In an attempt to both induce and maintain T-cell response, newer strategies combining checkpoint inhibitors with vaccine therapies are under investigation and hold promise in improving outcomes for patients with metastatic PDAC (NCT01693562, NCT01928394, NCT02243371, and NCT01473940).

CD40 AGONISTS

Another strategy to enhance antitumor immune response is by activation of CD40, a receptor member of tumor necrosis factor family, expressed by the tumor-associated macrophages. Activation of CD40 can cause $CD40^+$ macrophage infiltration into the tumor, depletion of the stroma, and tumor regression, as demonstrated in genetically engineered mouse model of PDAC.[107] A phase 1 study evaluating safety and antitumor activity of CP-870,893 (CD40 agonist) in combination with gemcitabine has provided evidence of potential efficacy of these agents in patients with advanced PDAC.[108]

Other immune therapies, in early phases of development, include inhibitors of immunosuppressive factor, indoleamine 2,3-dioxygenase, adoptive transfer of chimeric antigen receptor T cells, and targeting cancer-associated fibroblasts.[109–111]

Role of Ca 19-9 as a Biomarker and Therapeutic Target

Despite recent advances in available therapeutic options, lack of a validated prognostic or predictive marker to guide therapeutic decision-making remains a hindrance in further improving outcomes in PDAC.

CA 19-9, overexpressed in greater than 90% pancreatic cancer cases, is widely used in clinical practice. For screening purposes, CA 19-9 is a poor biomarker because of its low positive predictive value, false-negative result in Lewis antigen–negative individuals, and false elevation in biliary diseases.[112,113] In the metastatic disease setting, data suggest the potential role of CA 19-9 as a prognostic marker.[114–116] Generally, higher levels at baseline and increasing levels during treatment are associated with poorer outcomes.[116] Recently, a retrospective analysis of PRODIGE4/ACCORD11 study reported that patients who had greater than 20% decline in CA 19-9 at week 8 have longer median OS compared with those with less than 20% decline in both treatment arms (13.5 months vs 12 months in FOLFIRINOX arm, 8.6 months vs 7.6 months in gemcitabine arm).[117] More recently, similar prognostic role of CA 19-9 was demonstrated in the exploratory analysis of MPACT trial. Investigators reported that any decline in CA 19-9 level at 8 weeks of treatment was associated with improved OS and RR, regardless of the treatment arm.[118] These results support the utility of CA 19-9 as an early surrogate marker for treatment efficacy in patients with metastatic PDAC. Additionally, therapeutic targeting of CA 19-9 has now entered clinics in the form of a monoclonal antibody, MVT-5873 (HuMab 5B1), being evaluated for safety as a single agent, in combination with standard cytotoxic therapy, and as a radioconjugate label for imaging in PDAC (NCT02672917).

SUPPORTIVE AND PALLIATIVE CARE

A significant number of patients with metastatic PDAC require early and frequent palliative interventions, with the objective of alleviating/preventing suffering and achieving optimal QOL. Commonly encountered challenges include the need for decompression of biliary ducts to relieve jaundice, addressing anticoagulation for treatment of venous thromboembolism, pain control, and nutritional support to prevent cancer anorexia-cachexia syndrome. Moreover, treatment-induced side effects and the significant psychosocial distress incurred by the disease can be debilitating and need careful attention. Therefore, early multidisciplinary consultation is essential. This topic is reviewed in detail elsewhere in this issue.

SUMMARY

Progress in metastatic PDAC treatment has been slow, yet meaningful gains have accrued over the past several years. After decades of gemcitabine monotherapy as a standard option, 2 more effective regimens, FOLFIRINOX and gemcitabine/nab-paclitaxel, have emerged as new standard therapies in patients with advanced PDAC. Moreover, recent approval of MM-398 for gemcitabine-progressing disease has advanced the therapeutic landscape of metastatic PDAC. Nonetheless, despite these new therapies, most patients with metastatic disease die within a year of diagnosis, necessitating a major continued focus on new drug development. In addition, development of reliable and validated prognostic and predictive biomarkers is imperative to optimize therapeutics. Given the growing understanding of molecular oncogenesis and the diverse array of novel therapeutics currently being investigated, there is a sense of optimism that outcomes will improve in the coming years.

REFERENCES

1. American Cancer Society; Facts and figures.
2. SEER Stat Fact Sheets: Pancreas Cancer. 2015. Available at: http://seer.cancer.gov/statfacts/html/pancreas.html. Accessed April 15, 2016.
3. Rahib L, Smith BD, Aizenberg R, et al. Projecting cancer incidence and deaths to 2030: the unexpected burden of thyroid, liver, and pancreas cancers in the United States. Cancer Res 2014;74(11):2913–21.
4. Siegel RL, Miller KD, Jemal A. Cancer statistics, 2015. CA Cancer J Clin 2015; 65(1):5–29.
5. Von Hoff DD, Ervin T, Arena FP, et al. Increased survival in pancreatic cancer with nab-paclitaxel plus gemcitabine. N Engl J Med 2013;369(18):1691–703.
6. Conroy T, Desseigne F, Ychou M, et al. FOLFIRINOX versus gemcitabine for metastatic pancreatic cancer. N Engl J Med 2011;364(19):1817–25.
7. Raderer M, Kornek GV, Hejna MH, et al. Treatment of advanced pancreatic cancer with epirubicin, 5-fluorouracil and 1-leucovorin: a phase II study. Ann Oncol 1997;8(8):797–9.
8. Bruckner HW, Storch JA, Brown JC, et al. Phase II trial of combination chemotherapy for pancreatic cancer with 5-fluorouracil, mitomycin C, and hexamethylmelamine. Oncology 1983;40(3):165–9.
9. Huang P, Chubb S, Hertel LW, et al. Action of 2',2'-difluorodeoxycytidine on DNA synthesis. Cancer Res 1991;51(22):6110–7.
10. Burris HA, Moore MJ, Andersen J, et al. Improvements in survival and clinical benefit with gemcitabine as first-line therapy for patients with advanced pancreas cancer: a randomized trial. J Clin Oncol 1997;15(6):2403–13.

11. Grunewald R, Abbruzzese JL, Tarassoff P, et al. Saturation of 2',2'-difluorodeox-ycytidine 5'-triphosphate accumulation by mononuclear cells during a phase I trial of gemcitabine. Cancer Chemother Pharmacol 1991;27(4):258–62.
12. Poplin E, Feng Y, Berlin J, et al. Phase III, randomized study of gemcitabine and oxaliplatin versus gemcitabine (fixed-dose rate infusion) compared with gemcitabine (30-minute infusion) in patients with pancreatic carcinoma E6201: a trial of the Eastern Cooperative Oncology Group. J Clin Oncol 2009;27(23):3778–85.
13. Heinemann V, Boeck S, Hinke A, et al. Meta-analysis of randomized trials: evaluation of benefit from gemcitabine-based combination chemotherapy applied in advanced pancreatic cancer. BMC Cancer 2008;8:82.
14. Sultana A, Tudur Smith C, Cunningham D, et al. Meta-analyses of chemotherapy for locally advanced and metastatic pancreatic cancer: results of secondary end points analyses. Br J Cancer 2008;99(1):6–13.
15. Heinemann V, Labianca R, Hinke A, et al. Increased survival using platinum analog combined with gemcitabine as compared to single-agent gemcitabine in advanced pancreatic cancer: pooled analysis of two randomized trials, the GERCOR/GISCAD intergroup study and a German multicenter study. Ann Oncol 2007;18(10):1652–9.
16. Reni M, Cordio S, Milandri C, et al. Gemcitabine versus cisplatin, epirubicin, fluorouracil, and gemcitabine in advanced pancreatic cancer: a randomised controlled multicentre phase III trial. Lancet Oncol 2005;6(6):369–76.
17. Moore MJ, Goldstein D, Hamm J, et al. Erlotinib plus gemcitabine compared with gemcitabine alone in patients with advanced pancreatic cancer: a phase III trial of the National Cancer Institute of Canada Clinical Trials Group. J Clin Oncol 2007;25(15):1960–6.
18. da Cunha Santos G, Dhani N, Tu D, et al. Molecular predictors of outcome in a phase 3 study of gemcitabine and erlotinib therapy in patients with advanced pancreatic cancer: National Cancer Institute of Canada Clinical Trials Group Study PA.3. Cancer 2010;116(24):5599–607.
19. Van Cutsem E, Li CP, Nowara E, et al. Dose escalation to rash for erlotinib plus gemcitabine for metastatic pancreatic cancer: the phase II RACHEL study. Br J Cancer 2014;111(11):2067–75.
20. Gourgou-Bourgade S, Bascoul-Mollevi C, Desseigne F, et al. Impact of FOLFIRINOX compared with gemcitabine on quality of life in patients with metastatic pancreatic cancer: results from the PRODIGE 4/ACCORD 11 randomized trial. J Clin Oncol 2013;31(1):23–9.
21. Peddi PF, Lubner S, McWilliams R, et al. Multi-institutional experience with FOLFIRINOX in pancreatic adenocarcinoma. JOP 2012;13(5):497–501.
22. Goncalves PH, Ruch JM, Byer J, et al. Multi-institutional experience using 5-fluorouracil, leucovorin, irinotecan, and oxaliplatin (FOLFIRINOX) in patients with pancreatic cancer (PCA). J Clin Oncol 2012;30(15_suppl):e14519.
23. Faris JE, Blaszkowsky LS, McDermott S, et al. FOLFIRINOX in locally advanced pancreatic cancer: the Massachusetts General Hospital Cancer Center experience. Oncologist 2013;18(5):543–8.
24. Mahaseth H, Brutcher E, Kauh J, et al. Modified FOLFIRINOX regimen with improved safety and maintained efficacy in pancreatic adenocarcinoma. Pancreas 2013;42(8):1311–5.
25. Gunturu KS, Yao X, Cong X, et al. FOLFIRINOX for locally advanced and metastatic pancreatic cancer: single institution retrospective review of efficacy and toxicity. Med Oncol 2013;30(1):361.

26. James ES, YX, Cong X, et al. Interim analysis of a phase II study of dose-modified FOLFIRINOX (mFOLFIRINOX) in locally advanced (LAPC) and metastatic pancreatic cancer (MPC). ASCO Meeting Abstr 2014;32(Suppl. 3):256.

27. Neuzillet C, Tijeras-Raballand A, Cros J, et al. Stromal expression of SPARC in pancreatic adenocarcinoma. Cancer Metastasis Rev 2013;32(3–4):585–602.

28. Infante JR, Matsubayashi H, Sato N, et al. Peritumoral fibroblast SPARC expression and patient outcome with resectable pancreatic adenocarcinoma. J Clin Oncol 2007;25(3):319–25.

29. Frese KK, Neesse A, Cook N, et al. nab-Paclitaxel potentiates gemcitabine activity by reducing cytidine deaminase levels in a mouse model of pancreatic cancer. Cancer Discov 2012;2(3):260–9.

30. Von Hoff DD, Ramanathan RK, Borad MJ, et al. Gemcitabine plus nab-paclitaxel is an active regimen in patients with advanced pancreatic cancer: a phase I/II trial. J Clin Oncol 2011;29(34):4548–54.

31. Goldstein D, El-Maraghi RH, Hammel P, et al. nab-Paclitaxel plus gemcitabine for metastatic pancreatic cancer: long-term survival from a phase III trial. J Natl Cancer Inst 2015;107(2):413–9.

32. Hidalgo M, Plaza C, Musteanu M, et al. SPARC Expression Did Not Predict Efficacy of nab-Paclitaxel plus Gemcitabine or Gemcitabine Alone for Metastatic Pancreatic Cancer in an Exploratory Analysis of the Phase III MPACT Trial. Clin Cancer Res 2015;21(21):4811–8.

33. Cereda S, Reni M. Weekly docetaxel as salvage therapy in patients with gemcitabine-refractory metastatic pancreatic cancer. J Chemother 2008;20(4): 509–12.

34. Oettle H, Arnold D, Esser M, et al. Paclitaxel as weekly second-line therapy in patients with advanced pancreatic carcinoma. Anticancer Drugs 2000;11(8): 635–8.

35. Hosein PJ, de Lima Lopes G, Pastorini VH, et al. A phase II trial of nab-Paclitaxel as second-line therapy in patients with advanced pancreatic cancer. Am J Clin Oncol 2013;36(2):151–6.

36. Xiong HQ, Varadhachary GR, Blais JC, et al. Phase 2 trial of oxaliplatin plus capecitabine (XELOX) as second-line therapy for patients with advanced pancreatic cancer. Cancer 2008;113(8):2046–52.

37. Neuzillet C, Hentic O, Rousseau B, et al. FOLFIRI regimen in metastatic pancreatic adenocarcinoma resistant to gemcitabine and platinum-salts. World J Gastroenterol 2012;18(33):4533–41.

38. Boeck S, Weigang-Köhler K, Fuchs M, et al. Second-line chemotherapy with pemetrexed after gemcitabine failure in patients with advanced pancreatic cancer: a multicenter phase II trial. Ann Oncol 2007;18(4):745–51.

39. Lee S, Oh SY, Kim BG, et al. Second-line treatment with a combination of continuous 5-fluorouracil, doxorubicin, and mitomycin-C (conti-FAM) in gemcitabine-pretreated pancreatic and biliary tract cancer. Am J Clin Oncol 2009;32(4): 348–52.

40. Yi SY, Park YS, Kim HS, et al. Irinotecan monotherapy as second-line treatment in advanced pancreatic cancer. Cancer Chemother Pharmacol 2009;63(6): 1141–5.

41. Kozuch P, Grossbard ML, Barzdins A, et al. Irinotecan combined with gemcitabine, 5-fluorouracil, leucovorin, and cisplatin (G-FLIP) is an effective and non-crossresistant treatment for chemotherapy refractory metastatic pancreatic cancer. Oncologist 2001;6(6):488–95.

42. Assaf E, Verlinde-Carvalho M, Delbaldo C, et al. 5-fluorouracil/leucovorin combined with irinotecan and oxaliplatin (FOLFIRINOX) as second-line chemotherapy in patients with metastatic pancreatic adenocarcinoma. Oncology 2011;80(5–6):301–6.

43. Berk V, Ozdemir N, Ozkan M, et al. XELOX vs. FOLFOX4 as second line chemotherapy in advanced pancreatic cancer. Hepatogastroenterology 2012;59(120): 2635–9.

44. Zaniboni A, Aitini E, Barni S, et al. FOLFIRI as second-line chemotherapy for advanced pancreatic cancer: a GISCAD multicenter phase II study. Cancer Chemother Pharmacol 2012;69(6):1641–5.

45. Pelzer U, Schwaner I, Stieler J, et al. Best supportive care (BSC) versus oxaliplatin, folinic acid and 5-fluorouracil (OFF) plus BSC in patients for second-line advanced pancreatic cancer: a phase III-study from the German CONKO-study group. Eur J Cancer 2011;47(11):1676–81.

46. Oettle H, Riess H, Stieler JM, et al. Second-line oxaliplatin, folinic acid, and fluorouracil versus folinic acid and fluorouracil alone for gemcitabine-refractory pancreatic cancer: outcomes from the CONKO-003 trial. J Clin Oncol 2014; 32(23):2423–9.

47. Gill S, Ko YJ, Cripps MC, et al. PANCREOX: a randomized phase 3 study of 5FU/LV with or without oxaliplatin for second-line advanced pancreatic cancer (APC) in patients (pts) who have received gemcitabine (GEM)-based chemotherapy (CT). J Clin Oncol 2014;32(Suppl):4022 [abstract].

48. Drummond DC, Noble CO, Guo Z, et al. Development of a highly active nanoliposomal irinotecan using a novel intraliposomal stabilization strategy. Cancer Res 2006;66(6):3271–7.

49. Kalra AV, Kim J, Klinz SG, et al. Preclinical activity of nanoliposomal irinotecan is governed by tumor deposition and intratumor prodrug conversion. Cancer Res 2014;74(23):7003–13.

50. Wang-Gillam A, Li CP, Bodoky G, et al. Nanoliposomal irinotecan with fluorouracil and folinic acid in metastatic pancreatic cancer after previous gemcitabine-based therapy (NAPOLI-1): a global, randomised, open-label, phase 3 trial. Lancet 2016;387(10018):545–57.

51. Portal A, Pernot S, Tougeron D, et al. Nab-paclitaxel plus gemcitabine for metastatic pancreatic adenocarcinoma after Folfirinox failure: an AGEO prospective multicentre cohort. Br J Cancer 2015;113(7):989–95.

52. Zhang Y, Hochster H, Stein S, et al. Gemcitabine plus nab-paclitaxel for advanced pancreatic cancer after first-line FOLFIRINOX: single institution retrospective review of efficacy and toxicity. Exp Hematol Oncol 2015;4:29.

53. Yachida S, Jones S, Bozic I, et al. Distant metastasis occurs late during the genetic evolution of pancreatic cancer. Nature 2010;467(7319):1114–7.

54. Yachida S, Iacobuzio-Donahue CA. Evolution and dynamics of pancreatic cancer progression. Oncogene 2013;32(45):5253–60.

55. Cowan RW, Maitra A. Genetic progression of pancreatic cancer. Cancer J 2014; 20(1):80–4.

56. Caldas C, Kern SE. K-ras mutation and pancreatic adenocarcinoma. Int J Pancreatol 1995;18(1):1–6.

57. Hezel AF, Kimmelman AC, Stanger BZ, et al. Genetics and biology of pancreatic ductal adenocarcinoma. Genes Dev 2006;20(10):1218–49.

58. Biankin AV, Waddell N, Kassahn KS, et al. Pancreatic cancer genomes reveal aberrations in axon guidance pathway genes. Nature 2012;491(7424):399–405.

59. Jones S, Zhang X, Parsons DW, et al. Core signaling pathways in human pancreatic cancers revealed by global genomic analyses. Science 2008; 321(5897):1801–6.

60. di Magliano MP, Logsdon CD. Roles for KRAS in pancreatic tumor development and progression. Gastroenterology 2013;144(6):1220–9.

61. Ko AH, Bekaii-Saab T, Van Ziffle J, et al. A multicenter, open-label phase II clinical trial of combined MEK plus EGFR inhibition for chemotherapy-refractory advanced pancreatic adenocarcinoma. Clin Cancer Res 2016;22(1):61–8.

62. Kordes S, Klümpen HJ, Weterman MJ, et al. Phase II study of capecitabine and the oral mTOR inhibitor everolimus in patients with advanced pancreatic cancer. Cancer Chemother Pharmacol 2015;75(6):1135–41.

63. Javle MM, Shroff RT, Xiong H, et al. Inhibition of the mammalian target of rapamycin (mTOR) in advanced pancreatic cancer: results of two phase II studies. BMC Cancer 2010;10:368.

64. Mullendore ME, Koorstra JB, Li YM, et al. Ligand-dependent Notch signaling is involved in tumor initiation and tumor maintenance in pancreatic cancer. Clin Cancer Res 2009;15(7):2291–301.

65. Sjölund J, Manetopoulos C, Stockhausen MT, et al. The Notch pathway in cancer: differentiation gone awry. Eur J Cancer 2005;41(17):2620–9.

66. Wang Z, Zhang Y, Li Y, et al. Down-regulation of Notch-1 contributes to cell growth inhibition and apoptosis in pancreatic cancer cells. Mol Cancer Ther 2006;5(3):483–93.

67. Wang Z, Zhang Y, Banerjee S, et al. Notch-1 down-regulation by curcumin is associated with the inhibition of cell growth and the induction of apoptosis in pancreatic cancer cells. Cancer 2006;106(11):2503–13.

68. Yen WC, Fischer MM, Hynes M, et al. Anti-DLL4 has broad spectrum activity in pancreatic cancer dependent on targeting DLL4-Notch signaling in both tumor and vasculature cells. Clin Cancer Res 2012;18(19):5374–86.

69. Yen WC, Fischer MM, Axelrod F, et al. Targeting Notch signaling with a Notch2/Notch3 antagonist (tarextumab) inhibits tumor growth and decreases tumor-initiating cell frequency. Clin Cancer Res 2015;21(9):2084–95.

70. O'Reilly EM, Smith LS, Bendell JC, et al. Phase 1b of anticancer stem cell antibody omp-59r5 (anti-notch 2/3) in combination with nab-paclitaxel and gemcitabine in patients with untreated metastatic pancreatic cancer. J Clin Oncol 2014; 32(suppl 3):220a.

71. OncoMed. OncoMed Provides Update on Tarextumab Phase 2 Pancreatic Cancer ALPINE Trial.

72. Springuel L, Renauld JC, Knoops L. JAK kinase targeting in hematologic malignancies: a sinuous pathway from identification of genetic alterations towards clinical indications. Haematologica 2015;100(10):1240–53.

73. Thomas SJ, Snowden JA, Zeidler MP, et al. The role of JAK/STAT signalling in the pathogenesis, prognosis and treatment of solid tumours. Br J Cancer 2015; 113(3):365–71.

74. Lili LN, Matyunina LV, Walker LD, et al. Evidence for the importance of personalized molecular profiling in pancreatic cancer. Pancreas 2014;43(2):198–211.

75. Denley SM, Jamieson NB, McCall P, et al. Activation of the IL-6R/Jak/stat pathway is associated with a poor outcome in resected pancreatic ductal adenocarcinoma. J Gastrointest Surg 2013;17(5):887–98.

76. Hurwitz HI, Uppal N, Wagner SA, et al. Randomized, double-blind, phase ii study of ruxolitinib or placebo in combination with capecitabine in patients

with metastatic pancreatic cancer for whom therapy with gemcitabine has failed. J Clin Oncol 2015;33(34):4039–47.

77. Incyte. Incyte Announces Decision to Discontinue JANUS Studies of Ruxolitinib plus Capecitabine in Patients with Advanced or Metastatic Pancreatic Cancer.

78. Stromnes IM, DelGiorno KE, Greenberg PD, et al. Stromal reengineering to treat pancreas cancer. Carcinogenesis 2014;35(7):1451–60.

79. Rucki AA, Zheng L. Pancreatic cancer stroma: understanding biology leads to new therapeutic strategies. World J Gastroenterol 2014;20(9):2237–46.

80. Mahadevan D, Von Hoff DD. Tumor-stroma interactions in pancreatic ductal adenocarcinoma. Mol Cancer Ther 2007;6(4):1186–97.

81. Bachem MG, Schünemann M, Ramadani M, et al. Pancreatic carcinoma cells induce fibrosis by stimulating proliferation and matrix synthesis of stellate cells. Gastroenterology 2005;128(4):907–21.

82. Provenzano PP, Cuevas C, Chang AE, et al. Enzymatic targeting of the stroma ablates physical barriers to treatment of pancreatic ductal adenocarcinoma. Cancer Cell 2012;21(3):418–29.

83. Toole BP, Slomiany MG. Hyaluronan: a constitutive regulator of chemoresistance and malignancy in cancer cells. Semin Cancer Biol 2008;18(4):244–50.

84. Jacobetz MA, Chan DS, Neesse A, et al. Hyaluronan impairs vascular function and drug delivery in a mouse model of pancreatic cancer. Gut 2013;62(1): 112–20.

85. Hingorani SR, Harris WP, Seery TE. Interim results of a randomized phase II study of PEGPH20 added to nab-paclitaxel/gemcitabine in patients with stage IV previously untreated pancreatic cancer. J Clin Oncol 2016;34(suppl 4S) [abstract 439].

86. Sun JD, Liu Q, Wang J, et al. Selective tumor hypoxia targeting by hypoxia-activated prodrug TH-302 inhibits tumor growth in preclinical models of cancer. Clin Cancer Res 2012;18(3):758–70.

87. Duan JX, Jiao H, Kaizerman J, et al. Potent and highly selective hypoxia-activated achiral phosphoramidate mustards as anticancer drugs. J Med Chem 2008;51(8):2412–20.

88. Van Cutsem E, Lenz HJ, Furuse J, et al. Evofosfamide (TH-302) in combination with gemcitabine in previously untreated patients with metastatic or locally advanced unresectable pancreatic ductal adenocarcinoma: Primary analysis of the randomized, double-blind phase III MAESTRO study. J Clin Oncol 2016;34(suppl 4S) [abstract 193].

89. Turner N, Tutt A, Ashworth A. Hallmarks of 'BRCAness' in sporadic cancers. Nat Rev Cancer 2004;4(10):814–9.

90. Turner N, Tutt A, Ashworth A. Targeting the DNA repair defect of BRCA tumours. Curr Opin Pharmacol 2005;5(4):388–93.

91. Jasin M, Rothstein R. Repair of strand breaks by homologous recombination. Cold Spring Harb Perspect Biol 2013;5(11):a012740.

92. Helleday T, Bryant HE, Schultz N. Poly(ADP-ribose) polymerase (PARP-1) in homologous recombination and as a target for cancer therapy. Cell Cycle 2005; 4(9):1176–8.

93. Cavallo F, Graziani G, Antinozzi C, et al. Reduced proficiency in homologous recombination underlies the high sensitivity of embryonal carcinoma testicular germ cell tumors to Cisplatin and poly (adp-ribose) polymerase inhibition. PLoS One 2012;7(12):e51563.

94. Lowery MA, Kelsen DP, Stadler ZK, et al. An emerging entity: pancreatic adeno-carcinoma associated with a known BRCA mutation: clinical descriptors, treatment implications, and future directions. Oncologist 2011;16(10):1397–402.

95. Kaufman B, Shapira-Frommer R, Schmutzler RK, et al. Olaparib monotherapy in patients with advanced cancer and a germline BRCA1/2 mutation. J Clin Oncol 2015;33(3):244–50.

96. Niccolai E, Prisco D, D'Elios MM, et al. What is recent in pancreatic cancer immunotherapy? Biomed Res Int 2013;2013:492372.

97. Bellone G, Turletti A, Artusio E, et al. Tumor-associated transforming growth factor-beta and interleukin-10 contribute to a systemic Th2 immune phenotype in pancreatic carcinoma patients. Am J Pathol 1999;155(2):537–47.

98. Hiraoka N, Onozato K, Kosuge T, et al. Prevalence of FOXP3+ regulatory T cells increases during the progression of pancreatic ductal adenocarcinoma and its premalignant lesions. Clin Cancer Res 2006;12(18):5423–34.

99. Sideras K, Braat H, Kwekkeboom J, et al. Role of the immune system in pancreatic cancer progression and immune modulating treatment strategies. Cancer Treat Rev 2014;40(4):513–22.

100. Kraman M, Bambrough PJ, Arnold JN, et al. Suppression of antitumor immunity by stromal cells expressing fibroblast activation protein-alpha. Science 2010; 330(6005):827–30.

101. Lutz E, Yeo CJ, Lillemoe KD, et al. A lethally irradiated allogeneic granulocyte-macrophage colony stimulating factor-secreting tumor vaccine for pancreatic adenocarcinoma. A Phase II trial of safety, efficacy, and immune activation. Ann Surg 2011;253(2):328–35.

102. Bernhardt SL, Gjertsen MK, Trachsel S, et al. Telomerase peptide vaccination of patients with non-resectable pancreatic cancer: A dose escalating phase I/II study. Br J Cancer 2006;95(11):1474–82.

103. Buanes T, Maurel J, Liauw W. A randomized phase III study of gemcitabine (G) versus GV1001 in sequential combination with G in patients with unresectable and metastatic pancreatic cancer (PC). J Clin Oncol 2009;27(suppl):15s [abstract 4601].

104. Le DT, Brockstedt DG, Nir-Paz R, et al. A live-attenuated Listeria vaccine (ANZ-100) and a live-attenuated Listeria vaccine expressing mesothelin (CRS-207) for advanced cancers: phase I studies of safety and immune induction. Clin Cancer Res 2012;18(3):858–68.

105. Le DT, Wang-Gillam A, Picozzi V, et al. Safety and survival with GVAX pancreas prime and Listeria Monocytogenes-expressing mesothelin (CRS-207) boost vaccines for metastatic pancreatic cancer. J Clin Oncol 2015;33(12):1325–33.

106. Royal RE, Levy C, Turner K, et al. Phase 2 trial of single agent Ipilimumab (anti-CTLA-4) for locally advanced or metastatic pancreatic adenocarcinoma. J Immunother 2010;33(8):828–33.

107. Beatty GL, Chiorean EG, Fishman MP, et al. CD40 agonists alter tumor stroma and show efficacy against pancreatic carcinoma in mice and humans. Science 2011;331(6024):1612–6.

108. Beatty GL, Torigian DA, Chiorean EG, et al. A phase I study of an agonist CD40 monoclonal antibody (CP-870,893) in combination with gemcitabine in patients with advanced pancreatic ductal adenocarcinoma. Clin Cancer Res 2013; 19(22):6286–95.

109. Beatty GL, Moon EK. Chimeric antigen receptor T cells are vulnerable to immunosuppressive mechanisms present within the tumor microenvironment. Oncoimmunology 2014;3(11):e970027.

110. Rosenberg SA, Restifo NP. Adoptive cell transfer as personalized immunotherapy for human cancer. Science 2015;348(6230):62–8.
111. Manuel ER, Chen J, D'Apuzzo M, et al. Salmonella-Based Therapy Targeting Indoleamine 2,3-Dioxygenase Coupled with Enzymatic Depletion of Tumor Hyaluronan Induces Complete Regression of Aggressive Pancreatic Tumors. Cancer Immunol Res 2015;3(9):1096–107.
112. Tempero MA, Uchida E, Takasaki H, et al. Relationship of carbohydrate antigen 19-9 and Lewis antigens in pancreatic cancer. Cancer Res 1987;47(20):5501–3.
113. Ballehaninna UK, Chamberlain RS. The clinical utility of serum CA 19-9 in the diagnosis, prognosis and management of pancreatic adenocarcinoma: An evidence based appraisal. J Gastrointest Oncol 2012;3(2):105–19.
114. Ishii H, Okada S, Sato T, et al. CA 19-9 in evaluating the response to chemotherapy in advanced pancreatic cancer. Hepatogastroenterology 1997;44(13):279–83.
115. Halm U, Schumann T, Schiefke I, et al. Decrease of CA 19-9 during chemotherapy with gemcitabine predicts survival time in patients with advanced pancreatic cancer. Br J Cancer 2000;82(5):1013–6.
116. Boeck S, Stieber P, Holdenrieder S, et al. Prognostic and therapeutic significance of carbohydrate antigen 19-9 as tumor marker in patients with pancreatic cancer. Oncology 2006;70(4):255–64.
117. Robert M, Jarlier M, Conroy T, et al. Retrospective analysis of CA19-9 decrease in patients with metastatic pancreatic carcinoma (MPC) treated with FOLFIRINOX or gemcitabine (gem) in a randomized phase III study (ACCORD11/PRODIGE4). J Clin Oncol 2014;32(15_suppl (May 20 Supplement)):4115 [2014 ASCO Annual Meeting Abstracts].
118. Chiorean EG, Von Hoff DD, Reni M, et al. CA19–9 decrease at 8 weeks as a predictor of overall survival in a randomized phase III trial (MPACT) of weekly nab-paclitaxel plus gemcitabine vs gemcitabine alone in patients with metastatic pancreatic cancer. Ann Oncol 2016;27(4):654–60.
119. Berlin JD, Catalano P, Thomas JP, et al. Phase III study of gemcitabine in combination with fluorouracil versus gemcitabine alone in patients with advanced pancreatic carcinoma: Eastern Cooperative Oncology Group Trial E2297. J Clin Oncol 2002;20(15):3270–5.
120. Rocha Lima CM, Green MR, Rotche R, et al. Irinotecan plus gemcitabine results in no survival advantage compared with gemcitabine monotherapy in patients with locally advanced or metastatic pancreatic cancer despite increased tumor response rate. J Clin Oncol 2004;22(18):3776–83.
121. Louvet C, Labianca R, Hammel P, et al. Gemcitabine in combination with oxaliplatin compared with gemcitabine alone in locally advanced or metastatic pancreatic cancer: results of a GERCOR and GISCAD phase III trial. J Clin Oncol 2005;23(15):3509–16.
122. Oettle H, Richards D, Ramanathan RK, et al. A phase III trial of pemetrexed plus gemcitabine versus gemcitabine in patients with unresectable or metastatic pancreatic cancer. Ann Oncol 2005;16(10):1639–45.
123. Abou-Alfa GK, Letourneau R, Harker G, et al. Randomized phase III study of exatecan and gemcitabine compared with gemcitabine alone in untreated advanced pancreatic cancer. J Clin Oncol 2006;24(27):4441–7.
124. Heinemann V, Quietzsch D, Gieseler F, et al. Randomized phase III trial of gemcitabine plus cisplatin compared with gemcitabine alone in advanced pancreatic cancer. J Clin Oncol 2006;24(24):3946–52.

125. Herrmann R, Bodoky G, Ruhstaller T, et al. Gemcitabine plus capecitabine compared with gemcitabine alone in advanced pancreatic cancer: a randomized, multicenter, phase III trial of the Swiss Group for Clinical Cancer Research and the Central European Cooperative Oncology Group. J Clin Oncol 2007; 25(16):2212–7.

126. Cunningham D, Chau I, Stocken DD, et al. Phase III randomized comparison of gemcitabine versus gemcitabine plus capecitabine in patients with advanced pancreatic cancer. J Clin Oncol 2009;27(33):5513–8.

127. Colucci G, Labianca R, Di Costanzo F, et al. Randomized phase III trial of gemcitabine plus cisplatin compared with single-agent gemcitabine as first-line treatment of patients with advanced pancreatic cancer: the GIP-1 study. J Clin Oncol 2010;28(10):1645–51.

128. Ueno H, Ioka T, Ikeda M, et al. Randomized phase III study of gemcitabine plus S-1, S-1 alone, or gemcitabine alone in patients with locally advanced and metastatic pancreatic cancer in Japan and Taiwan: GEST study. J Clin Oncol 2013; 31(13):1640–8.

129. Bramhall SR, Schulz J, Nemunaitis J, et al. A double-blind placebo-controlled, randomised study comparing gemcitabine and marimastat with gemcitabine and placebo as first line therapy in patients with advanced pancreatic cancer. Br J Cancer 2002;87(2):161–7.

130. Van Cutsem E, van de Velde H, Karasek P, et al. Phase III trial of gemcitabine plus tipifarnib compared with gemcitabine plus placebo in advanced pancreatic cancer. J Clin Oncol 2004;22(8):1430–8.

131. Philip PA, Benedetti J, Corless CL, et al. Phase III study comparing gemcitabine plus cetuximab versus gemcitabine in patients with advanced pancreatic adenocarcinoma: Southwest Oncology Group-directed intergroup trial S0205. J Clin Oncol 2010;28(22):3605–10.

132. Infante JR, Somer BG, Park JO, et al. A randomised, double-blind, placebo-controlled trial of trametinib, an oral MEK inhibitor, in combination with gemcitabine for patients with untreated metastatic adenocarcinoma of the pancreas. Eur J Cancer 2014;50(12):2072–81.

133. Van Cutsem E, Vervenne WL, Bennouna J, et al. Phase III trial of bevacizumab in combination with gemcitabine and erlotinib in patients with metastatic pancreatic cancer. J Clin Oncol 2009;27(13):2231–7.

134. Kindler HL, Niedzwiecki D, Hollis D, et al. Gemcitabine plus bevacizumab compared with gemcitabine plus placebo in patients with advanced pancreatic cancer: phase III trial of the Cancer and Leukemia Group B (CALGB 80303). J Clin Oncol 2010;28(22):3617–22.

135. Kindler HL, Ioka T, Richel DJ, et al. Axitinib plus gemcitabine versus placebo plus gemcitabine in patients with advanced pancreatic adenocarcinoma: a double-blind randomised phase 3 study. Lancet Oncol 2011;12(3):256–62.

136. Gonçalves A, Gilabert M, François E, et al. BAYPAN study: a double-blind phase III randomized trial comparing gemcitabine plus sorafenib and gemcitabine plus placebo in patients with advanced pancreatic cancer. Ann Oncol 2012; 23(11):2799–805.

137. Rougier P, Riess H, Manges R, et al. Randomised, placebo-controlled, double-blind, parallel-group phase III study evaluating aflibercept in patients receiving first-line treatment with gemcitabine for metastatic pancreatic cancer. Eur J Cancer 2013;49(12):2633–42.

Palliative Care for Pancreatic and Periampullary Cancer

Jennifer A. Perone, MD[a], Taylor S. Riall, MD, PhD[b],*,
Kelly Olino, MD[a]

KEYWORDS

- Palliative care • Supportive care • Obstructive jaundice • Gastric outlet obstruction
- Palliative triangle • Celiac block • Biliary-enteric bypass • Endoscopic biliary stent

KEY POINTS

- In considering palliative options in pancreatic cancer, the physician must consider the performance status of the patient, the prognosis of the cancer, the availability and success of both surgical and nonsurgical management options, and the patient preferences.
- Endoscopic biliary stenting with self-expanding metal stents is currently the preferred palliation method for malignant biliary obstruction in pancreatic cancer.
- Surgical exploration should not be performed solely for the purpose of operative palliation of jaundice or gastric outlet obstruction.
- Advances in endoscopic stenting have made endoscopic palliation of gastric outlet obstruction a viable option.

INTRODUCTION

Pancreatic cancer remains a highly lethal disease, with nearly 80% of patients presenting with metastatic or locally advanced disease.[1–3] Modern first-line chemotherapy for metastatic disease (FOLFIRINOX: 5-fluorouracil, leucovorin, irinotecan, and oxaliplatin), improves median survival from 2 to 4 months to approximately 11 months in phase III trials,[4–7] while patients with unresectable locally advanced disease who receive treatment with chemoradiation have median survival ranging from 11 to 15 months.[4,8–11] The highest median survival rates are 22 to 26 months

The authors have nothing to disclose.

Funding: Supported by grants from the UTMB Clinical and Translational Science Award #UL1TR000071, NIH T-32 Grant # 5T32DK007639, AHRQ Grant #1R24HS022134, and Cancer Prevention and Research Institute Grant #RP140020.

[a] Department of Surgery, The University of Texas Medical Branch, 301 University Boulevard, Galveston, TX 77555, USA; [b] Department of Surgery, Banner-University Medical Center, University of Arizona, 1501 North Campbell Avenue, Tucson, AZ 85724, USA

* Corresponding author. Banner-University Medical Center, University of Arizona, 1501 North Campbell Avenue, Room 4327b, PO Box 245131, Tucson, AZ 85274-5131.

E-mail address: tsriall@surgery.arizona.edu

Surg Clin N Am 96 (2016) 1415–1430
http://dx.doi.org/10.1016/j.suc.2016.07.012
0039-6109/16/© 2016 Elsevier Inc. All rights reserved.

in patients who are candidates to undergo surgical resection, with the addition of neo-adjuvant or adjuvant therapy further improving survival.[12–15] More recent studies evaluating the impact of neoadjuvant therapy on highly selected patients with resectable disease have yielded median survival times as long as 44 months in patients with R0, node-negative disease.[16–18]

Despite these moderate improvements in survival, the overall prognosis remains poor, and treatment is associated with the inherent risks of surgery, radiation, and chemotherapy. Given this, multidisciplinary management and shared decision making are needed at every stage of disease in order to evaluate the prognosis, the performance status of the patient, the availability and success of both surgical and nonsurgical management options, and an individual patient's preferences.

The pendulum has shifted away from operative palliation in the last 2 decades. However, as both systemic therapy for metastatic pancreatic cancer and nonsurgical palliative options continue to evolve, the effectiveness of palliative therapy options with respect to both the quantity and quality of life must be continually re-evaluated as new therapeutic options are made available.

This article will first focus on the modern concept of palliative care and then discuss the options and outcomes for palliation in pancreatic cancer, focusing on 3 common problems: (1) relief of obstructive jaundice, (2) relief of duodenal or gastric outlet obstruction, and (3) relief of pain due to invasion of the celiac plexus. Finally, the article discusses issues related to nutrition and managing the sequelae of venous thromboembolic (VTE) disease.

GOALS AND OUTCOMES OF PALLIATIVE CARE

Palliative care is described by the World Health Organization (WHO) as: "The total active care of patients whose disease is not responsive to curative treatment. Control of pain, other symptoms, and psychological, social, and spiritual problems, is paramount. The goal of palliative care is achievement of the best quality of life for patients and their families."[19]

Palliative care aims to provide treatment that extends beyond the traditional goals of addressing physical symptoms and survival by integrating the psychosocial and spiritual aspects of patient care. Far from hastening death, early intervention with palliative care results in improved quality of life and at times prolonged survival compared with standard treatment alone.[20] As such, palliative care should be viewed more broadly as part of the spectrum of survivorship and supportive care (**Fig. 1**). Therefore, to be most effective, the concept of palliative care should be introduced early in the course of an illness, in conjunction with active disease treatment.

Given the high risks and poor outcomes of palliation in advanced-stage pancreatic cancer, appropriate risk stratification is essential. In addition, treatment decisions must be made in conjunction with the patient and his or her family, keeping the patient's goals and priorities in mind. Although conceptually intuitive, ascertaining this information can be difficult.

Models such as the palliative care triangle, first published by Thomas Miner in 2002, can serve as a rubric for physicians to learn how to assess the patient's and family's concerns, values, and emotions when evaluating the risks and benefits with available medical and surgical treatment options (**Fig. 2**).[21,22] Use of this model fosters strong relationships among all parties involved in treatment decisions, allowing for shared decision making and clear expectations as various treatment options are chosen.

When used in conjunction with risk stratification, the palliative care model helps treating physicians understand a patient's disease characteristics, prognosis, expectations,

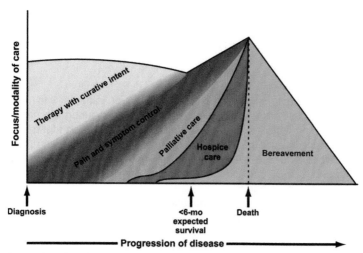

Fig. 1. Enhanced model of palliative care. Palliative care and hospice are crucial components along the spectrum of disease and ultimately death. From the time of diagnosis to the point of death, the focus and modality of care change from curative treatments to comfort care and hospice. Palliation is a crucial bridge between these 2 modalities, providing not only palliation for pain and symptoms, but also continuing to seek curative therapies.

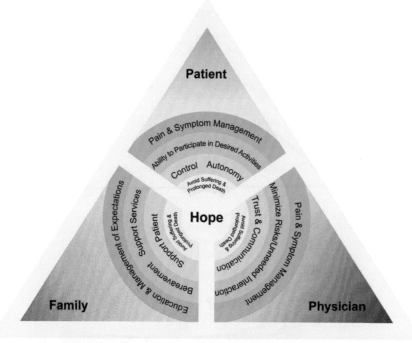

Fig. 2. Palliative triangle. The palliative triangle emphasizes the equal involvement between the physician, the patient, and the family. Each participant brings his or her own goals and desires to the conversation, and it is these individual desires and factors that help guide the treatment decisions. Ultimately, the triangle aims to unify all the participants in their desire for the good of the patient.

and goals of treatment in order to choose the best treatment when considering the various options available for the management of the most common sequelae of advanced pancreatic cancer: obstructive jaundice, gastric outlet obstruction, and pain.

OBSTRUCTIVE JAUNDICE

Jaundice is a presenting symptom in 51% to 72% of patients with unresectable pancreatic cancer and develops in over 80% of patients during the natural history of their disease.[2,3,23,24] Obstructive jaundice results in pruritus and fat malabsorption due to decreased excretion of bile acids into the duodenum, causing anorexia and diarrhea, and worsening malnutrition and cachexia. Fat malabsorption also decreases the ability to absorb fat-soluble vitamins, including vitamin K, leading to coagulopathy and increased risk of bleeding.[25]

Unrelieved cholestasis can lead to hepatic dysfunction and even liver failure. Patients with biliary obstruction are at increased risk for cholangitis, particularly if the biliary tree was previously instrumented and not appropriately drained. In 1 series, up to 38% of patients without any palliative treatment died from complications of biliary obstruction.[3]

Planned Operative and Endoscopic Palliation

Historically, operative biliary–enteric bypass was standard practice for locally advanced, unresectable disease (**Fig. 3**). Options including Roux-en-Y hepatico- or

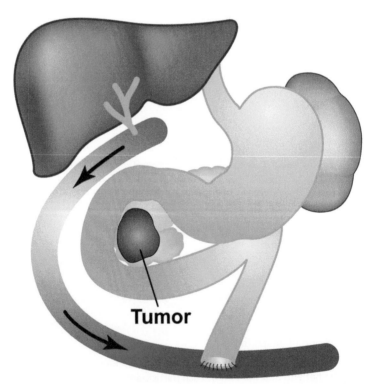

Fig. 3. Operative palliation for biliary obstruction involves the formation of a Roux-en-y hepaticojejunostomy or choledochojejunostomy with or without formation of a gastrojejunostomy to palliate gastric outlet obstruction.

choledochojejunostomy, were most commonly performed. Surgical palliation with cholecystojejunostomy or choledochoduodenostomy fell out of favor due to a high probability of cystic duct, duodenal, or gastric outlet obstruction by the tumor over time, as well as the possibility of bile reflux into the stomach.

In the 1990s, endoscopic interventions for the diagnosis and palliation of obstructive jaundice became more widely available. Currently, the placement of endoscopic biliary stents during endoscopic retrograde cholangiopancreatography (ERCP) is the preferred method for palliation of obstructive jaundice in patients with unresectable or metastatic pancreatic cancer. Advances in endoscopic technology have led to successful stent placement in more than 90% of patients during ERCP with equal efficacy, but less morbidity and mortality when compared to surgical palliation with biliary–enteric bypass.[3,26,27] Although less invasive than surgical palliation, endostent placement has associated risks including cholangitis (35%), acute pancreatitis (29%), bleeding (23%), perforation (6%), and early stent migration (3%).[3,27]

There are several different endostents available, each with its own benefits and limitations. Self-expanding metal stents (SEMS) have a longer patency, with covered metal stents lasting 7 to 10 months owing to their ability to withstand tumor ingrowth.[3,25,27] Stent migration occurs up to 20% of the time and can occur with any stent type.[3,27] Compared with covered metal stents, uncovered metal stents migrate less frequently,[28] but can theoretically be occluded by tumor ingrowth (shown in **Fig. 4**). Recent innovations in stent technology have led to the development of covered and uncovered SEMS with low axial force and flared ends. A 2013 randomized multicenter trial utilizing these newer stents showed no evidence of stent migration and longer periods without stent dysfunction in the covered stent cohort.[29]

Plastic stents are small and prone to obstruction secondary to biliary sludge and bacterial overgrowth, with a median patency of only 2 to 4 months.[3,25,27] Although plastic stents are significantly less expensive than metal stents, overall costs become lower with SEMS if a patient survives greater than 4 months due to fewer repeat procedures and hospitalizations, so selection should depend upon a patient's prognosis.[3] Therefore, in general it is recommended that patients with expected survival greater than 4 months have SEMS placed (**Fig. 5**).

As survival improves with newer chemotherapeutic agents, the role of operative biliary–enteric bypass may change. Although the previously discussed studies reported lower early complication rates with endoscopic stenting compared with operative bypass, stented patients have higher rates of later complications such as recurrent jaundice (36% vs 2%) requiring reintervention.[30] In these patients who remain unresectable but have a good performance status, operative intervention can be considered in the setting of repeated episodes of stent-associated complications. However, studies still show that most patients who are stented have an improved quality of life, even with the need for multiple stent changes and higher rates of recurrence.

Unresectable disease found at laparotomy

Prior to the development of thin-cut cross-sectional imaging in the 1990s, nearly 30% to 40% of patients undergoing surgical exploration for resection were found to have locally advanced or metastatic disease.[2,3] In these cases, surgical palliation included a hepaticojejunostomy and gastrojejunostomy (double bypass) in combination with ethanol ablation of the celiac neural plexus (chemical splanchnicectomy). Although improvements in preoperative imaging and staging have decreased the number of unresectable patients identified at exploration, up to 10% of patients are still found to have locally advanced or metastatic disease at the time of operation.[2,3]

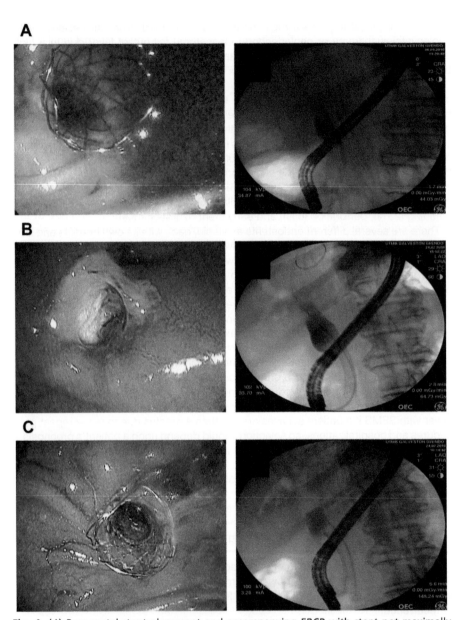

Fig. 4. (*A*) Bare metal stent placement and accompanying ERCP with stent not maximally expanded. (*B*) Tumor ingrowth through the stent including necrotic debris. ERCP shows fully expanded metal stent with proximal dilated biliary tree due to stent occlusion. (*C*) Covered metal stent placed with completion ERCP showing patent stent and well-draining biliary tree.

The management of the obstructed biliary tree in the setting of unexpected metastatic or locally advanced disease is controversial. Options include proceeding with operative palliation or closing the abdomen and pursuing endoscopic interventions if the patient did not already undergo preoperative biliary drainage. Unfortunately, there are no definitive data describing survival and quality of life of patients undergoing

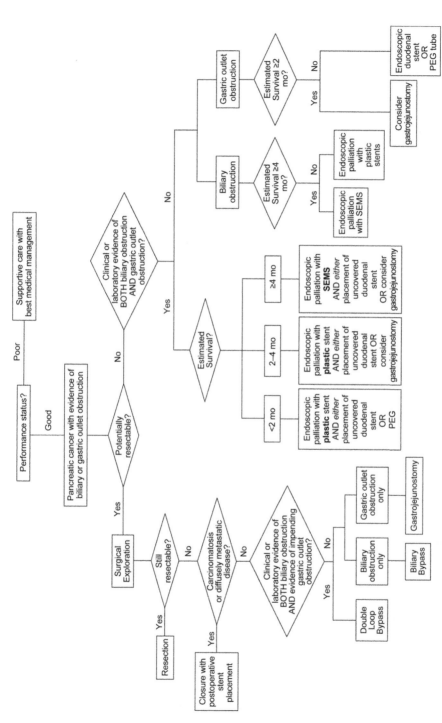

Fig. 5. Algorithm for the management of biliary and/or gastric outlet obstruction in pancreatic adenocarcinoma.

surgical bypass versus closure and rapid placement of endoscopic stents. For this reason, when faced with this decision, the surgeon's understanding of a patient's symptoms, functional status, and projected survival are crucial. In the setting of carcinomatosis or multifocal metastatic disease, regardless of performance status, endoscopic intervention should be favored because of the short median survival. However, in those patients with good functional status and low-volume metastatic disease or locally advanced disease, operative bypass is a reasonable option. **Fig. 5** provides an algorithm for the management of pancreatic malignancy.

Special Cases Requiring Percutaneous Transhepatic Palliation of Obstructive Jaundice

When endoscopic stent placement is unsuccessful or when anatomic constraints make endoscopic biliary cannulation difficult (ie, previous gastric bypass surgery or recurrence following pancreaticoduodenectomy), a transhepatic biliary catheter or metal stent can be placed by accessing the bile ducts with a needle percutaneously through the liver parenchyma. A wire is then advanced past the obstruction, allowing for the placement of biliary drains or metallic stents similar to those placed endoscopically. If a lesion cannot be traversed, a catheter(s) can be left proximal to the obstruction to drain the biliary tree. This approach is often required in the setting of recurrent tumor at the hepaticojejunostomy after pancreaticoduodenectomy.

GASTRIC OUTLET OBSTRUCTION

Ten percent to 25% of patients with pancreatic cancer will develop signs and symptoms of gastric outlet obstruction (GOO) requiring intervention prior to their death,[3,25,31,32] and an estimated 20% of patients will die with symptoms of duodenal obstruction.[32] Patients experience nausea and vomiting, resulting in decreased oral intake, electrolyte disturbances, and subsequent malnutrition and cachexia. Because of the impact on quality of life, addressing this is paramount, although obtaining symptom resolution is challenging once the disease has progressed to this extent.

Surgical Palliation—Gastrojejunostomy

Historically, the gold standard for management of GOO was the creation of a gastrojejunostomy. The procedure is performed by bringing up a loop of jejunum approximately 20 to 30 cm distal to the ligament of Treitz and performing a 3 to 4 cm side-to-side gastrojejunal anastomosis. This can be performed ante- or retrocolic, although the former is usually easier and also prevents obstruction of the loop by metastatic adenopathy at the root of the mesentery. If possible, the anastomosis should be performed on the posterior aspect of the stomach in order to improve emptying except in the case of large bulky tumors, where the anastomosis should be made on the anterior surface of the stomach to prevent reobstruction. The most common complication associated with creation of a gastrojejunostomy is delayed gastric emptying, which occurs in up to 30% to 50% of patients, leaving them with ongoing nausea, vomiting, and difficulty eating.[33,34]

There are limited data directly comparing laparoscopic to open gastrojejunostomy for malignant GOO. However, in a small cohort of 24 patients with malignant GOO randomized to laparoscopic or open gastrojejunostomy, Navarra and colleagues[35] found the laparoscopic approach resulted in decreased time to oral intake (4.08 vs 6.25 days) and a trend toward decreased rates of delayed gastric emptying and length of stay.

Prophylactic Gastrojejunostomy

Although it is generally accepted that a completely asymptomatic patient would not be explored to perform a prophylactic gastrojejunostomy, controversy exists on whether to perform a gastrojejunostomy in the absence of symptoms when metastatic or locally advanced disease is discovered during the time of exploration. Two prospective, randomized trials evaluated the role of prophylactic gastrojejunostomy in patients found to be unresectable at the time of surgery without symptoms of GOO preoperatively. Prophylactic gastrojejunostomy was associated with a decreased incidence of late GOO with no difference in postoperative complications and length of stay between the 2 groups.[36,37] Similarly, a 2013 Cochrane review concluded that routine prophylactic gastrojejunostomy was indicated in patients with unresectable periampullary cancer already undergoing exploratory laparotomy (with or without biliary bypass).[38] However, caution in the interpretation of these studies must be exercised, as these studies have an inherent selection bias. The overall survival and outcomes for patients who have not yet developed GOO are superior to those patients with symptomatic locally advanced disease. Also, it is unclear how many of these asymptomatic patients actually would have gone on to develop symptoms requiring intervention. Therefore, the universal adoption of prophylactic gastrojejunostomy is not recommended, but instead should be determined on a case-by-case basis (see **Fig. 5**). Similar to hepaticojejunostomy, the presence of carcinomatosis or metastatic disease should discourage surgeons from performing gastrojejunostomy in asymptomatic patients. As always, treatment decisions need to weigh the operative risks, duration of survival, and effectiveness of the intervention.

Endoscopic Palliation

With advances in endoscopic techniques, management of gastric outlet obstruction can be performed endoscopically, with placement of large self-expanding stents, typically 20 to 22 mm in diameter, and 60 to 90 mm in length. Stents are successful in 92% to 100% of cases, allowing patients to resume oral intake in as little as 24 hours in 73% to 93% of patients.[3,27] Although patients can manage their own salivary secretions and drink liquids, stent occlusion often occurs with solid food. Early complications occur in 2% to 12% of cases[27,31] and include perforation, gastrointestinal (GI) hemorrhage, aspiration pneumonia, or jaundice and potential cholangitis from compression of the common bile duct.[27] Overall complications occur in 26% of patients, including late complications such as stent failure and migration.[3] Stent placement should be reserved for symptomatic patients, as there is a high risk of migration if the stent is placed in noncritical stenosis.[27]

Endoscopic Stenting Versus Gastrojejunostomy

The decision to proceed with stenting or surgery for malignant GOO depends in large part on the patient's predicted survival time and functional status. Early studies reported similar success rates between stenting and surgery. Stented patients had fewer complications, faster return to oral intake, and shorter hospitalizations.[39–42] However, the surgical gastrojejunostomy or endoscopic stent placement for the palliation of malignant gastric outlet obstruction (SUSTENT) trial, a multicenter randomized control trial comparing stenting with surgery, found that although endoscopic palliation showed a quicker return to oral intake (5 vs 8 days) at 30 and 60 days, the surgical group had significantly better oral intake. After adjusting for survival, surgery was associated with more total days tolerating oral intake; therefore is recommended for patients with a life expectancy of 2 months or longer (see **Fig. 5**).[43] However, many surgeons would advocate for reserving operative intervention for those patients with a life expectancy of at least 4 months and a good functional status.

In the authors' experience, even when a technically sound anastomosis is performed, or a patent stent is in place, a stomach that has been chronically obstructed may not fully recover function. As there are no data predicting which patient populations will benefit, expectations of any intervention need to be tempered. Additionally, when a patient with poor functional status presents with a malignant gastric outlet obstruction from pancreatic cancer, outcomes with either procedure are routinely poor, with a median survival of 2 months.[44] In this setting, another option that should be considered is placement of a decompressive percutaneous endoscopic gastrostomy (PEG) to allow for pleasure feeds, or direct consultation of hospice services for symptom control.

PAIN MANAGEMENT

Seventy-five percent of patients will present with abdominal and/or back pain, and 80% of patients with advanced pancreatic cancer will experience severe pain prior to death, commonly associated with malignant invasion of the celiac plexus.[1,25,45] Although many patients are treated with oral and transdermal analgesics, there is evidence that patients who undergo early regional neurolysis of the celiac plexus experience improved quality of life.[3,45] A 2011 Cochrane meta-analysis of 6 randomized controlled trials found that celiac plexus block (chemical splanchnicectomy) results in a small but significant decrease in pain at 4 and 8 weeks postprocedure. Additionally, a durable decrease was found in overall opioid consumption and associated adverse effects.[46]

There are 4 ways to perform a celiac block: intraoperatively, percutaneously, endoscopically, or thoracoscopically. Intraoperative celiac block is performed by injecting ethanol or a local anesthetic to either side of the aorta at the level of celiac axis. In a double-blind randomized control trial by Lillemoe and colleagues,[47] intraoperative celiac block (chemical splanchnicectomy) produced a statistically significant decrease in pain and opioid consumption when compared with saline control. In a meta-analysis from 2009, patients undergoing endoscopic ultrasound-guided celiac plexus blocks had an 85% response rate to therapy (measured by improvement in pain score) and a low complication rate.[48] Similar response rates have been seen in small series evaluating thoracoscopic celiac blocks.[3]

Celiac plexus blocks can result in urinary retention, back pain, and diarrhea occurring in about 38% of patients, resulting from unopposed parasympathetic tone.[49,50] Patients can also experience transient orthostatic hypotension secondary to vasodilation (1%–3%), which can last almost a week.[49] More serious, but rare complications include transient or permanent paraplegia, abdominal aortic dissection, or retroperitoneal hemorrhage.[49,50]

OTHER ISSUES IN PANCREATIC CANCER
Nutrition and Pancreatic Exocrine Insufficiency

Pancreatic cancer patients experience cachexia caused by appetite loss, malnutrition, and hypercatabolism of lean tissue, leading to weakness, fatigue, and a poor quality of life. One modifiable factor is pancreatic exocrine insufficiency, resulting from pancreatic duct obstruction or replacement of the pancreatic parenchyma by malignant cells, gland fibrosis, or atrophy.[25] Sixty-five percent of patients with pancreatic cancer will experience symptoms of fat malabsorption, and 50% of patients will also have protein malabsorption.[1,50] Treatment of patients with pancreatic enzyme replacement has been found to improve malabsorption, bloating, and diarrhea, as well as prevent further weight loss.[1,25,51] In a randomized controlled trial, patients with unresectable pancreatic cancer who took enzyme replacements for 8 weeks were found to have a 1.2% increase in body weight, compared with placebo patients, who had a 3.7% decrease in body weight.[51]

Thromboembolic Disease

A 2004 analysis of the Medicare claims database showed that pancreatic cancer patients have one of the highest incidences of deep venous thrombosis (DVT) or pulmonary embolism (PE), with rates ranging from 17% to 57%, with a relative risk of VTE of 8.8 (95% confidence interval [CI] 3.5–22.4; $P = -.001$). This high rate was seen even when excluding patients with vascular access thrombosis or direct tumor-related vascular invasion.[52]

Although the presence of thromboembolic disease is associated with a worse prognosis, treatment can improve longevity and symptomatology. Patients with acute portal vein thrombosis (PVT) (symptoms <14 days prior to presentation) can be selectively treated with portal thrombolytic therapy, as propagation to the superior mesenteric vein can be deadly. Otherwise, treatment for all acute VTE disease includes treatment with low weight molecular heparin (LWMH), unfractionated heparin, or oral anticoagulation. The use of oral anticoagulants such as warfarin must be carefully considered, as factors such as malnutrition, liver dysfunction, chemotherapy, and antibiotics can all disrupt the vitamin K metabolism, making it difficult to achieve steady levels in these patients. The 2003 CLOT study (Randomized Comparison of Low-Molecular-Weight Heparin vs Oral Anticoagulant Therapy for the Prevention of Recurrent Venous Thromboembolism in Patients with Cancer Study) compared the use of LMWH to oral anticoagulation (dalteparin vs a warfarin derivative) in patients with acute DVT and malignancy. They found no difference in bleeding complications between the 2 groups, but patients on the warfarin derivative had an increased risk of recurrent thromboembolic disease compared with those on dalteparin (17% vs 9%, hazard ratio [HR] = 0.48, $P=.002$). Additionally, patients on the warfarin derivative had an international normalized ratio (INR) in the therapeutic range for only 46% of the 6-month study time.[53] Newer-generation oral anticoagulants are currently being studied for their use in this patient population. Once diagnosed with VTE, many patients will remain on anticoagulation until reaching the end of life.

END-OF-LIFE CARE AND THE ROLE OF HOSPICE

The aggressive nature and particularly poor prognosis associated with pancreatic adenocarcinoma can leave patients and families feeling blind-sided when suddenly faced with end-of-life decisions. Therefore, it is crucial to clarify the patient's and family's goals from the onset and address misconceptions they have about the various treatment options and survival. These conversations can be the most time-consuming and difficult portions of patient care, but establishing clear goals early on avoids unnecessary complications, cost, and conflict, especially as goals and attitudes evolve with changing prognosis. When discussing potential interventions, it is critical to discuss not only prognosis, but also the potential benefits and harms of every option. Unfortunately, little information is available on outcomes such as quality of life, time spent in the hospital, and other outcomes that may be important to patients, thereby limiting physicians' ability to help patients make informed decisions.

Analysis of the Surveillance, Epidemiology, and End Results (SEER)-Medicare linked data of 25,476 patients with pancreatic cancer from 1992 to 2005 found that across all treatment groups, hospital days increased at the end of life, suggesting the significant use of resources when they are least likely to benefit patients. Furthermore, in a population-based study of end-of-life care in pancreatic cancer patients, Sheffield and colleagues[54] found an increase in aggressive care in the last month of life, with an increase in intensive care unit (ICU) admission from 15.5% in 1992 to 1994 to 19.6% in 2004 to 2006 (P<.0001) and an increase in receipt of chemotherapy from 8.1% to 16.4% (P<.0001). This suggests that aggressive care, in addition to being linked to worse quality of life for patients, and worse bereavement adjustment for their care-givers,[55–58] results in increased costs with little survival benefit.

Despite the fact that enrollment in hospice care has been associated with lower Medicare costs and improved quality of life, including improved pain, less fatigue, and lower depression and anxiety rates, it is grossly underutilized.[59–61] In the same population-based study of end-of -life care in pancreatic cancer patients, only 56% of patients were enrolled in hospice prior to death, with only 35.9% of hospice users enrolled for 4 weeks or more, suggesting that more than half of patients with pancreatic cancer are not receiving the full benefit of hospice care. Furthermore, among patients with loco-regional disease, those who underwent resection were less likely to enroll in hospice before death, supporting the need for early discussion of palliative care and hospice care regardless of stage at diagnosis.[54]

The early introduction of hospice care can help normalize the concept to patients and families and give them ample time to clarify any misconceptions. Moreover, it is possible that a paradigm shift may occur where the receipt of hospice care may no longer mean having to forgo potentially curative therapies. An ongoing pilot study among Medicare patients with advanced cancer allows patients to receive potentially curative treatment in conjunction with hospice care and supportive services.[62] Results of pilot studies such as these may positively impact care on many levels, leading to more time spent with family at the end of life instead of in the hospital.

SUMMARY

The involvement of patients, families, physicians, and advocacy groups throughout the care process beginning at the time of diagnosis and utilizing the palliative care triangle to clarify a patient's and family's goals allow for the interpretation of potential outcomes in ways that are meaningful to all stakeholders. This allows patients with pancreatic cancer and their physicians to choose the right treatment, for the right patient, in the right setting. More importantly, these discussions provide an opportunity to reframe how patients and families think of hope, which is central to all who are dealing with cancer. Instead of creating a situation in which families feel robbed of hope when cure can no longer be offered, early discussions can focus on ways to empower patients to create new achievable goals. For some, this will be to die in the comfort of their home or to feel well enough to attend an important family event, instead of continuing treatment that will ultimately not change their overall outcome. When given new goals to focus on, hope is reborn, and patients, families, and providers benefit.

REFERENCES

1. el-Kamar FG, Grossbard ML, Kozuch PS. Metastatic pancreatic cancer: emerging strategies in chemotherapy and palliative care. Oncologist 2003;8(1):18–34.
2. Kneuertz PJ, Cunningham SC, Cameron JL, et al. Palliative surgical management of patients with unresectable pancreatic adenocarcinoma: trends and lessons learned from a large, single institution experience. J Gastrointest Surg 2011; 15(11):1917–27.

3. Stark A, Hines OJ. Endoscopic and operative palliation strategies for pancreatic ductal adenocarcinoma. Semin Oncol 2015;42(1):163–76.

4. Loehrer PJ Sr, Feng Y, Cardenes H, et al. Gemcitabine alone versus gemcitabine plus radiotherapy in patients with locally advanced pancreatic cancer: an Eastern Cooperative Oncology Group trial. J Clin Oncol 2011;29:4105–12.

5. Gourgou-Bourgade S, Bascoul-Mollevi C, Desseigne F, et al. Impact of FOLFIRINOX compared with gemcitabine on quality of life in patients with metastatic pancreatic cancer: results from the PRODIGE 4/ACCORD 11 randomized trial. J Clin Oncol 2013;31(1):23–9.

6. Singhal MK, Kapoor A, Bagri PK, et al. A phase III trial comparing FOLFIRINOX versus gemcitabine for metastatic pancreatic cancer. Ann Oncol 2014; 25(Suppl 4):iv210–1.

7. Conroy T, Desseigne F, Ychou M, et al. FOLFIRINOX versus gemcitabine for metastatic pancreatic cancer. N Engl J Med 2011;364(19):1817–25.

8. Moertel CG, Frytak S, Hahn RG, et al. Therapy of locally unresectable pancreatic carcinoma: a randomized comparison of high dose (6000 rads) radiation alone, moderate dose radiation (4000 rads + 5-fluorouracil), and high dose radiation + 5-fluorouracil: The Gastrointestinal Tumor Study Group. Cancer 1981;48(8): 1705–10.

9. Shinchi H, Takao S, Noma H, et al. Length and quality of survival after external-beam radiotherapy with concurrent continuous 5-fluorouracil infusion for locally unresectable pancreatic cancer. Int J Radiat Oncol Biol Phys 2002;53(1):146–50.

10. Sultana A, Tudur Smith C, Cunningham D, et al. Systematic review, including meta-analyses, on the management of locally advanced pancreatic cancer using radiation/combined modality therapy. Br J Cancer 2007;96(8):1183–90.

11. Hammel P, Huguet F, Van Laethem J, et al. Comparison of chemoradiotherapy (CRT) and chemotherapy (CT) in patients with a locally advanced pancreatic cancer (LAPC) controlled after 4 months of gemcitabine with or without erlotinib: final results of the inter- national phase III LAP 07 study. J Clin Oncol 2013; 31(Suppl) [abstract: LBA4003].

12. Winter JM, Brennan MF, Tang LH, et al. Survival after resection of pancreatic adenocarcinoma: results from a single institution over three decades. Ann Surg Oncol 2012;19(1):169–75.

13. Konstantinidis IT, Warshaw AL, Allen JN, et al. Pancreatic ductal adenocarcinoma: is there a survival difference for R1 resections versus locally advanced unresectable tumors? What is a "true" R0 resection? Ann Surg 2013;257(4):731–6.

14. Stathis A, Moore MJ. Advanced pancreatic carcinoma: current treatment and future challenges. Nat Rev Clin Oncol 2010;7(3):163–72.

15. Dimou F, Sineshaw H, Parmar AD, et al. Trends in receipt and timing of multimodality therapy in early-stage pancreatic cancer. J Gastrointest Surg 2016;20(1): 93–103.

16. Evans DB, Varadhachary GR, Crane CH, et al. Preoperative gemcitabine-based chemoradiation for patients with resectable adenocarcinoma of the pancreatic head. J Clin Oncol 2008;26(21):3496–502.

17. Varadhachary GR, Wolff RA, CRane CH, et al. Preoperative gemcitabine and cisplatin followed by gemcitabine-based chemoradiation for resectable adenocarcinoma of the pancreatic head. J Clin Oncol 2008;26(21):3487–95.

18. Christians KK, Heimler JW, George B, et al. Survival of patients with resectable pancreatic cancer who received neoadjuvant therapy. Surgery 2016;159(3): 893–900.

19. World Health Organization. World Health Organization. Available at: http://www.who.int/cancer/palliative/definition/en/. Accessed December 12, 2015.

20. Temel JS, Greer JA, Muzikansky A, et al. Early palliative care for patients with metastatic non-small-cell lung cancer. N Engl J Med 2010;363(8):733–42.

21. Miner TJ, Cohen J, Charpentier K, et al. The palliative triangle: improved patient selection and outcomes associated with palliative operations. Arch Surg 2011; 146(5):517–22.

22. Miner TJ. Communication skills in palliative surgery: skill and effort are key. Surg Clin North Am 2011;91(2):355–66, ix.

23. Lyons JM, Karkar A, Correa-Gallego CC, et al. Operative procedures for unresectable pancreatic cancer: does operative bypass decrease requirements for postoperative procedures and in-hospital days? HPB (Oxford) 2012;14(7): 469–75.

24. Crippa S, Dominguez I, Rodriguez JR, et al. Quality of life in pancreatic cancer: analysis by stage and treatment. J Gastrointest Surg 2008;12(5):783–93 [discussion: 793–4].

25. Nakakura EK, Warren RS. Palliative care for patients with advanced pancreatic and biliary cancers. Surg Oncol 2007;16(4):293–7.

26. House MG, Choti MA. Palliative therapy for pancreatic/biliary cancer. Surg Clin North Am 2005;85(2):359–71.

27. Maire F, Sauvanet A. Palliation of biliary and duodenal obstruction in patients with unresectable pancreatic cancer: endoscopy or surgery? J Visc Surg 2013;150(3 Suppl):S27–31.

28. Almadi MA, Barkun AN, Martel M. No benefit of covered vs uncovered self-expandable metal stents in patients with malignant distal biliary obstruction: a meta-analysis. Clin Gastroenterol Hepatol 2013;11(1):27–37.e1.

29. Kitano M, Yamashita Y, Tanaka K, et al. Covered self-expandable metal stents with an anti-migration system improve patency duration without increased complications compared with uncovered stents for distal biliary obstruction caused by pancreatic carcinoma: a randomized multicenter trial. Am J Gastroenterol 2013;108(11):1713–22.

30. Smith AC, Dowsett JF, Russell RC, et al. Randomised trial of endoscopic stenting versus surgical bypass in malignant low bileduct obstruction. Lancet 1994; 344(8938):1655–60.

31. Schmidt C, Gerdes H, Hawkins W, et al. A prospective observational study examining quality of life in patients with malignant gastric outlet obstruction. Am J Surg 2009;198(1):92–9.

32. Sohn TA, Lillemoe KD, Cameron JL, et al. Surgical palliation of unresectable periampullary adenocarcinoma in the 1990s. J Am Coll Surg 1999;188(6):658–66 [discussion: 666–9].

33. Oida T, Mimatsu K, Kawasaki A, et al. A novel technique of laparoscopic gastrojejunostomy-modified Devine exclusion with vertical stomach reconstruction-for gastric outlet obstruction to preventing blow-out of the distal gastric remnant and delayed in return of gastric emptying. Hepatogastroenterology 2009;56(89): 282–4.

34. Usuba T, Misawa T, Toyama Y, et al. Is modified Devine exclusion necessary for gastrojejunostomy in patients with unresectable pancreatobiliary cancer? Surg Today 2011;41(1):97–100.

35. Navarra G, Musolino C, Venneri A, et al. Palliative antecolic isoperistaltic gastrojejunostomy: a randomized controlled trial comparing open and laparoscopic approaches. Surg Endosc 2006;20(12):1831–4.

36. Lillemoe KD, Cameron JL, Hardacre JM, et al. Is prophylactic gastrojejunostomy indicated for unresectable periampullary cancer? A prospective randomized trial. Ann Surg 1999;230(3):322–8 [discussion: 328–30].

37. Van Heek NT, DeCastro SM, van Eijck CH, et al. The need for a prophylactic gastrojejunostomy for unresectable periampullary cancer: a prospective randomized multicenter trial with special focus on assessment of quality of life. Ann Surg 2003;238(6):894–902 [discussion: 902–5].

38. Gurusamy KS, Kumar S, Davidson BR. Prophylactic gastrojejunostomy for unresectable periampullary carcinoma. Cochrane Database Syst Rev 2013;(2):CD008533.

39. Fiori E, Lamazza A, Volpino P, et al. Palliative management of malignant antropyloric strictures. Gastroenterostomy vs. endoscopic stenting. A randomized prospective trial. Anticancer Res 2004;24(1):269–71.

40. Gaidos JK, Draganov PV. Treatment of malignant gastric outlet obstruction with endoscopically placed self-expandable metal stents. World J Gastroenterol 2009;15(35):4365–71.

41. Chandrasegaram MD, Eslick GH, Mansfield CO, et al. Endoscopic stenting versus operative gastrojejunostomy for malignant gastric outlet obstruction. Surg Endosc 2012;26(2):323–9.

42. Rudolph HU, Post S, Schlüter M, et al. Malignant gastroduodenal obstruction: retrospective comparison of endoscopic and surgical palliative therapy. Scand J Gastroenterol 2011;46(5):583–90.

43. Jeurnink SM, Steyerberg EW, van Hooft JE, et al. Surgical gastrojejunostomy or endoscopic stent placement for the palliation of malignant gastric outlet obstruction (SUSTENT study): a multicenter randomized trial. Gastrointest Endosc 2010; 71(3):490–9.

44. Oh SY, Edwards A, Mandelson M, et al. Survival and clinical outcome after endoscopic duodenal stent placement for malignant gastric outlet obstruction: comparison of pancreatic cancer and nonpancreatic cancer. Gastrointest Endosc 2015;82(3):460–8.e2.

45. Wong GY, Schroeder DR, Carns PE, et al. Effect of neurolytic celiac plexus block on pain relief, quality of life, and survival in patients with unresectable pancreatic cancer: a randomized controlled trial. JAMA 2004; 291(9):1092–9.

46. Arcidiacono PG, Calori G, Carrara S, et al. Celiac plexus block for pancreatic cancer pain in adults. Cochrane Database Syst Rev 2011;(3):CD007519.

47. Lillemoe KD, Caneron JL, Kaufman HS, et al. Chemical splanchnicectomy in patients with unresectable pancreatic cancer. A prospective randomized trial. Ann Surg 1993;217(5):447–55 [discussion: 456–7].

48. Puli SR, Reddy JB, Bechtold ML, et al. EUS-guided celiac plexus neurolysis for pain due to chronic pancreatitis or pancreatic cancer pain: a meta-analysis and systematic review. Dig Dis Sci 2009;54(11):2330–7.

49. Erdek MA, King LM, Ellsworth SG. Pain management and palliative care in pancreatic cancer. Curr Probl Cancer 2013;37(5):266–72.

50. Fazal S, Saif MW. Supportive and palliative care of pancreatic cancer. JOP 2007; 8(2):240–53.

51. Bruno MJ, Haverkort EB, Tijssen GP, et al. Placebo controlled trial of enteric coated pancreatin microsphere treatment in patients with unresectable cancer of the pancreatic head region. Gut 1998;42(1):92–6.

52. Khorana AA, Fine RL. Pancreatic cancer and thromboembolic disease. Lancet Oncol 2004;5(11):655–63.

53. Lee AY, Levine MN, Baker RI, et al. Low-molecular-weight heparin versus a coumarin for the prevention of recurrent venous thromboembolism in patients with cancer. N Engl J Med 2003;349(2):146–53.

54. Sheffield KM, Boyd CA, Benarroch-Gampel J, et al. End-of-life care in Medicare beneficiaries dying with pancreatic cancer. Cancer 2011;117(21):5003–12.

55. Wright AA, Zhang B, Ray A, et al. Associations between end-of-life discussions, patient mental health, medical care near death, and caregiver bereavement adjustment. JAMA 2008;300(14):1665–73.

56. Wright AA, Keating NL, Balboni TA, et al. Place of death: correlations with quality of life of patients with cancer and predictors of bereaved caregivers' mental health. J Clin Oncol 2010;28(29):4457–64.

57. Earle CC, Park ER, Lai B, et al. Identifying potential indicators of the quality of end-of-life cancer care from administrative data. J Clin Oncol 2003;21(6):1133–8.

58. Grunfeld E, Urquhart R, Mykhalovskiy E, et al. Toward population-based indicators of quality end-of-life care: testing stakeholder agreement. Cancer 2008; 112(10):2301–8.

59. Bischoff K, Weinberg V, Rabow MW. Palliative and oncologic co-management: symptom management for outpatients with cancer. Support Care Cancer 2013; 21(11):3031–7.

60. Mitchell SL, Kiely DK, Miller SC, et al. Hospice care for patients with dementia. J Pain Symptom Manage 2007;34(1):7–16.

61. Greer DS, Mor V, Morris JN, et al. An alternative in terminal care: results of the National Hospice Study. J Chronic Dis 1986;39(1):9–26.

62. Centers for Medicare & Medicaid Services. Centers for Medicare & Medicaid Services. Available at: https://innovation.cms.gov/initiatives/medicare-care-choices/. Accessed December 20, 2015.

Intraductal Papillary Mucinous Neoplasm of the Pancreas

Zhi Ven Fong, MD, Carlos Fernández-del Castillo, MD*

KEYWORDS

- Intraductal papillary mucinous neoplasm • Pancreas • Biology
- Clinical management

KEY POINTS

- Intraductal papillary mucinous neoplasms (IPMNs) of the pancreas are categorized as main-duct (MD) and branch-duct (BD) lesions, with MD-IPMNs associated with a higher risk of malignancy and warranting surgical resection.
- Most BD-IPMNs are biologically indolent, with obstructive jaundice and radiographic features, such as presence of mural nodule or main pancreatic duct dilation greater than 10 mm, indicating higher risks lesions that should prompt consideration for resection.
- IPMN is a disease associated with a field defect. For multilesion disease, every cyst should be risk-stratified individually, and cyst-specific segmental resection performed when indicated. Follow-up after resection should be pursued, even if it was for benign IPMNs, given the risk of recurrence in the remnant gland.
- There are no high-level data supporting the use of adjuvant chemotherapy or radiation for invasive IPMNs. However, IPMNs with even small foci of invasion are associated with lymph node metastasis that poses a significant recurrence risk, suggesting the use of adjuvant therapy is appropriate in selected settings.

INTRODUCTION

The incidence of intraductal papillary mucinous neoplasms (IPMNs) of the pancreas has been on a rise in the past 2 decades, driven mainly by the widespread use of cross-sectional imaging.[1,2] IPMNs are defined as intraductal mucin-producing neoplasms that involve the main pancreatic duct or its side branches and lack the ovarian stroma typically seen in mucinous cystic neoplasms. Most IPMNs are discovered incidentally and remain asymptomatic, making it difficult to estimate their true prevalence, which has been described to be as low as 0.0008%, and as high as 10% in patients

Department of Surgery, Massachusetts General Hospital, Harvard Medical School, 15 Parkman Street, Boston, MA 02114-3117, USA
* Corresponding author. Department of Surgery, Massachusetts General Hospital, 15 Parkman Street, Boston, MA 02114-3117.
E-mail address: cfernandez@partners.org

Surg Clin N Am 96 (2016) 1431–1445
http://dx.doi.org/10.1016/j.suc.2016.07.009
0039-6109/16/© 2016 Elsevier Inc. All rights reserved.

older than 70 years.[3,4] IPMNs follow a classic spectrum of dysplastic changes and can be classified as low, moderate, or high-grade dysplasia and invasive cancer. Based on experience and clinical evidence from the past 30 years, the International Association of Pancreatology (IAP) released consensus guidelines in 2006 and 2012 providing clinical algorithms based on IPMN features and risk of malignancy.[5,6] In this article, we review the different classifications of IPMNs, their natural history, and clinical management and address recent controversies in the literature.

BIOLOGY OF INTRADUCTAL PAPILLARY MUCINOUS NEOPLASMS
Duct Involvement

IPMNs are morphologically classified into 2 main subtypes based on the location of pancreatic duct involvement: main duct (MD) and branch duct (BD). This morphologic classification has important biologic implications; MD-IPMNs have been associated with a malignancy rate of 57% to 92%, whereas BD-IPMNs have a more indolent natural history, with a malignancy risk ranging from 6% to 46%.[7-14] However, these malignancy rates are based solely on resected lesions, suggesting that the true malignancy risk is lower for both MD-IPMNs and particularly so for BD-IPMNs.

There is a third group, IPMNs with mixed-duct involvement, which historically has been treated akin to MD involvement with regard to its malignancy risk. This concept has recently been challenged, with the Heidelberg group demonstrating that 29% (n = 512) of suspected BD-IPMNs revealed histologic involvement of the MD that was not evident on preoperative imaging.[15] However, in an analysis of our own data at the Massachusetts General Hospital (n = 404), we found that the risk of high-grade dysplasia and invasive carcinoma in these minimal-mixed IPMNs was 11% and 6%, respectively, which more closely resembles the natural history of BD-IPMNs.[16] This subset of minimal-mixed IPMNs is clearly biologically different from those with grossly mixed involvement, which has been reported to have malignancy rates of up to 72% (**Fig. 1**).[17]

Histologic and Cytologic Classification

In recent years, IPMNs have been further classified into the following categories based on their histologic characteristics and specific mucin expression: intestinal, pancreatobiliary, gastric, and oncocytic subtype (**Fig. 2**). When IPMNs progress to invasive cancer, they can be of the tubular or colloid subtype, and rarely oncocytic.[18-21] These subtypes have important implications and show that IPMN is a heterogeneous disease.

BD-IPMNs have been shown to be most commonly associated with the gastric subtype, which has the least likelihood of tumor invasion (10%) and tumor recurrence (9%) among all subtypes. However, when carcinoma does occur, they are usually of the tubular subtype, which is associated with an increased risk of vascular invasion, perineural invasion, and nodal metastasis, portending a poorer prognosis similar to that of conventional ductal adenocarcinoma.[18,21] Conversely, MD-IPMNs more commonly exhibit intestinal-type epithelium, which has a high likelihood of progressing to carcinoma but generally is of the biologically less aggressive colloid type.[21] The pancreatobiliary and oncocytic subtypes are both less common but very contrasting in their biological behavior. IPMNs exhibiting pancreatobiliary epithelium are associated with the highest rate of tumor invasion (68%) and transformation to tubular carcinoma (82%).[18,21] Oncocytic IPMNs, on the other hand, have a very indolent biology. In a review of 18 patients with oncocytic IPMN, Marchegiani and colleagues[22] reported that most patients (67%) were asymptomatic, and although they had a 10-year recurrence

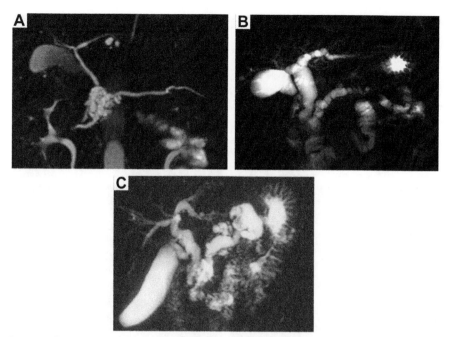

Fig. 1. Radiographic appearance of (*A*) BD, (*B*) MD, and (*C*) mixed-type IPMNs. (*Adapted from* Tanaka M. International consensus on the management of intraductal papillary mucinous neoplasm of the pancreas. Ann Transl Med 2015;3:286; with permission.)

rate of 46% (of which half underwent completion total pancreatectomy) there was no disease-specific death at a median follow-up of 7 years.

Field-Defect Concept

IPMNs are increasingly recognized as a disease associated with a "field defect" because of their propensity toward multifocality, which places the entire pancreatic gland at risk for neoplasia. The rate of synchronously occurring IPMN lesions has been reported to be as high as 83%,[23] and the risk of developing clinically significant metachronous lesions is approximately 8%.[24] Each lesion should be individually risk stratified, and cyst-specific segmental resection performed when indicated. More importantly, the rate of concomitantly occurring ductal adenocarcinoma has been reported to be approximately 4% and that of metachronous development of ductal adenocarcinoma as high as 11%. Although these rates are lower than that of invasive cancer arising from IPMNs, they have implications for postoperative surveillance and risk stratification (**Table 1**).[25–30] It is also important to differentiate pancreatic ductal adenocarcinoma occurring concomitantly with IPMN (also known as distinct) from carcinoma arising within an IPMN for risk stratification studies; the former is reflective of the risk of the entire pancreatic gland, and the latter defines the malignancy risk of BD-IPMNs, which guides recommendations for resection based on the cyst characteristics.

DIAGNOSIS
Imaging

The focus of diagnostics in IPMNs is in detecting specific cyst characteristics that are predictive of malignancy, specifically MD involvement and presence of mural nodule.

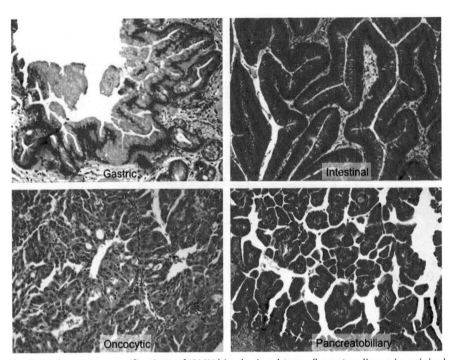

Fig. 2. High-power magnifications of IPMN histologic subtypes (hematoxylin-eosin, original magnification ×200). (*Adapted from* Fong ZV, Ferrone CR, Lillemoe KD, et al. Intraductal papillary mucinous neoplasm of the pancreas: current state of the art and ongoing controversies. Ann Surg 2016;263(5):908–17; with permission.)

Mural nodule, a solid protrusion of the internal lining of the cyst, is challenging to identify, as mucin globules can frequently mimic its appearance. Although there are no studies correlating the size of mural nodule with the risk of malignancy, the generally accepted size threshold used in the literature is 5 mm.[31–33] Most IPMNs are discovered incidentally when patients are imaged for an unrelated indication. Historically, a pancreas-protocol computed tomography (CT) scan or gadolinium-enhanced MRI with magnetic resonance cholangiopancreatography (MRCP) are the modalities of choice, with studies demonstrating similar diagnostic performance in detecting suspicious cyst features that guides clinical management.[34] However, MRI is preferred in practice, given its superior contrast resolution in delineating MD involvement and detecting mural nodules (**Fig. 3**), and it avoids repeated radiation exposure for patients requiring long-term surveillance. Although more invasive, endoscopic ultrasound (EUS) has a higher sensitivity and better detects mural nodules within IPMNs. However, it is less specific, and often picks up mucin globules, which may inadvertently lead to unnecessary resections.[35] Contrast-enhanced EUS, on the other hand, is better able to distinguish between both entities by detecting blood flow signals that are present in mural nodules, and has a specificity of more than 90%.[36]

Cyst Fluid Analysis

EUS also provides the opportunity for fine-needle aspiration (FNA) to sample the cyst fluid for analysis. This should be reserved for centers with appropriate local expertise, because the aspirated cyst fluid is often insufficient for accurate cytopathologic

Table 1
Summary of studies in the literature reporting on recurrence after resection of benign intraductal papillary mucinous neoplasm

First Author, Year	n	Median Follow-up, mo	Recurrence Rate, %	Recurrence Rate with Invasion, %	Time to Recurrence, mo	5-y Survival, %
Chari et al,[67] 2002	60	37	8.3	3.3	40	85
Sohn et al,[14] 2004	84	—	8.3	5.9	—	77
Wada et al,[68] 2005	75	—	1.3	0	—	100
Salvia et al,[69] 2009	80	31	1.0	0	—	100
Raut et al,[70] 2006	28	34	0	0	—	100
White et al,[71] 2007	78	40	7.7	5.1	22	87
Fujii et al,[72] 2010	103	—	9.7	7.8	—	—
Miller et al,[73] 2011	191	—	20	2	35	83
He et al,[60] 2013	130	38	17	4	46	81
Kang et al,[59] 2014	298	44	5.4	2.3	47	—
Marchegiani et al,[28] 2015	316	58	9	5	48	—

Data from Refs.[14,28,59,60,67–73]

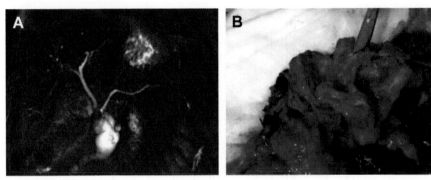

Fig. 3. (A) MRCP showing a large BD-IPMN associated with a mural nodule, with the (B) correlating specimen after surgical resection.

analysis and the specimen is often contaminated by cells from the gastric or duodenal wall. However, when performed well, cyst fluid analysis can differentiate mucinous from nonmucinous cysts with a sensitivity and specificity of 67% to 80% and 85% to 88%, respectively.[37–39] The most commonly used cyst fluid marker has been carcinoembryonic antigen (CEA), with studies suggesting a cutoff of 192 ng/mL was most accurate in the diagnosis of IPMN, although it cannot distinguish benign from malignant cysts.[40] Additionally, it is also equally elevated in mucinous cystic neoplasms (MCNs) and is low in approximately 30% of cases.[41] The 2 most common mutations tested for, KRAS and GNAS, are still investigational. KRAS can be found in approximately 50% of IPMNs but is also present in MCNs. GNAS is specific to IPMNs and is found in approximately 60% of cases. Both KRAS and GNAS also cannot differentiate benign from malignant disease.[42–44] Other promising biomarkers and mutations currently being investigated include monoclonal antibodies Das-1, SMAD4, TP53, P16, and BRAF.[45]

CLINICAL MANAGEMENT
The International Association of Pancreatology Guidelines

Given that we still are unable to reliably determine extent of MD involvement preoperatively, the current IAP guidelines recommend surgical resection for both MD-IPMNs and mixed-type IPMNs. Location-dependent segmental resection (pancreaticoduodenectomy for head lesions, distal pancreatectomy for body and tail lesions) should be performed, with lymph node dissection. Recently, parenchymal-sparing resections, such as enucleation and middle pancreatectomy, have been increasingly used. They are associated with a greater short-term complication rate, but preserve pancreatic exocrine and endocrine function.[46,47] This is especially appealing to younger patients who are better able to tolerate upfront morbidity for a longer-term benefit. Conversely, there also have been suggestions that total pancreatectomy should be recommended for younger patients with multifocal disease given their higher cumulative lifetime risk of malignancy; this should be balanced against the morbidity of a total pancreatectomy and the metabolic consequences of an apancreatic state.

The management of BD-IPMNs embraces a more tailored approach, given their indolent natural history. The 2006 IAP guidelines recommend that BD-IPMNs that are symptomatic, asymptomatic but larger than 3 cm, with main pancreatic duct dilatation to greater than 6 mm, or presence of a mural nodule be resected, given that these features represent harbingers for malignancy.[5,48] However, subsequent evaluation of the guideline has found that although these criteria yield a high negative predictive value, they have a low positive predictive value, indicating that resection is overused.[49–51] The IAP has since revised the guidelines, liberalizing the size threshold for resection and introduced 2 new categories: "high-risk stigmata," which is an indication for resection, and "worrisome features," which recommends further investigation (**Fig. 4**).[6] A review of 563 patients with BD-IPMNs at our institution revealed that liberalization of the size criteria with the new IAP guideline would have doubled the rate of missed high-grade dysplasia (8.8%) and would have missed one case of invasive cancer.[52] Other studies corroborate the concerns, reporting a higher risk of malignancy with increasing cyst size on interval follow-up imaging.[53,54] To further address this concern, Crippa and colleagues[55] reviewed 281 patients with worrisome features or high-risk stigmata who did not undergo surgical resection secondary to physician recommendation, patients' personal choice, or comorbidities precluding surgery. At a median follow-up of 51 months, invasive cancer developed in 12% of patients; the 5-year disease-free survival was 95%. Taken together, although the new IAP guidelines are safe, caution should be exercised in younger patients, given their higher cumulative lifetime risk of progression. Conversely, conservative management in elderly, frail patients is appropriate and should be offered as a treatment option.

The American Gastroenterology Association Guidelines

In 2015, the American Gastroenterology Association (AGA)'s Clinical Practice Guideline Committee released their official guidelines on the management of asymptomatic neoplastic pancreatic cysts (**Box 1**).[56] The guidelines were based on an extensive review of 1500 articles on the topic, and notably recommended the following: (1) surgery for an asymptomatic patient only if a cyst has 2 of the 3 concerning features (presence of nodule, size >3 cm, or duct dilation) and EUS shows malignancy, (2) surveillance interval of 2 years regardless of size of the cyst, and (3) discontinuation of surveillance after 5 years of no significant change or after resection of the cyst. These recommendations contradict the IAP's guidelines and take a drastically more conservative approach. The basis of their recommendations is their analysis of the Surveillance, Epidemiology, and End Results (SEER) database that revealed only 1137 identified cases of mucinous pancreatic adenocarcinoma amidst an estimated 3.5 million cysts in the population, suggesting an exceedingly low risk of cancer. However, mucinous adenocarcinoma arises from MCNs and is indeed a rare entity; invasive cancer arising from IPMN is indistinguishable from the coded pancreatic cancer and is impossible to be identified from the SEER database. Additionally, their recommendations ignore a decade's long evidence of IPMNs being a disease with a field defect, disregarding the risks of metachronously occurring IPMNs and ductal adenocarcinomas, as detailed in **Table 1**. The current criteria for resection and surveillance set by the IAP represent possibly the only chance of early intervention in pancreatic cancer, and in our opinions, the AGA guidelines need to be further vetted before they can be safely recommended to practitioners.

FOLLOW-UP STRATEGY
Surveillance of the Nonresected Intraductal Papillary Mucinous Neoplasm

Given that all MD-IPMNs should be resected, this section pertains to patients with BD-IPMNs. The intensity of surveillance depends on the initial size and feature of the IPMN and the interval progression of the lesion. In smaller lesions (0–2 cm), it is recommended that imaging (CT or MRCP) be performed every 2 years, and interval can be

1438

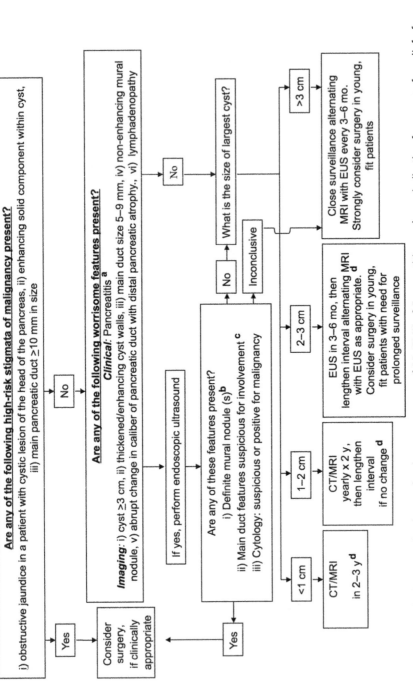

Fig. 4. Clinical algorithm put forth in 2012 by the IAP for the management of BD-IPMNs. [a] Pancreatitis may be an indication for surgery for relief of symptoms. [b] Differential diagnosis includes mucin. Mucin can move with change in patient position, may be dislodged on cyst lavage and does not have doppler flow. Features of true tumor nodule include lack of mobility, presence of doppler flow and FNA of nodule showing tumor tissue. [c] Presence of any one of thickened walls, intraductal mucin or mural nodules is suggestive of main duct involvement. In their absence main duct involvement is incolclusive. [d] Studies from Japan suggest that on follow-up of subjects with suspected BD-IPMN there is increased incidence of pancreatic ductal adenocarcinoma unrelated to malignant transformation of the BD-IPMN(s) being followed. However, it is unclear if imaging surveillance can detect early ductal adenocarcinoma, and, if so, at what interval surveillance imaging should be performed.

Box 1
Recommendations put forth by the American Gastroenterology Association (AGA) on the diagnosis and management of patients with intraductal papillary mucinous neoplasms

Recommendations from the AGA Guidelines

1. Before starting any pancreatic cyst surveillance program, patients should have a clear understanding of the risks and benefits.

2. Patients with pancreatic cysts smaller than 3 cm without a solid component or dilated pancreatic duct undergo MRI for surveillance in 1 year followed by every 2 years for a total of 5 years.

3. Pancreatic cysts with at least 2 high-risk features, such as size ≥3 cm, a dilated main pancreatic duct, or the presence of an associated solid component, should be examined with endoscopic ultrasound–fine-needle aspiration (EUS-FNA).

4. Patients without concerning EUS-FNA results should undergo MRI surveillance after 1 year and then every 2 years to ensure no change in risk of malignancy.

5. Significant changes in the characteristics of the cyst (solid component, increasing size of pancreatic duct, and/or diameter ≥3 cm) are indications for EUS-FNA.

6. Recommend against continued surveillance of pancreatic cysts if there has been no significant change in the characteristics of the cyst after 5 years of surveillance or if the patient is no longer a surgical candidate.

7. Patients with both a solid component and a dilated pancreatic duct and/or concerning features on EUS-FNA should undergo surgery to reduce the risk of mortality from carcinoma.

8. If surgery is considered, patients are referred to a center with demonstrated expertise in pancreatic surgery.

9. Patients with invasive cancer/dysplasia in a cyst that has been resected should undergo MRI surveillance of any remaining pancreas every 2 years.

10. Recommend against routine surveillance of pancreatic cysts without high-grade dysplasia or malignancy at surgical resection.

Adapted from Vege SS, Ziring B, Jain R, et al. American Gastroenterological Association institute guideline on the diagnosis and management of asymptomatic neoplastic pancreatic cysts. Gastroenterology 2015;148(4):819–22; [quiz: 12–3]; with permission.

lengthened if a pattern of stability has been established. In lesions larger than 2 cm, imaging along with EUS is recommended every 3 to 6 months, and lengthening of interval alternating MRCP with EUS if there has been no change on follow-up.[6] It should be noted that the degree of interval lengthening is entirely subjective, given that these recommendations are based on expert consensus. The degree of interval lengthening probably does not matter as much as the consistency; patients should be referred to and enrolled in a dedicated pancreatic cyst clinic with an established surveillance program and followed in a standardized manner. Surveillance of patients with low-risk IPMNs also can cause patient anxiety and poses a significant burden on health care cost and resources. Hence, physicians should exercise clinical judgment in balancing continued surveillance against the patients' accumulative lifetime risk of malignancy and fitness for surgery.

Follow-up of the Resected Intraductal Papillary Mucinous Neoplasm

For patients with invasive cancer arising from their resected IPMN, postoperative surveillance should follow that of ductal adenocarcinoma, given the similarly overwhelming risk of systemic and local recurrence.[57,58] The recurrence pattern for resected benign IPMNs is different and would be a reflection of the risk of synchronous, low-risk lesions left behind and the development of metachronous lesions in the healthy remnant gland as a result of the field defect with which IPMNs are associated.

The rate of synchronous disease has been reported to be as high as 83%,[23] and the risk of developing metachronous disease is approximately 8%.[24] Of patients undergoing resection for benign IPMNs, the recurrence rate ranges from 5.4% to 9.0%, of which 2.3% to 5.0% are invasive recurrences, occurring from 22 to 46 months from the index surgery (see **Table 1**).[28,59] The Johns Hopkins group analyzed 130 patients who underwent resection for benign IPMNs and reported 1-year, 5-year, and 10-year risks of developing invasive cancer being 0%, 7%, and 38%, respectively. At a median follow-up of 60 months, those patients who underwent completion pancreatectomy for recurrent invasive disease remained alive with no evidence of recurrent disease. These data imply that long-term surveillance is necessary, as recurrence can occur up to 4 years after resection of benign IPMNs, further reaffirming the danger of the AGA guidelines that would potentially deprive patients of the opportunity at early surgical intervention that has a positive impact on long-term survival.

Better understanding cohorts at higher risk of developing recurrences can guide postoperative surveillance strategies and maximize efficiency. A family history of pancreatic cancer has been shown to be associated with a higher likelihood of developing recurrence (23% vs 7%, $P<.05$),[60] concurrently occurring ductal adenocarcinoma (11.1% vs 2.9%, $P = .02$), and extrapancreatic malignancies (35.6% vs 20.1%, $P = .03$) after resection of benign IPMNs.[61] Patients with a positive margin have been shown to have a significantly higher rate of recurrence (25% vs 14%, $P = .008$) and a positive margin was the strongest independent predictor of survival (hazard ratio 2.6, $P = .0046$).[17] Finally, high-grade dysplasia in the primary lesion, despite negative margins, also has been shown to be a strong predictor of recurrence, portending an eightfold increase in the risk of developing invasive recurrence.[62]

The current IAP guidelines recommend performing a history/physical examination and MRCP surveillance at 2 years and 5 years after resection of noninvasive IPMNs, with a gradual lengthening of the follow-up interval once a pattern of stability has been determined.[6] Based on the evidence presented previously, the guidelines may not be sufficient. Caution must be exercised, particularly in patients with a family history of pancreatic cancer or high-grade dysplasia found in the primary lesion or surgical margin. For selected elderly patients with significant comorbidities in whom life expectancy is short or who cannot tolerate a pancreatectomy, follow-up could potentially be avoided altogether, especially if the aforementioned risk factors are absent.

ADJUVANT THERAPY

The role of adjuvant chemotherapy and radiation in patients with invasive IPMNs has not been well defined. Current studies in the literature are retrospective reviews confounded by patient selection,[63–65] and a randomized controlled trial is not feasible given the heterogeneity of the morphologic and histopathological subtypes. In a recent analysis of patients with IPMNs with small (<2 cm) invasive components, 19% were found to have lymph node metastases, which was highly predictive of recurrence rates (24%) and overall survival.[66] This suggests that IPMNs associated with invasive cancer should be treated similarly to conventional pancreatic adenocarcinoma, but the implication of malignancy morphology (tubular vs colloid) is still unknown. There are currently no formal recommendations regarding the use of adjuvant therapy in patients with invasive IPMN, but treatment certainly would be appropriate in the right context.

SUMMARY

It has been 3 decades since the initial discovery of IPMNs, and our understanding of the disease is still evolving. Although it may represent the only window of opportunity of early intervention in pancreatic cancer, we must be cautious and strike a judicious balance to prevent overutilization of surgical resection and avoid unnecessary morbidity and mortality. Presently, the IAP guidelines are safe and should be used as the gold standard for the management of patients with IPMNs, and clinical judgment should be exercised when treating younger and older/frail patients depending on their cumulative lifetime risk of progression. Efforts focusing on the development of serum and cyst fluid biomarkers that can better distinguish benign from malignant lesions and guide clinical management are under way.

REFERENCES

1. Valsangkar NP, Morales-Oyarvide V, Thayer SP, et al. 851 resected cystic tumors of the pancreas: a 33-year experience at the Massachusetts General Hospital. Surgery 2012;152:S4–12.
2. Winter JM, Cameron JL, Lillemoe KD, et al. Periampullary and pancreatic incidentaloma: a single institution's experience with an increasingly common diagnosis. Ann Surg 2006;243:673–80 [discussion: 680–3].
3. Laffan TA, Horton KM, Klein AP, et al. Prevalence of unsuspected pancreatic cysts on MDCT. AJR Am J Roentgenol 2008;191:802–7.
4. Lee KS, Sekhar A, Rofsky NM, et al. Prevalence of incidental pancreatic cysts in the adult population on MR imaging. Am J Gastroenterol 2010;105:2079–84.
5. Tanaka M, Chari S, Adsay V, et al. International consensus guidelines for management of intraductal papillary mucinous neoplasms and mucinous cystic neoplasms of the pancreas. Pancreatology 2006;6:17–32.
6. Tanaka M, Fernandez-del Castillo C, Adsay V, et al. International consensus guidelines 2012 for the management of IPMN and MCN of the pancreas. Pancreatology 2012;12:183–97.
7. Kobari M, Egawa S, Shibuya K, et al. Intraductal papillary mucinous tumors of the pancreas comprise 2 clinical subtypes: differences in clinical characteristics and surgical management. Arch Surg 1999;134:1131–6.
8. Terris B, Ponsot P, Paye F, et al. Intraductal papillary mucinous tumors of the pancreas confined to secondary ducts show less aggressive pathologic features as compared with those involving the main pancreatic duct. Am J Surg Pathol 2000;24:1372–7.
9. Doi R, Fujimoto K, Wada M, et al. Surgical management of intraductal papillary mucinous tumor of the pancreas. Surgery 2002;132:80–5.
10. Matsumoto T, Aramaki M, Yada K, et al. Optimal management of the branch duct type intraductal papillary mucinous neoplasms of the pancreas. J Clin Gastroenterol 2003;36:261–5.
11. Choi BS, Kim TK, Kim AY, et al. Differential diagnosis of benign and malignant intraductal papillary mucinous tumors of the pancreas: MR cholangiopancreatography and MR angiography. Korean J Radiol 2003;4:157–62.
12. Kitagawa Y, Unger TA, Taylor S, et al. Mucus is a predictor of better prognosis and survival in patients with intraductal papillary mucinous tumor of the pancreas. J Gastrointest Surg 2003;7:12–8 [discussion: 18–9].

13. Sugiyama M, Izumisato Y, Abe N, et al. Predictive factors for malignancy in intraductal papillary-mucinous tumours of the pancreas. Br J Surg 2003;90:1244–9.

14. Sohn TA, Yeo CJ, Cameron JL, et al. Intraductal papillary mucinous neoplasms of the pancreas: an updated experience. Ann Surg 2004;239:788–97 [discussion: 797–9].

15. Fritz S, Klauss M, Bergmann F, et al. Pancreatic main-duct involvement in branch-duct IPMNs: an underestimated risk. Ann Surg 2014;260:848–55 [discussion: 855–6].

16. Sahora K, Fernandez-del Castillo C, Dong F, et al. Not all mixed-type intraductal papillary mucinous neoplasms behave like main-duct lesions: implications of minimal involvement of the main pancreatic duct. Surgery 2014;156:611–21.

17. Marchegiani G, Mino-Kenudson M, Sahora K, et al. IPMN involving the main pancreatic duct: biology, epidemiology, and long-term outcomes following resection. Ann Surg 2015;261:976–83.

18. Koh YX, Zheng HL, Chok AY, et al. Systematic review and meta-analysis of the spectrum and outcomes of different histologic subtypes of noninvasive and invasive intraductal papillary mucinous neoplasms. Surgery 2015;157:496–509.

19. Mino-Kenudson M, Fernandez-del Castillo C, Baba Y, et al. Prognosis of invasive intraductal papillary mucinous neoplasm depends on histological and precursor epithelial subtypes. Gut 2011;60:1712–20.

20. Fong ZV, Ferrone CR, Lillemoe KD, et al. Intraductal papillary mucinous neoplasm of the pancreas: current state of the art and ongoing controversies. Ann Surg 2016;263(5):908–17.

21. Distler M, Kersting S, Niedergethmann M, et al. Pathohistological subtype predicts survival in patients with intraductal papillary mucinous neoplasm (IPMN) of the pancreas. Ann Surg 2013;258:324–30.

22. Marchegiani G, Mino-Kenudson M, Ferrone CR, et al. Oncocytic-type intraductal papillary mucinous neoplasms: a unique malignant pancreatic tumor with good long-term prognosis. J Am Coll Surg 2015;220:839–44.

23. Bendix Holme J, Jacobsen NO, Rokkjaer M, et al. Total pancreatectomy in six patients with intraductal papillary mucinous tumour of the pancreas: the treatment of choice. HPB (Oxford) 2001;3:257–62.

24. Matthaei H, Norris AL, Tsiatis AC, et al. Clinicopathological characteristics and molecular analyses of multifocal intraductal papillary mucinous neoplasms of the pancreas. Ann Surg 2012;255:326–33.

25. Yamaguchi K, Kanemitsu S, Hatori T, et al. Pancreatic ductal adenocarcinoma derived from IPMN and pancreatic ductal adenocarcinoma concomitant with IPMN. Pancreas 2011;40:571–80.

26. Ideno N, Ohtsuka T, Kono H, et al. Intraductal papillary mucinous neoplasms of the pancreas with distinct pancreatic ductal adenocarcinomas are frequently of gastric subtype. Ann Surg 2013;258:141–51.

27. Ohtsuka T, Kono H, Tanabe R, et al. Follow-up study after resection of intraductal papillary mucinous neoplasm of the pancreas; special references to the multifocal lesions and development of ductal carcinoma in the remnant pancreas. Am J Surg 2012;204:44–8.

28. Marchegiani G, Mino-Kenudson M, Ferrone CR, et al. Patterns of recurrence after resection of IPMN: who, when, and how? Ann Surg 2015;262(6):1108–14.

29. Miyasaka Y, Ohtsuka T, Tamura K, et al. Predictive factors for the metachronous development of high-risk lesions in the remnant pancreas after partial pancreatectomy for intraductal papillary mucinous neoplasm. Ann Surg 2016;263(6):1180–7.

30. Ingkakul T, Sadakari Y, Ienaga J, et al. Predictors of the presence of concomitant invasive ductal carcinoma in intraductal papillary mucinous neoplasm of the pancreas. Ann Surg 2010;251:70–5.

31. Hirono S, Tani M, Kawai M, et al. The carcinoembryonic antigen level in pancreatic juice and mural nodule size are predictors of malignancy for branch duct type intraductal papillary mucinous neoplasms of the pancreas. Ann Surg 2012;255:517–22.

32. Okabayashi T, Kobayashi M, Nishimori I, et al. Clinicopathological features and medical management of intraductal papillary mucinous neoplasms. J Gastroenterol Hepatol 2006;21:462–7.

33. Ohno E, Itoh A, Kawashima H, et al. Malignant transformation of branch duct-type intraductal papillary mucinous neoplasms of the pancreas based on contrast-enhanced endoscopic ultrasonography morphological changes: focus on malignant transformation of intraductal papillary mucinous neoplasm itself. Pancreas 2012;41:855–62.

34. Seo N, Byun JH, Kim JH, et al. Validation of the 2012 International Consensus Guidelines using computed tomography and magnetic resonance imaging: branch duct and main duct intraductal papillary mucinous neoplasms of the pancreas. Ann Surg 2016;263(3):557–64.

35. Anand N, Sampath K, Wu BU. Cyst features and risk of malignancy in intraductal papillary mucinous neoplasms of the pancreas: a meta-analysis. Clin Gastroenterol Hepatol 2013;11:913–21 [quiz: e59–60].

36. Ohno E, Hirooka Y, Itoh A, et al. Intraductal papillary mucinous neoplasms of the pancreas: differentiation of malignant and benign tumors by endoscopic ultrasound findings of mural nodules. Ann Surg 2009;249:628–34.

37. Ono J, Yaeger KA, Genevay M, et al. Cytological analysis of small branch-duct intraductal papillary mucinous neoplasms provides a more accurate risk assessment of malignancy than symptoms. Cytojournal 2011;8:21.

38. Kubo H, Nakamura K, Itaba S, et al. Differential diagnosis of cystic tumors of the pancreas by endoscopic ultrasonography. Endoscopy 2009;41:684–9.

39. Genevay M, Mino-Kenudson M, Yaeger K, et al. Cytology adds value to imaging studies for risk assessment of malignancy in pancreatic mucinous cysts. Ann Surg 2011;254:977–83.

40. Brugge WR, Lewandrowski K, Lee-Lewandrowski E, et al. Diagnosis of pancreatic cystic neoplasms: a report of the cooperative pancreatic cyst study. Gastroenterology 2004;126:1330–6.

41. Correa-Gallego C, Warshaw AL, Fernandez-del Castillo C. Fluid CEA in IPMNs: a useful test or the flip of a coin? Am J Gastroenterol 2009;104:796–7.

42. Tan MC, Basturk O, Brannon AR, et al. GNAS and KRAS mutations define separate progression pathways in intraductal papillary mucinous neoplasm-associated carcinoma. J Am Coll Surg 2015;220:845–54.e1.

43. Wu J, Matthaei H, Maitra A, et al. Recurrent GNAS mutations define an unexpected pathway for pancreatic cyst development. Sci Transl Med 2011;3:92ra66.

44. Fritz S, Fernandez-del Castillo C, Mino-Kenudson M, et al. Global genomic analysis of intraductal papillary mucinous neoplasms of the pancreas reveals significant molecular differences compared to ductal adenocarcinoma. Ann Surg 2009;249:440–7.

45. Das KK, Xiao H, Geng X, et al. mAb Das-1 is specific for high-risk and malignant intraductal papillary mucinous neoplasm (IPMN). Gut 2014;63(10):1626–34.

46. Sauvanet A, Gaujoux S, Blanc B, et al. Parenchyma-sparing pancreatectomy for presumed noninvasive intraductal papillary mucinous neoplasms of the pancreas. Ann Surg 2014;260:364–71.

47. Faitot F, Gaujoux S, Barbier L, et al. Reappraisal of pancreatic enucleations: a single-center experience of 126 procedures. Surgery 2015;158(1):201–10.

48. Tanaka M. International consensus on the management of intraductal papillary mucinous neoplasm of the pancreas. Ann Transl Med 2015;3:286.

49. Rodriguez JR, Salvia R, Crippa S, et al. Branch-duct intraductal papillary mucinous neoplasms: observations in 145 patients who underwent resection. Gastroenterology 2007;133:72–9 [quiz: 309–10].

50. Tang RS, Weinberg B, Dawson DW, et al. Evaluation of the guidelines for management of pancreatic branch-duct intraductal papillary mucinous neoplasm. Clin Gastroenterol Hepatol 2008;6:815–9 [quiz: 719].

51. Nagai K, Doi R, Ito T, et al. Single-institution validation of the international consensus guidelines for treatment of branch duct intraductal papillary mucinous neoplasms of the pancreas. J Hepatobiliary Pancreat Surg 2009;16:353–8.

52. Sahora K, Mino-Kenudson M, Brugge W, et al. Branch duct intraductal papillary mucinous neoplasms: does cyst size change the tip of the scale? A critical analysis of the revised international consensus guidelines in a large single-institutional series. Ann Surg 2013;258:466–75.

53. Kang MJ, Jang JY, Kim SJ, et al. Cyst growth rate predicts malignancy in patients with branch duct intraductal papillary mucinous neoplasms. Clin Gastroenterol Hepatol 2011;9:87–93.

54. Rautou PE, Levy P, Vullierme MP, et al. Morphologic changes in branch duct intraductal papillary mucinous neoplasms of the pancreas: a midterm follow-up study. Clin Gastroenterol Hepatol 2008;6:807–14.

55. Crippa S, Bassi C, Salvia R, et al. Low progression of intraductal papillary mucinous neoplasms with worrisome features and high-risk stigmata undergoing non-operative management: a mid-term follow-up analysis. Gut 2016. [Epub ahead of print].

56. Vege SS, Ziring B, Jain R, et al. American Gastroenterological Association institute guideline on the diagnosis and management of asymptomatic neoplastic pancreatic cysts. Gastroenterology 2015;148:819–22 [quiz: 12–3].

57. Yopp AC, Allen PJ. Prognosis of invasive intraductal papillary mucinous neoplasms of the pancreas. World J Gastrointest Surg 2010;2:359–62.

58. Fong ZV, Castillo CF. Intraductal papillary mucinous adenocarcinoma of the pancreas: clinical outcomes, prognostic factors, and the role of adjuvant therapy. Viszeralmedizin 2015;31:43–6.

59. Kang MJ, Jang JY, Lee KB, et al. Long-term prospective cohort study of patients undergoing pancreatectomy for intraductal papillary mucinous neoplasm of the pancreas: implications for postoperative surveillance. Ann Surg 2014;260(2):356–63.

60. He J, Cameron JL, Ahuja N, et al. Is it necessary to follow patients after resection of a benign pancreatic intraductal papillary mucinous neoplasm? J Am Coll Surg 2013;216:657–65 [discussion: 665–7].

61. Nehra D, Oyarvide VM, Mino-Kenudson M, et al. Intraductal papillary mucinous neoplasms: does a family history of pancreatic cancer matter? Pancreatology 2012;12:358–63.

62. Rezaee N, Barbon C, Zaki A. Intraductal papillary mucinous neoplasm (IPMN) with high grade dysplasia is a risk factor for the subsequent development of pancreatic ductal adenocarcinoma. HPB (Oxford) 2016;18(3):236–46.

63. Alexander BM, Fernandez-Del Castillo C, Ryan DP, et al. Intraductal papillary mucinous adenocarcinoma of the pancreas: clinical outcomes, prognostic factors, and the role of adjuvant therapy. Gastrointest Cancer Res 2011;4:116–21.

64. Swartz MJ, Hsu CC, Pawlik TM, et al. Adjuvant chemoradiotherapy after pancreatic resection for invasive carcinoma associated with intraductal papillary mucinous neoplasm of the pancreas. Int J Radiat Oncol Biol Phys 2010;76: 839–44.

65. Turrini O, Waters JA, Schnelldorfer T, et al. Invasive intraductal papillary mucinous neoplasm: predictors of survival and role of adjuvant therapy. HPB (Oxford) 2010; 12:447–55.

66. Winter JM, Jiang W, Basturk O, et al. Recurrence and survival after resection of small intraductal papillary mucinous neoplasm-associated carcinomas (</=20-mm invasive component): a multi-institutional analysis. Ann Surg 2016;263(4): 793–801.

67. Chari ST, Yadav D, Smyrk TC, et al. Study of recurrence after surgical resection of intraductal papillary mucinous neoplasm of the pancreas. Gastroenterology 2002;123:1500–7.

68. Wada K, Kozarek RA, Traverso LW. Outcomes following resection of invasive and noninvasive intraductal papillary mucinous neoplasms of the pancreas. Am J Surg 2005;189:632–6 [discussion: 637].

69. Salvia R, Partelli S, Crippa S, et al. Intraductal papillary mucinous neoplasms of the pancreas with multifocal involvement of branch ducts. Am J Surg 2009;198: 709–14.

70. Raut CP, Cleary KR, Staerkel GA, et al. Intraductal papillary mucinous neoplasms of the pancreas: effect of invasion and pancreatic margin status on recurrence and survival. Ann Surg Oncol 2006;13:582–94.

71. White R, D'Angelica M, Katabi N, et al. Fate of the remnant pancreas after resection of noninvasive intraductal papillary mucinous neoplasm. J Am Coll Surg 2007;204:987–93 [discussion: 993–5].

72. Fujii T, Kato K, Kodera Y, et al. Prognostic impact of pancreatic margin status in the intraductal papillary mucinous neoplasms of the pancreas. Surgery 2010;148: 285–90.

73. Miller JR, Meyer JE, Waters JA, et al. Outcome of the pancreatic remnant following segmental pancreatectomy for non-invasive intraductal papillary mucinous neoplasm. HPB (Oxford) 2011;13:759–66.

Surgical Management of Pancreatic Neuroendocrine Tumors

Jason B. Liu, MD[a], Marshall S. Baker, MD, MBA[a,b],*

KEYWORDS

• Pancreatic neuroendocrine tumor • PNET • Management • Surgery • Review

KEY POINTS

- Management of pancreatic neuroendocrine tumors (PNETs) is challenging because of their heterogeneous pathologic features and unpredictable clinical behaviors.
- Although most PNETs are nonfunctional, certain PNETs are functional and can present with classic endocrinopathies related to hormone excess.
- Surgery remains the cornerstone of management for localized disease, and operative approaches are customized to the clinical behavior of the particular PNET.
- Frequent evaluation of vague abdominal symptoms using axial imaging has led to an upsurge of incidentally detected, small, asymptomatic PNETs resulting in management controversies.

INTRODUCTION

Pancreatic neuroendocrine tumors (PNETs) are the second most common pancreatic neoplasm behind adenocarcinoma, with an overall incidence of approximately 5:1,000,000 and an estimated prevalence of 1:100,000.[1,2] PNETs are most frequently detected between the fourth and sixth decades of life. Approximately 10% to 30% of PNETs are associated with familial syndromes including multiple endocrine neoplasia type I (MEN I) and von Hippel-Lindau syndrome.[1–3] PNETs may overproduce certain hormones and present with classic endocrinopathies. Most, however, are nonfunctional incidentalomas detected on imaging obtained for unrelated reasons. With the increased use of axial imaging to evaluate vague abdominal symptoms, the rate of detection has increased fourfold to sevenfold since the year 2000, and the size of the tumors at time of diagnosis has markedly decreased.[4] PNETs have traditionally

Financial Disclosures: The authors have no financial disclosures to report or conflicts of interest related to this work.

[a] Department of Surgery, University of Chicago Hospitals, Chicago, IL, USA; [b] Division of Surgical Oncology, Department of Surgery, NorthShore University Health System, Evanston, IL, USA
* Corresponding author. 2650 Ridge Avenue, Walgreen Building, 2nd Floor, Evanston, IL 60201.
E-mail address: mbaker3@northshore.org

been thought to be biologically less aggressive than pancreatic adenocarcinomas but there has been increased recognition that the pathologic potential of PNETs is highly variable.[5,6] Many PNETs are indolent with a small proclivity to metastasize and with very favorable long-term prognoses, while others are high-grade tumors that demonstrate a relentless progression to early metastases that makes their biology seem more aggressive than typical for ductal adenocarcinomas.

Surgical resection remains the primary curative modality in the management of PNETs.[7] The current trend toward early incidental detection of the tumors combined with their heterogeneous and unpredictable pathology challenge optimal treatment decision making. In the current review, we discuss the surgical management of functional and nonfunctional PNETs with particular attention to the surgical management of small (≤2 cm) asymptomatic, nonfunctional PNETs (NF-PNETs).

PATHOPHYSIOLOGY

PNETs are neuroendocrine tumors arising from the cells that make up the pancreatic islets. The underlying etiology of PNETs is believed to be acquired and/or from congenital genetic alterations in the cell of origin, but there is no genetic mutation that has been consistently and definitively associated with the development of these tumors. The most frequently mutated genes found in PNETs involve chromatin-remodeling genes, such as *MEN I* (44%) and *DAXX/ATRX* (43%), and genes of the mammalian target of Rapamycin pathway (15%).[5,8] Well-differentiated PNETs lack the alterations in *KRAS*, *TP53*, *CDKN2A*, and *SMAD4* genes frequently encountered in pancreatic ductal adenocarcinomas, whereas poorly differentiated PNETs do exhibit genetic alterations found in pancreatic ductal adenocarcinomas.[9]

Functional PNETs by definition produce and secrete 1 or more active hormones. They must manifest the characteristic endocrinopathy to be considered functional. Hormones produced by PNETs include insulin, gastrin, glucagon, somatostatin, vasoactive intestinal peptide (VIP), pancreatic polypeptide, and cholecystokinin.[2,10,11] Additionally, both functional and NF-PNETs can express peptides characteristic of NETs in general, such as chromogranin A and synaptophysin. These are commonly used for purposes of diagnosis and surveillance as serologic and/or histologic markers of PNETs. Overproduction of chromogranin A and synaptophysin are not typically associated with characteristic endocrinopathies.

PNETs frequently express somatostatin receptors (SSTR1-5), which are normally present throughout the central nervous system, the gastrointestinal tract, and the endocrine and exocrine glands.[5,12] PNETs express a range of SSTRs, and synthetic somatostatin analogs, such as octreotide or lanreotide, have varying activity profiles against the range of SSTRs expressed by PNETs.

CLASSIFICATION AND STAGING

Tumors are first categorized as either functional or nonfunctional, as symptoms related to the tumor may be the primary driver for therapeutic intervention, particularly in small lesions. The vast majority of PNETs, as many as 90% in select series, are nonfunctional. Functional PNETs occur in approximately 10% of cases and are named based on their clinical endocrinopathy. They include insulinomas, gastrinomas, VIPomas, glucagonomas, and somatostatinomas (**Table 1**).[1,13] Functionality of PNETs appears to be independent of both grade and stage.

Among the various subtypes of functional tumors, insulinomas are generally less aggressive and rarely present with metastatic disease, whereas gastrinomas tend to have a higher proclivity for metastasis. In general, a loss in differentiation tends to

Table 1
Characteristics of functional pancreatic neuroendocrine tumors

Tumor Type	Frequency		Clinical Features	Diagnosis	Tumor Location	Surgical Recommendations[a]
	Sporadic	MEN I				
Insulinoma	30%–40%	10%–18%	Whipple triad, weight gain; likely benign	72-h fast; serum insulin, proinsulin, C-peptide, glucose; avoid SRS	Within pancreas	Enucleation Laparoscopic
Gastrinoma	20%–50%	30%–54%	Zollinger-Ellison syndrome; likely malignant	Secretin stimulation test	Gastrinoma triangle; often duodenum	Formal resection Intraoperative exploration Open
Glucagonoma	Rare	3%	Necrolytic migratory erythema, diabetes mellitus, anemia, weight loss, hypercoagulability	History and physical; serum glucagon	Tail of pancreas	Formal resection when possible
VIPoma	Rare	17%	Verner-Morrison syndrome; iron and vitamin B_{12} deficiency	Serum VIP	Tail of pancreas	Formal resection when possible
Somatostatinoma	Rare	<5%	Abdominal pain, weight loss, diabetes, cholelithiasis, diarrhea, steatorrhea	Serum somatostatin	Pancreas, ampulla, duodenum, jejunum	Formal resection when possible

Abbreviations: MEN I, multiple endocrine neoplasia, type 1; SRS, somatostatin receptor scintigraphy; VIP, vasoactive intestinal peptide.
[a] For sporadic cases; see text for MEN I management recommendations.

result in a loss of hormone production abilities and therefore are less likely to produce an endocrinopathy. However, the biology of these lesions is highly variable, and low-grade, localized lesions or high-grade, widely disseminated tumors may be hormonally active and cause an endocrinopathy.

Beyond functionality, PNETs are categorized by grade and pathologic stage. Recent international experience with PNETs has demonstrated that several of the pathologic features typically used to determine prognosis in cancers do not consistently predict the biologic behavior of PNETs and thus are imperfect determinants of which treatment modalities are best.[5] In these cases, lymph node involvement, large tumor size, and even presence of distant metastases do not necessarily correlate with either the length of disease-specific survival or the degree to which the functional health of the patient is compromised. Instead, the single most important determinant of prognosis is the histologic grade of the tumor. This observation has led to the development of a unique classification scheme for PNETs that differs substantially from traditional TNM staging systems used for most solid tumors. The most recent consensus classification system is the 2010 World Health Organization (WHO) classification, which has also been endorsed by the European Neuroendocrine Tumor Society (ENETS) (**Table 2**).[14,15] PNETs are generally assigned a WHO grade or class and a TNM stage. The WHO classification stratifies PNETs by the degree of differentiation and by histologic grade. The histologic grade is defined by the mitotic rate and/or Ki-67 index, with the higher of either the mitotic rate or Ki-67 index being used to determine the histologic grade of the tumor.[16,17] The pathologic staging system typically used for PNETs is outlined in the seventh edition of the American Joint Committee on Cancer (AJCC 2010) staging manual and is identical to that used for pancreatic ductal adenocarcinoma (**Table 3**).[18] Although PNETs have distinctly different tumor biology and in general have a better long-term survival than pancreatic ductal adenocarcinoma, the AJCC TNM system does provide useful stage discrimination that can aid in treatment decision making. Treating clinicians must bear in mind that histologic grade will tend to surpass stage in prognostic capability, meaning that patients with

---

Table 2
2010 European Neuroendocrine Tumor Society/World Health Organization nomenclature and grading system for pancreatic neuroendocrine tumors

Category	Differentiation	Grade	Mitotic Count	Ki-67 Index
Neuroendocrine tumor, Grade 1	Well differentiated	Low grade (G1)	<2 per 10 HPF	<3%
Neuroendocrine tumor, Grade 2		Intermediate grade (G2)	2–20 per 10 HPF	3%–20%
Neuroendocrine carcinoma, Grade 3, small cell	Poorly differentiated	High grade (G3)	>20 per 10 HPF	>20%
Neuroendocrine carcinoma, Grade 3, large cell				

Abbreviation: HPF, high-power microscopic fields.

Adapted from Falconi M, Bartsch DK, Eriksson B, et al. ENETS consensus guidelines for the management of patients with digestive neuroendocrine neoplasms of the digestive system: well-differentiated pancreatic non-functioning tumors. Neuroendocrinology 2012;95(2):122; and Rindi G, Arnold R, Bosman F, et al. Nomenclature and classification of neuroendocrine neoplasms of the digestive system. In: WHO classification of tumors of the digestive system, vol. 4. 2010. p. 13–4

Table 3			
AJCC seventh edition TNM staging system for exocrine and endocrine tumors of the pancreas			
Primary Tumor (T)			
TX	Primary tumor cannot be assessed		
T0	No evidence of primary tumor		
Tis	Carcinoma in situ*		
T1	Tumor limited to pancreas, 2 cm or smaller in greatest dimension		
T2	Tumor limited to the pancreas, larger than 2 cm in greatest dimension		
T3	Tumor extends beyond the pancreas but without involvement of the celiac axis or the superior mesenteric artery		
T4	Tumor involves the celiac axis or the superior mesenteric artery (unresectable primary tumor)		
Regional lymph nodes (N)			
NX	Regional lymph nodes cannot be assessed		
N0	No regional lymph node metastasis		
N1	Regional lymph node metastasis		
Distant metastasis (M)			
M0	No distant metastasis		
M1	Distant metastasis		
Anatomic stage/prognostic groups			
Stage 0	Tis	N0	M0
Stage IA	T1	N0	M0
Stage IB	T2	N0	M0
Stage IIA	T3	N0	M0
Stage IIB	T1	N1	M0
	T2	N1	M0
	T3	N1	M0
Stage III	T4	Any N	M0
Stage IV	Any T	Any N	M1

* Includes PanIN III.
Abbreviation: AJCC, American Joint Committee on Cancer.
From American Joint Committee on Cancer. AJCC cancer staging manual. 7th edition. Chicago: American College of Surgeons; 2010; with permission.

widespread distant metastasis may be asymptomatic for years, whereas others presenting with localized high-grade disease will frequently have early recurrence and succumb to the tumor within months of diagnosis.[19]

CLINICAL PRESENTATION AND DIAGNOSIS
Nonfunctional Pancreatic Neuroendocrine Tumors

NF-PETs present as pancreatic incidentalomas on imaging obtained for unrelated reasons, with symptoms related to local mass effect, or with metastatic disease. NF-PNETs either do not produce any hormone, produce amounts of hormone insufficient to cause an endocrinopathy, or produce hormones that do not cause an endocrinopathy (eg, chromogranins, synaptophysin, neuron-specific enolase or ghrelin).[7] Because of this, NF-PNETs tend to present at a later stage than functional tumors. Approximately 60% to 70% of patients have metastatic disease and 20% have locally advanced disease at time of diagnosis.[13] Symptoms are nonspecific and can include abdominal pain, back pain, weight loss, nausea, vomiting, anorexia, obstructive jaundice, and/or pancreatitis. NF-PNETs have male gender preponderance and most often occur in the fourth to sixth decades of life. There is no predilection for ethnicity.[2]

Biochemical Evaluation of Nonfunctional Pancreatic Neuroendocrine Tumors

The initial evaluation of NF-PNETs includes a biochemical evaluation for endocrinopathies as clinically indicated. Serum chromogranin A levels are elevated in more than 60% of patients with functional and NF-PNETs and may be used as a tumor marker in postoperative surveillance and for monitoring treatment effect.[7,17] Elevated levels have been associated with poor overall prognosis, and early decreases may be associated with favorable treatment outcomes. The specificity of chromogranin A is limited: 50% to 80%.[13,20] Falsely elevated serum chromogranin A levels can be caused by renal or hepatic failure, chronic atrophic gastritis, acute coronary syndrome, and the use of proton pump inhibitors (PPIs) or H_2 antagonists. The North American Neuroendocrine Tumor Society recommends following serum chromogranin A levels as surrogate markers of disease progression or response to therapy if abnormal at time of diagnosis.[21]

Imaging of Nonfunctional Pancreatic Neuroendocrine Tumors

Dedicated pancreas multiphasic computed tomography (CT) or MRI remains the first step in assessing the primary tumor site and extent of disease.[5,10] On triple-phase CT, NF-PNETs are well-circumscribed hypervascular lesions and best visualized in the late arterial or portal-venous inflow phase (**Fig. 1**).[12,22] Calcifications also may be present. Local invasion of vascular structures also can be assessed to determine resectability. CT has a sensitivity and specificity of 63% to 82% and 83% to 100%, respectively,

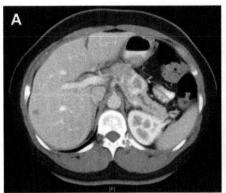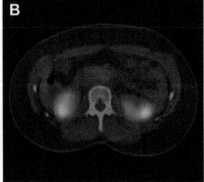

Fig. 1. Representative image (*A*) from contrast-enhanced CT for a 36-year-old woman presenting with vague abdominal pain demonstrating characteristic hyperenhancement on arterial phase typical of PNETs. The hypointense lesion in the right lobe of the liver was not visualized on octreotide scan, evaluated by MRI, and found to be a cyst. The pancreatic mass was managed by laparoscopic distal pancreatectomy with splenectomy. The patient is now 2 years post resection with no evidence of recurrence. Representative image (*B*) from octreotide scan for the same patient preoperatively. The image demonstrates mild octreotide binding typical of an NF-PNET.

varying with the size of the lesion. For liver metastases, the mean sensitivity and specificity are 82% and 92%, respectively. Approximately 10% of NF-PNETs appear as cystic lesions within the pancreas and can have a misdiagnosis rate of 43% from other cystic pancreatic lesions.[22,23] MRI has improved tissue contrast in evaluating the pancreas and the liver (**Fig. 2**). NF-PNETs are typically dark on T1-weighted images and bright on T2-weighted images. Sensitivity and specificity for MRI varies between 85% to 100% and 75% to 100%, respectively.[22] Mean detection rate is 73% for NF-PNETs and 82% for NET liver metastasis.[12] Magnetic resonance cholangiopancreatography (MRCP) can also be included during MRI for preoperative planning. MRI is most useful when monitoring developing or persistent hepatic lesions.

In addition to traditional axial imaging, 2 nuclear medicine modalities are available for evaluation of NF-PNETs: somatostatin receptor scintigraphy (SRS) and PET. Many PNETs express high levels of a number of SSTRs, particularly SSTR-2, and can therefore be imaged with radiolabeled somatostatin analogs (see **Fig. 1**), such as ^{111}In-pentetreotide (Octreoscan). SRS is more commonly available and often used for localizing NF-PNETs, staging these tumors, identifying sites of metastatic disease, surveying for recurrence, and assessing the effect of systemic therapy. There are few data, however, to support the contention that these tests provide information above that gained by high-quality CT or MR axial imaging. SRS is costly and can present a significant logistical burden for the patient.

Imaging using PET involves 2 types of radiotracers: those that bind to SSTRs and those that characterize tumor metabolism. Traditional fludeoxyglucose (FDG)-PET scanning may not visualize NF-PNETs well due to their low metabolic rate, but has been used to characterize highly metabolically active poorly differentiated PNETs. Compared with SRS, PET involving SSTRs allows improved contrast and can detect

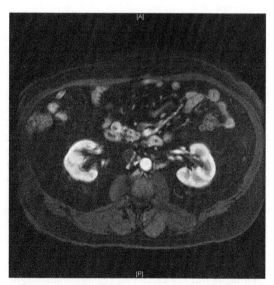

Fig. 2. Select images from contrast-enhanced axial MR imaging demonstrating a hyperenhancing mass in the pancreatic head. Endoscopic ultrasound with aspiration was consistent with a pancreatic neuroendocrine tumor. Biochemical workup was negative. This PNET was managed with enucleation. Margins were negative. The patient recovered without complication and is 2 years post resection with no evidence of disease recurrence on follow-up axial imaging.

tumors approximately 0.5 cm in size. Combined with CT, PET/CT has shown improvement in localization of both functional and NF-PNETs.[22] In one study, use of PET/CT changed treatment decisions in 59.6% of patients compared with CT or MRI alone.[24] Most patients in this study were characterized as well-differentiated, but functionality was not reported.

Functional Pancreatic Neuroendocrine Tumors

Functional PNETs are hormonally active tumors. Patients present with symptoms driven by the hormones the tumors produce: an endocrinopathy. Functional PNETs are typically detected at an earlier stage than nonfunctional tumors, although their detection can be delayed due to the rarity of the tumors, and the symptoms may be attributed to other potential etiologies. When suspicions are raised early, the tumors may be small and difficult to localize. Multiple radiologic modalities are used in the evaluation of these patients to localize the tumors before operative exploration. However, it is not uncommon for patients to be operatively explored before definitive radiographic localization given the certainty of the diagnosis.

Insulinoma

Insulinomas comprise approximately 35% to 40% of functional PNETs.[6] These are hormonally active tumors, produce symptoms early, are typically small (<2 cm in size), and are solitary lesions at the time of presentation. They may develop in any location within the pancreatic parenchyma but are found only within the pancreas. These are typically not metastatic at presentation, but invasive transformation has been reported.[25,26]

Insulinomas present with neuroglycopenic symptoms of palpations, tremors, diaphoresis, weakness, confusion, agitation, loss of consciousness, and/or seizures that are associated with hypoglycemia and relieved with oral intake or intravenous glucose infusion. The constellation of documented hypoglycemia, neuroglycopenic symptoms, and resolution of those symptoms with glucose intake is identified as the Whipple Triad. Combined with the anabolic effects of insulin, patients with insulinoma often will eat to manage their glycopenic symptoms and gain weight.[7]

Diagnosis is confirmed biochemically with the evaluation of serum insulin, proinsulin, C-peptide, and glucose levels to establish endogenous paradoxic hyperinsulinism occurring at times of hypoglycemia. Ninety percent to 95% of patients will develop hypoglycemia during a 48-hour observed fast, although a 72-hour observed fast is the gold standard.[7,27] Sulfonylurea metabolites also should be evaluated to exclude factitious hyperinsulinism. Patients have also been reported to demonstrate islet cell hyperplasia (nesidioblastosis) and, rarely, multifocal insulinomas months to years following Roux-en-Y gastric bypass.[28]

Once biochemically confirmed, most insulinomas can be localized with contrast-enhanced CT or MRI. These tumors are typically well-circumscribed. Endoscopic ultrasound (EUS) can aid in the diagnosis and localization of these tumors with identification of lesions as small as 2 to 5 mm. Compared with normal pancreatic parenchyma, insulinomas appear hypodense on ultrasound. Intraoperative ultrasound is also frequently used if these tumors cannot be localized preoperatively.

SRS is not helpful given the tumor's low expression of SSTR-2.[22,29] Interestingly, insulinomas overexpress glucagonlike peptide 1 (GLP-1) receptor, and radiolabeled GLP-1 analogs, such as exendin-3 and exendin-4, have been developed with promising results.[30] SRS is, however, useful to evaluate the burden of disease and to test the appropriateness of peptide receptor radiotherapy (PRRT).

Gastrinoma

Gastrinomas arise predominantly within the duodenum followed by the pancreas. Passaro[31] identified an anatomic triangle called the gastrinoma triangle, where most gastrinomas originate. This triangle is outlined by the junction of the cystic duct and common bile duct, the junction of the neck and body of the pancreas, and the lateral wall of the duodenum between the second and third portions. Up to 90% of these lesions are malignant with pancreatic gastrinomas often more aggressive than those found within the wall of the duodenum.[7] Patients present with the Zollinger-Ellison syndrome: severe refractory peptic ulcer disease, gastric acid hypersecretion, and diarrhea.[32] Metastatic disease is present in approximately 30% of patients with gastrinomas, and therefore symptoms associated with hepatic metastases may also be the presenting symptoms. Gastrinomas are the most common PNET in patients with MEN I occurring in up to 50% of cases.[3,33]

Gastrinomas that produce the Zollinger-Ellison syndrome can be biochemically diagnosed by measuring fasting serum gastrin concentration and/or performing a secretin stimulation test. Diagnosis, however, remains quite difficult due to the many conditions that can lead to hypergastrinemia, such as gastroesophageal reflux disease, gastric outlet obstruction, antral G-cell hyperplasia, and retained gastric antrum. In the presence of gastric acid production (ie, not due to secondary hypergastrinemia), a serum gastrin value of more than 1000 pg/mL is diagnostic, but this occurs in only 5% to 9% of patients. Two-thirds of patients have a fasting serum gastrin value that is less than 10 times the upper limit of normal, a nondiagnostic range.[34] Higher levels of gastrin are associated with pancreatic tumors, larger tumors, and metastatic disease.

A secretin stimulation test is used in instances in which a fasting serum gastrin is nondiagnostic and there is no mass lesion apparent on axial imaging. Patients taking PPIs can produce false-positive results. In these instances in which provocative testing is needed to secure a diagnosis, PPIs should be discontinued by tapering over 1 week before the test and switched to H_2 antagonists. Once this is done, baseline serum gastrin is measured, an ampule of secretin is given intravenously, and serum gastrin levels repeated sequentially over time. A change in fasting serum gastrin levels of 120 pg/mL or more is associated with a sensitivity and specificity of 94% and 100%, respectively.[35] This is biochemical proof of a gastrinoma. Selective venous sampling for gastrin of the drainage of the pancreas can be performed to localize the tumor preoperatively. Gastrinomas typically express SSRT-2, and SRS is another useful modality to localize gastrinomas before surgical exploration. Rarely, all efforts to localize the tumor preoperatively will fail, and operative exploration with intraoperative ultrasound and manual palpation of the wall of the duodenum will be indicated.

Other Functional Pancreatic Neuroendocrine Tumors

Other functional PNETs are exceptionally rare and include glucagonomas, VIPomas, and somatostatinomas. Glucagonomas classically present with weight loss, venous thrombosis, and necrolytic migratory erythema. VIPomas cause Verner-Morrison syndrome, also referred to as the WDHA (watery diarrhea, hypokalemia, achlorhydria) syndrome or pancreatic cholera. Patients with somatostatinomas can present with diabetes mellitus, cholelithiasis, diarrhea, and steatorrhea. Most of these functional PNETs are metastatic at presentation, and surgical management is limited.

SURGICAL MANAGEMENT
Principles of Surgical Management

Surgical resection remains the only potentially curative treatment for patients with PNETs.[36,37] Indeed, the goals are to prevent metastases and improve long-term survival. Surgery also may alleviate symptoms from hypersecretion of hormones by functional tumors or symptoms that may be due to nonfunctional tumors. According to the National Comprehensive Cancer Network guidelines, patients with localized PNETs should undergo resection except in those cases in which patients are unfit for surgery or have widely metastatic disease.[38] Several controversies remain, however, regarding the implementation of surgery in the management of PNETs. First, recent success with watchful waiting in elderly patients and patients with high perioperative risk that present with small NF-PNETs has led to the hypothesis that certain small PNETs are very indolent and exceedingly unlikely to represent a substantial threat to the patient during his or her lifetime. Yet, all pancreatic surgeons will have patients with high-grade localized tumors with early and aggressive recurrences after resection. These phenomena have driven recent recognition that there are tumors that present as localized disease but that should not be resected, either because they are not a threat to the patient or they are so aggressive that resection will provide no benefit. The second controversy in the field is with regard to the application of minimally invasive and pancreas-sparing operations (ie, enucleations and central pancreatectomies) to the treatment of PNETs. Last, there remains debate about the role and extent of surgery in patients with MEN I presenting with PNETs.[20,21]

Asymptomatic Small Pancreatic Neuroendocrine Tumors

The increased utilization of high-resolution axial imaging to evaluate vague abdominal symptoms has resulted in a significant increase in the diagnosis of asymptomatic NF-PNETs.[4] The surgical management of pancreatic neuroendocrine incidentalomas is a topic of active debate. There are no clear radiologic or histologic features that are in isolation definitively predictive of malignancy.[19,39,40] Tumor size has traditionally been thought to be directly related to malignant potential, with larger tumors thought to be more likely to behave aggressively and carry more risk of death from disease. Previous investigators, considering the substantial risk of perioperative morbidity and the potential for exocrine and endocrine pancreatic insufficiency after pancreatectomy, have proposed an "observation first" approach for small, incidentally detected tumors.[41,42] There is, however, increasing recognition that there exist small high-grade tumors with aggressive behavior.

The data in the literature currently are mixed on the appropriate management strategy for small, asymptomatic PNETs. In a recent study using data between 1993 and 2013 from Memorial Sloan Kettering Cancer Center's institutional cancer database, Sadot and colleagues[4] constructed a matched case-control study of patients with PNETs of 3 cm or smaller who were observed with those who underwent upfront resection. They found that of those tumors that were observed, 51% increased in size, 18% experienced no change in size, and 31% experienced a decrease in size with no difference in overall survival ($P = .3$) between groups. Within the limitations of their study, they concluded that a watchful waiting approach is justified in the management of small, asymptomatic NF-PNETs. Other studies have demonstrated similar results stating that observation is acceptable for patients with PNETs smaller than 2 cm. In a single-center retrospective study, Zhang and colleagues[43] found that the overall survival of patients with NF-PNETs was improved when managed surgically. The effect of surgery was particularly pronounced when tumors were larger than 1.5 cm in diameter, and observation was recommended for those tumors that were smaller. Similarly, Kishi and colleagues[44] found that NF-PNETs of 1.5 cm or smaller can be safely observed with imaging studies at 6-month intervals. Regenet and colleagues[45] examined the natural course of 66 patients with NF-PNETs of 2 cm or smaller managed operatively and 14 patients managed non-operatively. They found that a tumor size cutoff of 1.7 cm was 92% sensitive and 75% specific for predicting malignancy, and therefore recommended surgical resection for tumors larger than 1.7 cm. Because even small NF-PNETs can develop metastases in 7.7% to 29% of patients, size alone may not be an appropriate criterion in predicting their behavior. Scarpa and colleagues[46] suggested a Ki-67 cutoff of 5%, but this was not predictive in the study by Regenet and colleagues.[45] Contrary to the findings of these studies, in a large population study using the National Cancer Data Base, Sharpe and colleagues[47] examined 380 patients with NF-PNETs of 2 cm or smaller between 1998 and 2006. Eighty-one percent of the cohort underwent resection and 19% were observed. The 5-year overall survival was 73.6%, with a median follow-up of 5 years. Of those who underwent resection, their 5-year overall survival was 82.2% compared with a 5-year overall survival of 34.3% in those who underwent observation (P<.0001, **Fig. 3**). Surgical management continued to be strongly associated with survival even after accounting for tumor size, location, and lymph node status. Tumor grade was also strongly associated with overall survival, as surgical management continued to provide a benefit independent of tumor grade (**Fig. 4**).

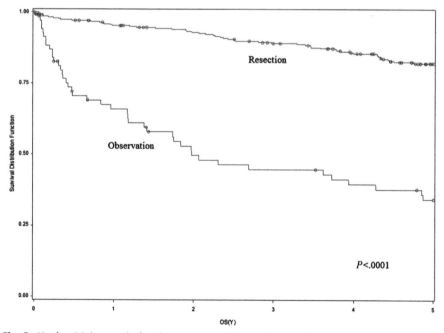

Fig. 3. Kaplan-Meier survival estimates comparing patients with PNETs ≤2 cm who underwent surgical resection or observation. (*From* Sharpe SM, In H, Winchester DJ, et al. Surgical resection provides an overall survival benefit for patients with small pancreatic neuroendocrine tumors. J Gastrointest Surg 2015;19(1):120. [discussion: 123]; with permission.)

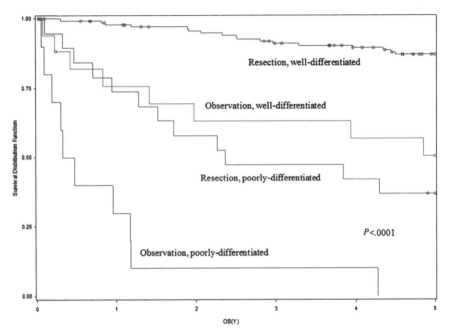

Fig. 4. Kaplan-Meier survival estimates comparing patients with PNETs ≤2 cm who underwent surgical resection or observation, by histologic grade. (*From* Sharpe SM, In H, Winchester DJ, et al. Surgical resection provides an overall survival benefit for patients with small pancreatic neuroendocrine tumors. J Gastrointest Surg 2015;19(1):122. [discussion: 123]; with permission.)

A novel strategy to the management of these small, incidentally discovered NF-PNETs is to obtain a tissue diagnosis with EUS and fine-needle aspiration (FNA), thereby aiding decision making based on cytopathology. Reliability between EUS-FNA cytopathology and surgical specimen histology is reportedly 70% to 80%.[48,49] Studies have previously demonstrated the additional benefit of EUS in localizing lesions not seen on CT but clinically suspected (eg, insulinoma), particularly for PNETs smaller than 2 cm.[50] The tissue sampling capabilities of EUS with FNA may be able to stratify patients with incidentally discovered small, asymptomatic NF-PNETs to surgery versus observation although specific studies in this population are lacking. Studies have argued that small (<2 cm) NF-PNETs with a WHO Grade 3 should be treated surgically, but cautioned the decision-making ability of those with WHO Grade 2.[51,52]

Our current approach to incidentally found NF-PNETs has been to pursue resection for tumors that are 2 cm in size or larger, unless there is evidence of significant metastatic disease or major comorbidity that would make resection untenable. For tumors that are smaller than 1 cm, we generally pursue observation with close interval surveillance. Our regimen involves repeat axial imaging 3 months following diagnosis and then at 6-month intervals for 1 year and yearly thereafter. We reconsider surgical resection if the tumor size changes substantially on surveillance imaging. For tumors between 1 and 2 cm, we tend to individualize treatment based on the age of the patient and location of the tumor. We will have a discussion with the patient regarding the risks and benefits in light of the location of the lesion and undergo a process of shared decision making with the understanding that either resection or close interval surveillance are reasonable.

The Role of Enucleation

There has been very little evidence that lymph node clearance provides any survival advantage in the management of PNETs. For this reason and because anatomic resections (pancreaticoduodenectomy and left pancreatectomy) carry significant risk of major perioperative morbidity, many prior investigators have suggested that PNETs might simply and effectively be managed by enucleation.[53–55] Patient selection is of the utmost importance when considering enucleation. Tumors that are likely to be benign, solitary, and are not abutting the pancreatic or biliary ducts are appropriate for enucleation.[7] Cauley and colleagues[56] compared the surgical outcomes of 45 patients undergoing enucleation with 90 patients undergoing pancreatectomy and found that enucleation was significantly associated with shorter operative times, lower blood loss, and lower rates of pancreatic insufficiency compared with patients undergoing pancreatectomy. Pitt and colleagues[53] compared patients undergoing enucleation versus pancreatectomy for localized PNETs, and found similar overall morbidity and 5-year survival rates between groups. Enucleation was associated with decreased blood loss, operative time, and hospital length of stay. Despite these positive results, pancreatic fistula was significantly greater in the enucleation group (38% vs 15%, $P<.01$). However, most pancreatic fistulas in the enucleation group were ISGPF (International Study Group on Pancreatic Fistula) grade A, whereas those in the resection group were ISGPF grade B. After appropriate patient selection, the data on this subject would suggest that enucleation is a safe and effective strategy for small PNETs, both functional and nonfunctional.

The Role of Central Pancreatectomy

Central pancreatectomy is an acceptable alternative to the management of PNETs when the lesion is not amenable to enucleation.[57] As a parenchyma-sparing operation, central pancreatectomy has the benefit of minimizing postoperative endocrine and exocrine insufficiency, and can be approached laparoscopically.[58] However, central pancreatectomy has been associated with longer operative times and higher rates of pancreatic fistula ($\sim$30%), despite having endocrine and exocrine preservation rates equivalent to traditional pancreatectomies.[59,60] Given the rarity of this operation, few studies have examined the impact of central pancreatectomy on outcomes specifically for PNETs. In a large single-center experience involving 100 total patients, 35 patients underwent central pancreatectomy for PNET (25 patients were WHO grade 1, 9 WHO grade 2, and 1 WHO grade 3).[61] Overall morbidity was 72%, and 63% of patients had pancreatic fistula. With a median follow-up of 36 months, one of the patients with PNET (3-cm lesion, WHO grade 2) developed recurrence. As with enucleation, appropriate patient selection is warranted when pursuing central pancreatectomy in light of the paucity of evidence.

Minimally Invasive Techniques

Minimally invasive approaches (ie, laparoscopy, robotics) have recently been more frequently applied to the management of both functional and NF-PNETs.[62,63] No consensus has been established regarding the indications of minimally invasive surgery, but laparoscopic surgery has been shown to be feasible and safe for appropriately selected PNETs.[64–66]

Laparoscopic enucleation can be accomplished successfully for well-circumscribed, small (<3 cm) PNETs with noninvasive features and without involvement of the main pancreatic duct or ampulla.[54,62] As such, laparoscopic enucleation is not limited to the location of the lesion, but rather by proximity to vessels and the pancreatic duct.[55] Intraoperative ultrasonography is often used to confirm tumor location and its relation to critical vasculature (eg, superior mesenteric artery and vein) and the main pancreatic duct (>2–3 mm) before proceeding with enucleation. Formal pancreatic resection is recommended when enucleation cannot be accomplished and is based on tumor location (ie, head, body, tail).

Laparoscopic distal pancreatectomy has been shown to be safe, and short-term outcomes may be favorable with this approach over an open approach.[63–65,67,68] Several techniques have been described including spleen-preserving (eg, Warshaw technique) and spleen-sacrificing methods of laparoscopic distal pancreatectomy.[69] Our approach is to pursue splenectomy for patients with ductal adenocarcinoma to produce an adequate lymphadenectomy.[66] For PNETs, the main factors that dictate the procedure chosen are the location of the tumor within the pancreatic body or tail and its relation to the splenic vessels and splenic hilum. Again, there has been little indication that lymph node clearance provides a survival advantage in PNET, and a strong argument can be made for splenic preservation in most cases in which the tumor is remote from the splenic hilum. Our approach in these patients is to be selective regarding splenectomy. In patients for whom there is evidence of lymphadenopathy on preoperative studies, we will pursue distal pancreatectomy with splenectomy. In patients for whom there is no evidence of significant lymphadenopathy on preoperative imaging and for whom spleen preservation is technically possible (tumor remote from the splenic hilum), we will perform laparoscopic distal pancreatectomy by means of the Warshaw spleen-preserving technique: saving the short gastric blood supply to the spleen while ligating the splenic artery and vein. Frozen sections are routinely sent to confirm adequate margin and to evaluate the grade of the tumor. If margins are involved or the tumor is high grade on frozen section, we continue with splenectomy to obtain an adequate lymphadenectomy.

Laparoscopic pancreaticoduodenectomy has been slow to gain popularity because of technical demands, long operative times, and increased cost.[70–73] Moreover, many surgeons have been reluctant to use the technique in the setting of malignancy, particularly pancreatic adenocarcinoma, because there are limited data regarding short-term and long-term oncologic outcomes. In patients with PNETs, there is additional potential complexity with regard to the reconstruction laparoscopically, as most patients with PNET will have normal-sized, small-caliber pancreatic ducts and soft glands. Both of these features contribute substantial difficulty to the pancreaticojejunostomy and garner increased risk of postoperative pancreatic fistula even under the best possible circumstances.

Robotic surgery has quickly evolved over the past decade, particularly fueled by patient preference. The robotic technique has been shown to be feasible for both distal pancreatectomy and pancreaticoduodenectomy, and short-term outcomes are encouraging.[74] Further studies are needed to assess the applicability of robotic surgery to PNETs.

Functional Pancreatic Neuroendocrine Tumors

Surgical management of functional PNETs varies depending on the tumor type, the tumor extent, and the underlying genetic etiology. Patients presenting with functional PNETs in the context of MEN I present several unique management problems and are discussed further in the next section. Insulinomas, either as part of MEN I or sporadic findings, are indolent tumors and rarely metastasize to regional lymph nodes. For these reasons, enucleation is often all that is needed for appropriate management.[75]

Sporadic gastrinomas have a greater potential for malignant behavior and can occur anywhere within the gastrinoma triangle, making localization challenging. Localization may need to be performed at the time of the operation using manual palpation and intraoperative ultrasonography, endoscopic duodenal transillumination, or duodenotomy.[7] The use of minimally invasive resection is thus controversial for these tumors. Because gastrinomas are more likely to be malignant, surgical management warrants formal pancreatic resection with regional lymphadenectomy. Norton and colleagues[33] reported the results of 151 patients with Zollinger-Ellison syndrome treated operatively as part of a prospective study of the National Institutes of Health. Twenty-eight patients had MEN I. Twenty-three patients had 2 operations, whereas 2 patients had 3 or more operations. The duodenum was the most common location of gastrinomas independent of MEN I status (74 patients, 49%). Five-year disease-free survival among patients with sporadic gastrinomas was 40% compared with 4% for patients with MEN I; however, the 5-year disease-specific survival for sporadic gastrinomas and MEN I were both 100%. Lymph nodes in the region of the head of the pancreas and duodenum should be routinely removed at surgery even if they appear normal because they may contain microscopic gastrinoma.

Surgical resection whenever possible is recommended for other functional PNETs, particularly for symptom control and chance of cure. Glucagonomas are typically large and advanced at the time of presentation.[76,77] As such, enucleation and minimally invasive approaches are not recommended. Similarly, up to 80% of patients with VIPomas and up to 75% of patients with somatostatinomas have metastatic disease at the time of diagnosis.[78–80] Cytoreductive surgery may have a role to play to improve hormonal control.[81,82]

Multiple Endocrine Neoplasia Type I

MEN I is an autosomal dominant disorder attributed to a mutation in the *MEN I* tumor suppressor gene located at chromosome 11q13. Patients with MEN I usually develop primary hyperparathyroidism (90%–100%), followed by PNETs that can be functional (20%–70%), of which gastrinoma is the most common, or nonfunctional (80%–100%), and pituitary adenomas (20%–65%).[3] Surgical management of MEN I primarily involves subtotal parathyroidectomy for the primary hyperparathyroidism.

The surgical management of PNETs in patients with MEN I is challenging, as tumors in MEN I are almost always diffuse and multifocal.[83] Most agree that surgical resection should be undertaken for patients with MEN I who develop insulinomas or other rare functional PNETs.[84] These tend to be indolent tumors and patients will typically have prolonged symptomatic improvement with resection of detectable pathology. Patients presenting with gastrinoma in the context of MEN I present a unique management problem. The lesions tend to be multiple, recurrence is common, and there is little survival benefit afforded by resection.[3,85] Patients with MEN I and gastrinoma will rarely be cleared of the disease by local resection. Symptoms associated with Zollinger-Ellison syndrome are now effectively managed with PPIs or H_2-antagonists. Incomplete resection is not beneficial, and surgery is not indicated when there are extensive metastases. Studies have shown that patients with MEN I with gastrinoma are more likely to die of other causes than their gastrinomas.[3]

Up to 60% of patients with MEN I will have NF-PNETs. These lesion can grow to sizes that cause symptoms in up to 12%.[3] Similar to the debate in sporadic cases, there is no consensus to the management of small NF-PNETs in those with MEN I. Several studies have shown that patients with NF-PNETs smaller than 2 cm have no difference in long-term survival compared with those with MEN I and no PNETs.[7,83,85,86] Others recommend surgery for those that are 1 cm.[87] Unfortunately, the rarity of the disease prevents adequate evidence-based conclusions. Nevertheless, surgical management is warranted when NF-PNETs are large (>2 cm) or symptomatic when they occur in patients with MEN I akin to recommendations for sporadic cases.[87]

Metastatic Disease

PNETs present with distant metastases in approximately 40% to 45% of cases. The liver is the most common site of metastasis.[88] Resection of metastatic disease undoubtedly has a role to play in select patients with metastatic PNETs.[7,89] There is little to no level-I evidence to aid decision making in these cases. The treatment decisions should be individualized based on the underlying general health of the patient, the tumor's underlying biology, and the pattern of metastasis. ENETS has developed a consensus opinion regarding the minimum requirements for hepatectomy for curative intent of metastatic disease: technically feasible, well-differentiated disease with an acceptable morbidity and less than 5% mortality, absence of right heart insufficiency, absence of extra-abdominal metastases, and absence of diffuse peritoneal carcinomatosis.[14] Multiple prior studies have shown increased survival when an R0 resection is achieved compared with an R1 resection. Significant controversy exists regarding the role of cytoreductive surgery.[89,90] Most consensus guidelines recommend considering cytoreductive surgery if more than 90% of the tumor burden can be removed, the patient is symptomatic from disease, and the tumor is indolent. Tumor debulking has been argued to prevent the development of symptoms or provide symptom control (eg, from mass effect), to facilitate liver-directed therapies, and to increase survival.[90–92]

Treatment methods used for colorectal liver metastases are also used for liver metastases in PNETs. Liver-directed therapies, such as radiofrequency ablation and transcatheter embolization/transcatheter chemoembolization, have been used when resection is not feasible with reasonable results.[7,81,89,93] Liver transplantation has also been applied to some patients with PNET and isolated diffuse liver metastasis.[94] Mazzaferro and colleagues[95] reported a 96% 5-year survival and an approximately 80% 5-year recurrence-free survival for 30 patients who underwent liver transplantation following stringent patient selection criteria (**Box 1**).

Box 1
Milan criteria for liver transplantation in patients with hepatic metastases from neuroendocrine tumors

Inclusion Criteria

1. Confirmed histology of carcinoid tumor (low-grade neuroendocrine tumors) with or without syndrome

2. Primary tumor drained by the portal system (pancreas and intermediate gut: from distal stomach to sigmoid colon) removed with a curative resection (pretransplant removal of all extrahepatic tumor deposits) through surgical procedures different and separate from transplantation

3. Metastatic diffusion to liver parenchyma ≤50%

4. Good response or stable disease for at least 6 months during the pretransplantation period

5. Age ≤55 years

Exclusion Criteria

1. Small-cell carcinoma and high-grade neuroendocrine carcinomas (noncarcinoid tumors)

2. Other medical/surgical conditions contraindicating liver transplantation, including previous tumors

3. Nongastrointestinal carcinoids or tumors not drained by the portal system

From Mazzaferro V, Pulvirenti A, Coppa J. Neuroendocrine tumors metastatic to the liver: how to select patients for liver transplantation? J Hepatol 2007;47(4):462; with permission.

SUMMARY

PNETs are a heterogeneous group of tumors within a spectrum of neuroendocrine disease. Endocrinopathies produced by roughly 10% of these tumors have been their historical allure. However, with the increasing use of high-resolution imaging, PNETs are more frequently found when smaller, and we do not yet understand their optimal management. Nevertheless, because of their potential for malignancy, surgical resection remains a foundation in their management.

REFERENCES

1. Lawrence B, Gustafsson BI, Chan A, et al. The epidemiology of gastroentero-pancreatic neuroendocrine tumors. Endocrinol Metab Clin North Am 2011; 40(1):1–18, vii.
2. Yao JC, Hassan M, Phan A, et al. One hundred years after "carcinoid": epidemiology of and prognostic factors for neuroendocrine tumors in 35,825 cases in the United States. J Clin Oncol 2008;26(18):3063–72.
3. Norton JA, Krampitz G, Jensen RT. Multiple endocrine neoplasia: genetics and clinical management. Surg Oncol Clin N Am 2015;24(4):795–832.
4. Sadot E, Reidy-Lagunes DL, Tang LH, et al. Observation versus resection for small asymptomatic pancreatic neuroendocrine tumors: a matched case-control study. Ann Surg Oncol 2016;23(4):1361–70.
5. Klimstra DS, Beltran H, Lilenbaum R, et al. The spectrum of neuroendocrine tumors: histologic classification, unique features and areas of overlap. Am Soc Clin Oncol Educ Book 2015;92–103.
6. Vortmeyer AO, Huang S, Lubensky I, et al. Non-islet origin of pancreatic islet cell tumors. J Clin Endocrinol Metab 2004;89(4):1934–8.
7. Clancy TE. Surgical management of pancreatic neuroendocrine tumors. Hematol Oncol Clin North Am 2016;30(1):103–18.
8. Jiao Y, Shi C, Edil BH, et al. DAXX/ATRX, MEN1, and mTOR pathway genes are frequently altered in pancreatic neuroendocrine tumors. Science 2011; 331(6021):1199–203.
9. Yachida S, Vakiani E, White CM, et al. Small cell and large cell neuroendocrine carcinomas of the pancreas are genetically similar and distinct from well-differentiated pancreatic neuroendocrine tumors. Am J Surg Pathol 2012;36(2): 173–84.
10. Kunz PL. Carcinoid and neuroendocrine tumors: building on success. J Clin Oncol 2015;33(16):1855–63.
11. Rehfeld JF, Federspiel B, Bardram L. A neuroendocrine tumor syndrome from cholecystokinin secretion. N Engl J Med 2013;368(12):1165–6.
12. van Essen M, Sundin A, Krenning EP, et al. Neuroendocrine tumours: the role of imaging for diagnosis and therapy. Nat Rev Endocrinol 2014;10(2):102–14.
13. McKenna LR, Edil BH. Update on pancreatic neuroendocrine tumors. Gland Surg 2014;3(4):258–75.
14. Falconi M, Bartsch DK, Eriksson B, et al. ENETS Consensus Guidelines for the management of patients with digestive neuroendocrine neoplasms of the digestive system: well-differentiated pancreatic non-functioning tumors. Neuroendocrinology 2012;95(2):120–34.
15. Rindi G, Arnold R, Bosman FT, et al. Nomenclature and classification of neuroendocrine neoplasms of the digestive system. In: Bosman FT, Carneiro F, Hruban RH, et al, editors. WHO classification of tumors of the digestive system. Lyon: IARC; 2010.

16. McCall CM, Shi C, Cornish TC, et al. Grading of well-differentiated pancreatic neuroendocrine tumors is improved by the inclusion of both Ki67 proliferative index and mitotic rate. Am J Surg Pathol 2013;37(11):1671–7.

17. Cherenfant J, Talamonti MS, Hall CR, et al. Comparison of tumor markers for predicting outcomes after resection of nonfunctioning pancreatic neuroendocrine tumors. Surgery 2014;156(6):1504–10 [discussion: 1510–1].

18. American Joint Committee on Cancer. AJCC cancer staging manual. 7th edition. Chicago: American College of Surgeons; 2010.

19. Cherenfant J, Stocker SJ, Gage MK, et al. Predicting aggressive behavior in nonfunctioning pancreatic neuroendocrine tumors. Surgery 2013;154(4):785–91 [discussion: 791–3].

20. Kunz PL, Reidy-Lagunes D, Anthony LB, et al. Consensus guidelines for the management and treatment of neuroendocrine tumors. Pancreas 2013;42(4):557–77.

21. Reid MD, Balci S, Saka B, et al. Neuroendocrine tumors of the pancreas: current concepts and controversies. Endocr Pathol 2014;25(1):65–79.

22. Kartalis N, Mucelli RM, Sundin A. Recent developments in imaging of pancreatic neuroendocrine tumors. Ann Gastroenterol 2015;28(2):193–202.

23. Baker MS, Knuth JL, DeWitt J, et al. Pancreatic cystic neuroendocrine tumors: preoperative diagnosis with endoscopic ultrasound and fine-needle immunocytology. J Gastrointest Surg 2008;12(3):450–6.

24. Frilling A, Sotiropoulos GC, Radtke A, et al. The impact of 68Ga-DOTATOC positron emission tomography/computed tomography on the multimodal management of patients with neuroendocrine tumors. Ann Surg 2010;252(5):850–6.

25. Armbruster S, Dorrance C, Voorhees P, et al. Malignant insulinoma: a rare presentation of a rare tumor. Gastrointest Endosc 2007;66(6):1228–9 [discussion: 1229].

26. Ferrer-Garcia JC, Iranzo Gonzalez-Cruz V, Navas-DeSolis S, et al. Management of malignant insulinoma. Clin Transl Oncol 2013;15(9):725–31.

27. Hirshberg B, Livi A, Bartlett DL, et al. Forty-eight-hour fast: the diagnostic test for insulinoma. J Clin Endocrinol Metab 2000;85(9):3222–6.

28. Service GJ, Thompson GB, Service FJ, et al. Hyperinsulinemic hypoglycemia with nesidioblastosis after gastric-bypass surgery. N Engl J Med 2005;353(3): 249–54.

29. Kisker O, Bartsch D, Weinel RJ, et al. The value of somatostatin-receptor scintigraphy in newly diagnosed endocrine gastroenteropancreatic tumors. J Am Coll Surg 1997;184(5):487–92.

30. Christ E, Wild D, Ederer S, et al. Glucagon-like peptide-1 receptor imaging for the localisation of insulinomas: a prospective multicentre imaging study. Lancet Diabetes Endocrinol 2013;1(2):115–22.

31. Stabile BE, Morrow DJ, Passaro E Jr. The gastrinoma triangle: operative implications. Am J Surg 1984;147(1):25–31.

32. Ellison EC, Johnson JA. The Zollinger-Ellison syndrome: a comprehensive review of historical, scientific, and clinical considerations. Curr Probl Surg 2009;46(1): 13–106.

33. Norton JA, Fraker DL, Alexander HR, et al. Surgery to cure the Zollinger-Ellison syndrome. N Engl J Med 1999;341(9):635–44.

34. Berna MJ, Hoffmann KM, Serrano J, et al. Serum gastrin in Zollinger-Ellison syndrome: I. Prospective study of fasting serum gastrin in 309 patients from the National Institutes of Health and comparison with 2229 cases from the literature. Medicine (Baltimore) 2006;85(6):295–330.

35. Berna MJ, Hoffmann KM, Long SH, et al. Serum gastrin in Zollinger-Ellison syndrome: II. Prospective study of gastrin provocative testing in 293 patients from

the National Institutes of Health and comparison with 537 cases from the literature. Evaluation of diagnostic criteria, proposal of new criteria, and correlations with clinical and tumoral features. Medicine (Baltimore) 2006;85(6):331–64.

36. Haugvik SP, Janson ET, Osterlund P, et al. Surgical treatment as a principle for patients with high-grade pancreatic neuroendocrine carcinoma: a nordic multi-center comparative study. Ann Surg Oncol 2016;23(5):1721–8.

37. Shiba S, Morizane C, Hiraoka N, et al. Pancreatic neuroendocrine tumors: a single-center 20-year experience with 100 patients. Pancreatology 2016;16(1):99–105.

38. National Comprehensive Cancer Network. Neuroendocrine tumors. 2015. Version 1.2015. Available at: http://www.nccn.org/professionals/physician_gls/pdf/neuroendocrine.pdf. Accessed February 15, 2016.

39. Rosenberg AM, Friedmann P, Del Rivero J, et al. Resection versus expectant management of small incidentally discovered nonfunctional pancreatic neuroendocrine tumors. Surgery 2016;159(1):302–9.

40. Sallinen V, Haglund C, Seppanen H. Outcomes of resected nonfunctional pancreatic neuroendocrine tumors: do size and symptoms matter? Surgery 2015;158(6): 1556–63.

41. Gaujoux S, Partelli S, Maire F, et al. Observational study of natural history of small sporadic nonfunctioning pancreatic neuroendocrine tumors. J Clin Endocrinol Metab 2013;98(12):4784–9.

42. Haynes AB, Deshpande V, Ingkakul T, et al. Implications of incidentally discovered, nonfunctioning pancreatic endocrine tumors: short-term and long-term patient outcomes. Arch Surg 2011;146(5):534–8.

43. Zhang IY, Zhao J, Fernandez-Del Castillo C, et al. Operative versus nonoperative management of nonfunctioning pancreatic neuroendocrine tumors. J Gastrointest Surg 2016;20(2):277–83.

44. Kishi Y, Shimada K, Nara S, et al. Basing treatment strategy for non-functional pancreatic neuroendocrine tumors on tumor size. Ann Surg Oncol 2014;21(9): 2882–8.

45. Regenet N, Carrere N, Boulanger G, et al. Is the 2-cm size cutoff relevant for small nonfunctioning pancreatic neuroendocrine tumors: a French multicenter study. Surgery 2016;159(3):901–7.

46. Scarpa A, Mantovani W, Capelli P, et al. Pancreatic endocrine tumors: improved TNM staging and histopathological grading permit a clinically efficient prognostic stratification of patients. Mod Pathol 2010;23(6):824–33.

47. Sharpe SM, In H, Winchester DJ, et al. Surgical resection provides an overall survival benefit for patients with small pancreatic neuroendocrine tumors. J Gastrointest Surg 2015;19(1):117–23 [discussion: 123].

48. Rustagi T, Farrell JJ. Endoscopic diagnosis and treatment of pancreatic neuroendocrine tumors. J Clin Gastroenterol 2014;48(10):837–44.

49. Khashab MA, Yong E, Lennon AM, et al. EUS is still superior to multidetector computerized tomography for detection of pancreatic neuroendocrine tumors. Gastrointest Endosc 2011;73(4):691–6.

50. James PD, Tsolakis AV, Zhang M, et al. Incremental benefit of preoperative EUS for the detection of pancreatic neuroendocrine tumors: a meta-analysis. Gastrointest Endosc 2015;81(4):848–56.e1.

51. Piani C, Franchi GM, Cappelletti C, et al. Cytological Ki-67 in pancreatic endocrine tumours: an opportunity for pre-operative grading. Endocr Relat Cancer 2008;15(1):175–81.

52. Weynand B, Borbath I, Bernard V, et al. Pancreatic neuroendocrine tumour grading on endoscopic ultrasound-guided fine needle aspiration: high

reproducibility and inter-observer agreement of the Ki-67 labelling index. Cytopathology 2014;25(6):389–95.

53. Pitt SC, Pitt HA, Baker MS, et al. Small pancreatic and periampullary neuroendocrine tumors: resect or enucleate? J Gastrointest Surg 2009;13(9):1692–8.

54. Dedieu A, Rault A, Collet D, et al. Laparoscopic enucleation of pancreatic neoplasm. Surg Endosc 2011;25(2):572–6.

55. Jilesen AP, van Eijck CH, Busch OR, et al. Postoperative outcomes of enucleation and standard resections in patients with a pancreatic neuroendocrine tumor. World J Surg 2016;40(3):715–28.

56. Cauley CE, Pitt HA, Ziegler KM, et al. Pancreatic enucleation: improved outcomes compared to resection. J Gastrointest Surg 2012;16(7):1347–53.

57. Lavu H, Knuth JL, Baker MS, et al. Middle segment pancreatectomy can be safely incorporated into a pancreatic surgeon's clinical practice. HPB (Oxford) 2008;10(6):491–7.

58. DiNorcia J, Ahmed L, Lee MK, et al. Better preservation of endocrine function after central versus distal pancreatectomy for mid-gland lesions. Surgery 2010; 148(6):1247–54 [discussion: 1254–6].

59. Shikano T, Nakao A, Kodera Y, et al. Middle pancreatectomy: safety and long-term results. Surgery 2010;147(1):21–9.

60. Roggin KK, Rudloff U, Blumgart LH, et al. Central pancreatectomy revisited. J Gastrointest Surg 2006;10(6):804–12.

61. Goudard Y, Gaujoux S, Dokmak S, et al. Reappraisal of central pancreatectomy a 12-year single-center experience. JAMA Surg 2014;149(4):356–63.

62. Fernandez Ranvier GG, Shouhed D, Inabnet WB 3rd. Minimally invasive techniques for resection of pancreatic neuroendocrine tumors. Surg Oncol Clin N Am 2016;25(1):195–215.

63. Baker MS, Bentrem DJ, Ujiki MB, et al. A prospective single institution comparison of peri-operative outcomes for laparoscopic and open distal pancreatectomy. Surgery 2009;146(4):635–43 [discussion: 643–5].

64. Baker MS, Bentrem DJ, Ujiki MB, et al. Adding days spent in readmission to the initial postoperative length of stay limits the perceived benefit of laparoscopic distal pancreatectomy when compared with open distal pancreatectomy. Am J Surg 2011;201(3):295–9 [discussion: 299–300].

65. Baker MS, Sherman KL, Stocker S, et al. Defining quality for distal pancreatectomy: does the laparoscopic approach protect patients from poor quality outcomes? J Gastrointest Surg 2013;17(2):273–80.

66. Sharpe SM, Talamonti MS, Wang E, et al. The laparoscopic approach to distal pancreatectomy for ductal adenocarcinoma results in shorter lengths of stay without compromising oncologic outcomes. Am J Surg 2015;209(3):557–63.

67. Xourafas D, Tavakkoli A, Clancy TE, et al. Distal pancreatic resection for neuroendocrine tumors: is laparoscopic really better than open? J Gastrointest Surg 2015;19(5):831–40.

68. Fronza JS, Bentrem DJ, Baker MS, et al. Laparoscopic distal pancreatectomy using radiofrequency energy. Am J Surg 2010;199(3):401–4 [discussion: 404].

69. Guerra F, Pesi B, Fatucchi LM, et al. Splenic preservation during open and minimally-invasive distal pancreatectomy. Surgery 2015;158(6):1743–4.

70. Kim SC, Song KB, Jung YS, et al. Short-term clinical outcomes for 100 consecutive cases of laparoscopic pylorus-preserving pancreatoduodenectomy: improvement with surgical experience. Surg Endosc 2013;27(1):95–103.

71. Waters JA, Canal DF, Wiebke EA, et al. Robotic distal pancreatectomy: cost effective? Surgery 2010;148(4):814–23.

72. Sharpe SM, Talamonti MS, Wang CE, et al. Early national experience with laparo-scopic pancreaticoduodenectomy for ductal adenocarcinoma: a comparison of laparoscopic pancreaticoduodenectomy and open pancreaticoduodenectomy from the National Cancer Data Base. J Am Coll Surg 2015;221(1):175–84.

73. Baker MS, Sharpe SM, Talamonti MS, et al. The learning curve is surmountable: in reply to Fong and colleagues. J Am Coll Surg 2016;222(2):210–1.

74. Zeh HJ 3rd, Bartlett DL, Moser AJ. Robotic-assisted major pancreatic resection. Adv Surg 2011;45:323–40.

75. Mehrabi A, Fischer L, Hafezi M, et al. A systematic review of localization, surgical treatment options, and outcome of insulinoma. Pancreas 2014;43(5):675–86.

76. van Beek AP, de Haas ER, van Vloten WA, et al. The glucagonoma syndrome and necrolytic migratory erythema: a clinical review. Eur J Endocrinol 2004;151(5):531–7.

77. Kindmark H, Sundin A, Granberg D, et al. Endocrine pancreatic tumors with glucagon hypersecretion: a retrospective study of 23 cases during 20 years. Med Oncol 2007;24(3):330–7.

78. Perry RR, Vinik AI. Clinical review 72: diagnosis and management of functioning islet cell tumors. J Clin Endocrinol Metab 1995;80(8):2273–8.

79. Soga J, Yakuwa Y. Somatostatinoma/inhibitory syndrome: a statistical evaluation of 173 reported cases as compared to other pancreatic endocrinomas. J Exp Clin Cancer Res 1999;18(1):13–22.

80. Doherty GM. Rare endocrine tumours of the GI tract. Best Pract Res Clin Gastro-enterol 2005;19(5):807–17.

81. Grandhi MS, Lafaro KJ, Pawlik TM. Role of locoregional and systemic ap-proaches for the treatment of patients with metastatic neuroendocrine tumors. J Gastrointest Surg 2015;19(12):2273–82.

82. Frilling A, Al-Nahhas A, Clift AK. Transplantation and debulking procedures for neuroendocrine tumors. Front Horm Res 2015;44:164–76.

83. Kouvaraki MA, Shapiro SE, Cote GJ, et al. Management of pancreatic endocrine tumors in multiple endocrine neoplasia type 1. World J Surg 2006;30(5):643–53.

84. Giudici F, Nesi G, Brandi ML, et al. Surgical management of insulinomas in mul-tiple endocrine neoplasia type 1. Pancreas 2012;41(4):547–53.

85. Lopez CL, Waldmann J, Fendrich V, et al. Long-term results of surgery for pancre-atic neuroendocrine neoplasms in patients with MEN1. Langenbecks Arch Surg 2011;396(8):1187–96.

86. Tomassetti P, Campana D, Piscitelli L, et al. Endocrine pancreatic tumors: factors correlated with survival. Ann Oncol 2005;16(11):1806–10.

87. Triponez F, Goudet P, Dosseh D, et al. Is surgery beneficial for MEN1 patients with small (< or = 2 cm), nonfunctioning pancreaticoduodenal endocrine tumor? An analysis of 65 patients from the GTE. World J Surg 2006;30(5):654–62 [discus-sion: 663–4].

88. Frilling A, Modlin IM, Kidd M, et al. Recommendations for management of pa-tients with neuroendocrine liver metastases. Lancet Oncol 2014;15(1):e8–21.

89. Frilling A, Clift AK. Therapeutic strategies for neuroendocrine liver metastases. Cancer 2015;121(8):1172–86.

90. Yuan CH, Wang J, Xiu DR, et al. Meta-analysis of liver resection versus nonsur-gical treatments for pancreatic neuroendocrine tumors with liver metastases. Ann Surg Oncol 2016;23(1):244–9.

91. Sarmiento JM, Heywood G, Rubin J, et al. Surgical treatment of neuroendocrine metastases to the liver: a plea for resection to increase survival. J Am Coll Surg 2003;197(1):29–37.

92. Capurso G, Rinzivillo M, Bettini R, et al. Systematic review of resection of primary midgut carcinoid tumour in patients with unresectable liver metastases. Br J Surg 2012;99(11):1480–6.
93. Castellano D, Grande E, Valle J, et al. Expert consensus for the management of advanced or metastatic pancreatic neuroendocrine and carcinoid tumors. Cancer Chemother Pharmacol 2015;75(6):1099–114.
94. Frilling A, Rogiers X, Malago M, et al. Liver transplantation in patients with liver metastases of neuroendocrine tumors. Transplant Proc 1998;30(7):3298–300.
95. Mazzaferro V, Pulvirenti A, Coppa J. Neuroendocrine tumors metastatic to the liver: how to select patients for liver transplantation? J Hepatol 2007;47(4):460–6.

Index

Note: Page numbers of article titles are in **boldface** type.

Surg Clin N Am 96 (2016) 1469–1481
http://dx.doi.org/10.1016/S0039-6109(16)52156-2
0039-6109/16

Moving?

Make sure your subscription moves with you!

To notify us of your new address, find your **Clinics Account Number** (located on your mailing label above your name), and contact customer service at:

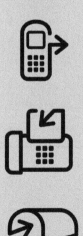

Email: journalscustomerservice-usa@elsevier.com

800-654-2452 (subscribers in the U.S. & Canada)
314-447-8871 (subscribers outside of the U.S. & Canada)

Fax number: 314-447-8029

Elsevier Health Sciences Division
Subscription Customer Service
3251 Riverport Lane
Maryland Heights, MO 63043

Printed and bound by CPI Group (UK) Ltd, Croydon, CR0 4YY

03/10/2024

01040391-0006